STUDY GUIDE FOR

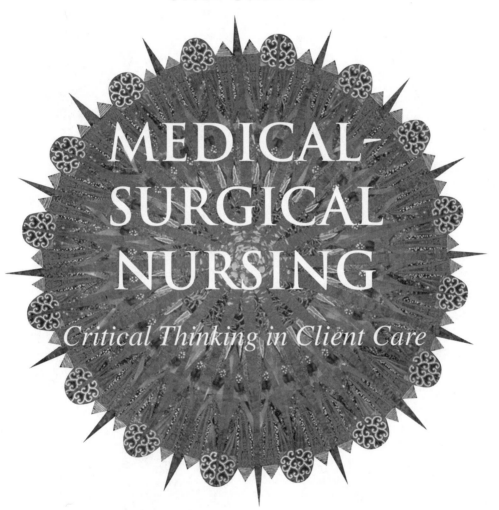

MEDICAL-SURGICAL NURSING

Critical Thinking in Client Care

LEMONE AND BURKE

STUDY GUIDE FOR

MEDICAL-
SURGICAL
NURSING

Critical Thinking in Client Care

FOURTH EDITION

CHRISTINA BAUMER, PHD, RN, CNOR, CHES
Division Chair, Continuing Education
Program Director, Surgical Technology
Lancaster General College of Nursing and Health Sciences
Lancaster, Pennsylvania

MICHELLE BUCHMAN, RN, BSN, BC
Educational Support Services, LLC
St. John's Marian Center
Chesterfield, Missouri

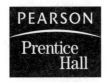

PEARSON
Prentice
Hall

Upper Saddle River, New Jersey

Copyright © 2008 by Pearson Education, Inc., Upper Saddle River, New Jersey 07458. Pearson Prentice Hall. All rights reserved. Printed in the United States of America. This publication is protected by Copyright and permission should be obtained from the publisher prior to any prohibited reproduction, storage in a retrieval system, or transmission in any form or by any means, electronic, mechanical, photocopying, recording, or likewise. For information regarding permission(s), write to: Rights and Permissions Department.

Pearson Prentice Hall™ is a trademark of Pearson Education, Inc.
Pearson® is a registered trademark of Pearson plc
Prentice Hall® is a registered trademark of Pearson Education, Inc.

Pearson Education Ltd.
Pearson Education Singapore Pte. Ltd.
Pearson Education Canada, Ltd.
Pearson Education—Japan
Pearson Education Australia Pty. Limited

Pearson Education North Asia Ltd.
Pearson Educación de Mexico, S. A. de C.V.
Pearson Education Malaysia Pte. Ltd.
Pearson Education, Upper Saddle River, NJ

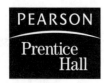

10 9 8 7 6 5 4 3 2 1
ISBN: 0-13-198570-1
ISBN-13: 978-0-13-198570-4

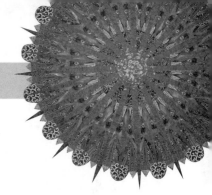

PREFACE

Students entering the field of nursing have a tremendous amount to learn in a very short time. This Study Guide that accompanies *Medical-Surgical Nursing, 4th edition* is designed to reinforce the knowledge that you—the student—has gained in each chapter and to help you master the critical concepts.

At the beginning of each chapter in this Study Guide, you will find a MediaLink box. Just as in the main textbook, this box identifies all the specific media resources and activities available for that chapter on the DVD-ROM in the main textbook, and the text's Companion Website. You will find references to animations from the DVD-ROM and case studies and care plans from the Companion Website to help you visualize and understand difficult concepts. Chapter by chapter, this MediaLink box hones your critical thinking skills and enables you to apply concepts from the book to practice.

In addition, each chapter includes a variety of questions and activities to help you understand difficult concepts and reinforce basic knowledge gained from textbook reading assignments. Following is a list of features included in this edition that will enhance your learning experience:

- **Learning Outcomes** summarize the objective of each chapter.
- **Multiple Choice** questions provide you with additional review on key topics.
- More exercises are in the **Focused Study Tips** section.
- **Case Studies** and **Care Plan Critical Thinking Activities** apply concepts from the textbook to real nursing scenarios.
- **NCLEX-RN® Review Questions** help you to practice for this exam.
- **Answers** are included in the Answer Key to provide immediate reinforcement and to allow you to check the accuracy of your work.

It is our hope that this Study Guide will serve as a valuable learning tool and will contribute to your success in the nursing profession.

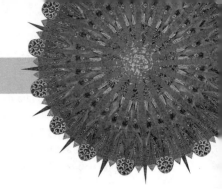

CONTENTS

LEMONE AND BURKE

Study Guide for

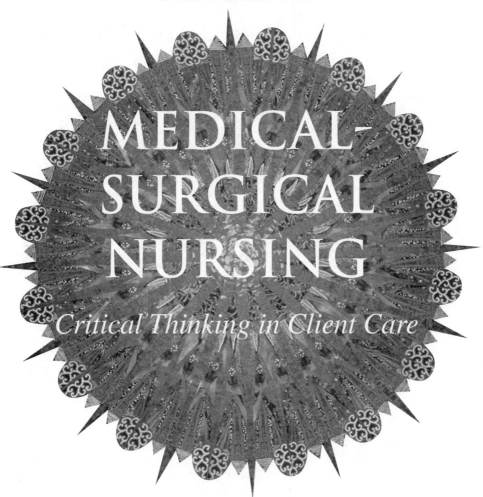

MEDICAL-SURGICAL NURSING

Critical Thinking in Client Care

CHAPTER 1

MEDICAL-SURGICAL NURSING

LEARNING OUTCOMES

After completing Chapter 1, you will be able to demonstrate the following objectives:

- Describe the core competencies for healthcare professionals: patient centered care, interdisciplinary teams, evidence-based practice, quality improvement, and informatics.
- Explain the importance of nursing codes and standards as guidelines for clinical nursing practice.
- Apply the attitudes, mental habits, and skills necessary for critical thinking when using the nursing process in client care.
- Explain the activities and characteristics of the nurse as caregiver, educator, advocate, leader and manager, and researcher.

CLINICAL COMPETENCIES

- Demonstrate critical thinking when using the nursing process to provide knowledgeable, safe client care.
- Provide clinical care within a framework that integrates, as appropriate, the medical-surgical nursing roles of caregiver, educator, advocate, leader/manager, and researcher.

KEY TERMS

advance directives
client
code of ethics
core competencies
critical pathway
critical thinking
delegation
dilemma
ethics
medical-surgical nursing
nursing process
standard
quality assurance

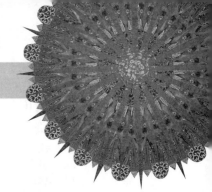

MediaLink

www.prenhall.com/lemone

Resources for this chapter can be found on the Prentice Hall Nursing MediaLink DVD accompanying this textbook, and on the Companion Website at http://www.prenhall.com/lemone. Click on Chapter 1 to select the activities for this chapter.

Prentice Hall Nursing MediaLink DVD-ROM
- Audio Glossary
- NCLEX-RN® Review

Companion Website
www.prenhall.com/lemone
- Audio Glossary
- NCLEX-RN® Review
- Care Plan Activity: Nursing Process
- Case Studies
  - Advance Directive
  - Critical Thinking in the Nursing Process
- MediaLink Applications
  - Medication and Healthcare Needs Assist Programs
  - Nursing Code of Ethics
- Links to Resources

CHAPTER OUTLINE

I. Core Competencies for Safe and Effective Health Care
II. Framework for Practice: Critical Thinking in the Nursing Process
    A. Critical Thinking
        1. Attitudes and Mental Habits Necessary for Critical Thinking
        2. Critical Thinking Skills
    B. The Nursing Process
        1. Assessment
        2. Diagnosis
        3. Planning
        4. Implementation
        5. Evaluation
        6. The Nursing Process in Clinical Practice
III. Guidelines for Nursing Practice
    A. Codes for Nurses
        1. The ICN Code
        2. The ANA Code
    B. Standards of Nursing Practice
IV. Legal and Ethical Dilemmas in Nursing
V. Roles of the Nurse in Medical-Surgical Nursing Practice
    A. The Nurse as Caregiver
    B. The Nurse as Educator
    C. The Nurse as Advocate
    D. The Nurse as Leader and Manager
        1. Models of Care Delivery
        2. Delegation
        3. Evaluating Outcomes of Nursing Care
    E. The Nurse as Researcher

FOCUSED STUDY TIPS

1. Contact your local state board of nursing and request a copy of the Nurse Practice Act. Review the information about student nurses. Make certain that you acquire a copy every year for each state in which you are licensed.

2. List the five stages of the nursing process. Briefly explain each stage. Do you use all five stages each day, for each clinical client?

    _____

    _____

    _____

    _____

    _____

3. Use your web browser to go to http://www.nursingworld.org/ethics/ecode.htm. You can either purchase the code of ethics or view the code in sections. How does the code of ethics match your thoughts about the practice of nursing?

    _____

    _____

    _____

    _____

CASE STUDY

66-year-old Jacob Amrah has been diagnosed with diabetes mellitus. He will require insulin fingersticks four times a day to maintain his blood sugar. Jacob has been caring for his wife of 44 years who has the early stages of Alzheimer's. Jacob states that he can't do anymore. He wants his advanced directive changed to refuse all heroic measures; Jacob is including the administration of insulin in the category of heroic measures. Jacob wants to move into an assisted living facility with his wife. The facility does have an Alzheimer's unit into which his wife could be moved as her disease progresses. Jacob will have to do his own blood sugar testing and insulin administration.

1. Explain the concept of heroic measures with regard to the administration of insulin. Does this constitute a dilemma for the nursing staff?

2. While Jacob's reaction to a new chronic diagnosis may be common, what is he really saying?

3. What role or roles might the nurse play in helping both Jacob and his wife at this time?

NCLEX REVIEW QUESTIONS

1. In 2001 the Institute of Medicine found that:
    1. Errors are common and are most often caused by nursing.
    2. Misuse of services is more common than errors.
    3. Errors occur often because of the nursing shortage.
    4. Lack of focus often causes life-threatening emergencies.
    5. Errors are often caused by system problems, not healthcare professionals.
2. Critical thinking:
    1. Focuses on specific client situations.
    2. Removes one's attitudes and prejudices from the process.
    3. Is an innate, inborn ability to make decisions.
    4. Restricts the nurse's domain of practice.
3. The components of critical thinking include:
    1. A focus on the specifics of a situation and discounts divergent opinions.
    2. Reflection as an essential criterion during all situations.
    3. Clarification as well as noting similarities and differences.
    4. The requirement of processing of independent information.
4. Which is not a part of client assessment in the nursing process?
    1. Developing nursing diagnoses based on NANDA guidelines
    2. Clarifying subjective data
    3. Developing a client care plan through assessment findings
    4. Evaluating measurable client outcomes
5. Which statement best describes nursing documentation?
    1. Documentation is most important in the implementation process.
    2. Documenting assessment findings is the most critical legal issue.
    3. Computer-assisted documentation limits charting options.
    4. Charting by exception is an accepted form of documentation.
6. Evaluation in the nursing process determines the effectiveness of
    1. Assessment.
    2. Diagnosis.
    3. Outcomes.
    4. Implementation.

7. If a nursing outcome was not met, what should be the nurse's best response?
   1. Modify the outcome.
   2. Recognize that she/he has not been successful and renegotiate the outcome.
   3. Recognize that the client has not been successful and modify the outcome.
   4. Continue with the plan.
8. Nursing standards:
   1. Protect client confidentiality.
   2. Facilitate prosecution of nurses who put the health and welfare of the client at risk.
   3. Protect the public.
   4. Establish procedures for handling nursing dilemmas.
9. The role of the nurse as educator:
   1. Focuses on keeping clients out of the hospital.
   2. Is more important because of shorter hospital days.
   3. Begins in the home after discharge.
   4. Assists the client in decision making.
10. The care delivery model that requires the greatest amount of delegation is:
    1. Primary nursing.
    2. Team nursing.
    3. Case management.
    4. Both 2 and 3.

CHAPTER 2
HEALTH AND ILLNESS IN THE ADULT CLIENT

LEARNING OUTCOMES

After completing Chapter 2, you will be able to demonstrate the following objectives:

- Define health, incorporating the health–illness continuum and the concept of high-level wellness.
- Explain factors affecting functional health status.
- Discuss the nurse's role in health promotion.
- Describe the primary, secondary, and tertiary levels of illness prevention.
- Describe characteristics of health, disease, and illness.
- Describe illness behaviors and needs of the client with acute illness and chronic illness.
- Compare and contrast the physical status, risks for alterations in health, assessment guidelines, and healthy behaviors of the young adult, middle adult, and older adult.
- Explain the definitions, functions, and developmental stages and tasks of the family.

CLINICAL COMPETENCIES

- Include knowledge of developmental levels and of activities to promote, restore, and maintain health when planning and implementing care for adult clients.
- Include family members in teaching to promote and maintain health of the adult client.

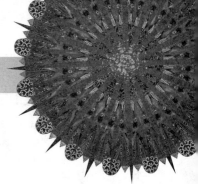

MediaLink

www.prenhall.com/lemone

Resources for this chapter can be found on the Prentice Hall Nursing MediaLink DVD accompanying this textbook, and on the Companion Website at http://www.prenhall.com/lemone. Click on Chapter 2 to select the activities for this chapter.

Prentice Hall Nursing MediaLink DVD-ROM
- Audio Glossary
- NCLEX-RN® Review

Companion Website
www.prenhall.com/lemone
- Audio Glossary
- NCLEX-RN® Review
- Care Plan Activity: Family-Centered Care in Chronic Illness
- Case Studies
  - Care Across the Lifespan
  - Developing Teaching Programs
- MediaLink Applications
- Links to Resources

KEY TERMS

acute illness	exacerbation	health–illness continuum	manifestations
chronic illness	family	holistic health care	remission
disease	health	illness	wellness

CHAPTER OUTLINE

I. The Health–Illness Continuum and High-Level Wellness
   A. Factors Affecting Health
      1. Genetic Makeup
      2. Cognitive Abilities and Educational Level
      3. Race, Ethnicity, and Cultural Background
      4. Age, Gender, and Developmental Level
      5. Lifestyle and Environment
      6. Socioeconomic Background
      7. Geographic Area
   B. Health Promotion and Maintenance
      1. Healthy Living
      2. National Health Promotion
   C. Disease and Illness
      1. Disease
      2. Illness
II. Meeting Health Needs of Adults
   A. The Young Adult
      1. Risks for Alterations in Health
      2. Assessment Guidelines
      3. Promoting Healthy Behaviors in the Young Adult
   B. The Middle Adult
      1. Risks for Alterations in Health
      2. Assessment Guidelines
      3. Promoting Healthy Behaviors in the Middle Adult
   C. The Older Adult
      1. Risks for Alterations in Health
      2. Assessment Guidelines
      3. Promoting Healthy Behaviors in the Older Adult
III. The Family of the Adult Client
   A. Definitions and Functions of the Family
   B. Family Developmental Stages and Tasks
      1. Couple
      2. Family with Infants and Preschoolers
      3. Family with School-Age Children
      4. Family with Adolescents and Young Adults
      5. Family with Middle Adults
      6. Family with Older Adults
   C. The Family of the Client with a Chronic Illness

FOCUSED STUDY TIPS

1. List and describe factors that affect health.

   a. _____

   b. _____

   c. _____

   d. _____

   e. _____

   f. _____

   g. _____

2. Identify the generally-accepted common causes of disease:

a. _____

b. _____

c. _____

d. _____

e. _____

f. _____

g. _____

h. _____

i. _____

3. Describe the difference between an acute and chronic illness.

_____

_____

_____

_____

_____

4. Give examples of primary, secondary, and tertiary illness prevention activities.

a. Primary Activities:

_____

_____

b. Secondary Activities:

_____

_____

c. Tertiary Activities:

_____

_____

CASE STUDY

Jacob is a 50-year-old black unemployed male with a history of past substance abuse who is being counseled about health promotion activities. Answer the following questions based on your knowledge of the middle aged adult and Jacob's history.

1. What alterations in health is Jacob at risk for developing as a middle aged adult?

2. What guidelines are useful in assessing the achievement of significant developmental tasks in the middle adult?

3. How can the nurse promote healthy behaviors in Jacob?

NCLEX REVIEW QUESTIONS

1. Identify the acute illness from those listed below.
   1. Influenza
   2. Cancer
   3. Hemophilia
   4. Sickle cell disease
2. An example of an altered response of health to lifestyle and environmental influences is the relationship of:
   1. Cigarette smoking to a sedentary lifestyle.
   2. Alcoholism to obesity.
   3. Obesity to hypertension.
   4. A sedentary lifestyle to chronic obstructive pulmonary disease.
3. Which of the following practices is not known to promote health and wellness?
   1. Sleeping five to six hours each day
   2. Smoking cessation
   3. Keeping sun exposure to a minimum
   4. Maintaining recommended immunizations
4. The client demonstrates behaviors of self-preoccupation during the initial assessment. This behavior is characteristic of what stage of illness?
   1. Experiencing symptoms
   2. Assuming a dependent role
   3. Achieving recovery and rehabilitation
   4. Assuming the sick role
5. Given that the client is 35 years old, the nurse knows that the client would fall into what stage of adulthood?
   1. Young adult
   2. Middle adult
   3. Older adult
   4. Young middle adult
6. Identify the cancer not commonly found in the middle adult.
   1. Lung
   2. Liver
   3. Reproductive
   4. Colon
7. All of the following are frequently-occurring conditions in the older adult except:
   1. Hypertension.
   2. Arthritis.
   3. Sinusitis.
   4. Obesity.
8. Identify the family developmental stage that focuses on transition.
   1. Family with infants and preschoolers
   2. Family with school-age children
   3. Family with adolescents and young adults
   4. Family with middle adults
9. The nurse is caring for a 45-year-old Chinese American client. The nurse is aware that the client is at risk for all of the following illnesses except:
   1. An eye disorder.
   2. A cardiovascular disorder.
   3. Obesity.
   4. Sexually-transmitted disease.
10. Identify the ineffective coping skill of a client with a chronic illness.
    1. Learning to adapt activities of daily living and self-care activities
    2. Denying the inevitability of death
    3. Complying with a medical treatment plan
    4. Maintaining a feeling of being in control

CHAPTER 3

COMMUNITY-BASED AND HOME CARE OF THE ADULT CLIENT

LEARNING OUTCOMES

After completing Chapter 3, you will be able to demonstrate the following objectives:

- Differentiate community-based care from community health care.
- Discuss selected factors affecting health in the community.
- Describe services and settings for healthcare consumers receiving community-based and home care.
- Describe the components of the home healthcare system, including agencies, clients, referrals, physicians, reimbursement, legal considerations, and nursing care.
- Compare and contrast the roles of the nurse providing home care with the roles of the nurse in medical-surgical nursing discussed in Chapter 1.
- Explain the purpose of rehabilitation in health care.

CLINICAL COMPETENCIES

- Provide client care in community-based settings and the home.
- Apply the nursing process to care of the client in the home.

KEY TERMS

community-based care
contracting
disability
handicap
home care
hospice care
impairment
parish nursing
referral source
rehabilitation
respite care

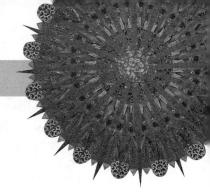

CHAPTER OUTLINE

I. Community-Based Nursing Care
   A. Factors Affecting Health in the Community
      1. Social Support Systems
      2. Community Healthcare Structure
      3. Environmental Factors
      4. Economic Resources
II. Community-Based Healthcare Services
   A. Community Centers and Clinics
   B. Day Care Programs
   C. Parish Nursing
   D. Meals-on-Wheels
III. Home Care
   A. Brief History of Home Care
   B. Hospice and Respite Care
   C. The Home Care System
      1. Types of Home Health Agencies
      2. Clients
      3. Referrals
      4. Physicians
      5. Reimbursement for Services
      6. Legal Considerations
   D. The Nursing Process in Home Care
      1. Assessment
      2. Diagnosis
      3. Planning
      4. Implementation
      5. Evaluation
   E. Roles of the Home Care Nurse
      1. Advocate
      2. Provider of Direct Care
      3. Educator
      4. Coordinator of Services
   F. Special Considerations in Home Care Nursing
   G. Nursing Interventions to Ensure Competent Home Care
      1. Establish Trust and Rapport
      2. Proceed Slowly
      3. Set Goals and Boundaries
      4. Assess the Home Environment
      5. Set Priorities
      6. Promote Learning
      7. Limit Distractions
      8. Put Safety First
      9. Make Do
      10. Control Infection
IV. Rehabilitation

FOCUSED STUDY TIPS

1. Knowing your resources is very important. Contact five community health agencies. Identify the target population and available services for each. Share this research with your peers to expand your database of community resources.

_____

_____

_____

_____

_____

2. List two nursing interventions that ensure good rapport between the client and the nurse in community home care.

_____

_____

_____

_____

_____

3. Safety issues often pose problems for both the client and the nurse. Find a neighbor, family friend, or family member, assess their home for common safety issues, and write your findings in chart below. Discuss the identified safety issues with the homeowner.

Safety Issue	Findings
Family or other support	
Stairs with hand-rails	
Smoke detector	
Bathroom issues	
Electrical hazards	
Throw rugs	
Clear walkways	
Medications (expired and storage)	
Poor-fitting shoes	
Inadequate food supply and access	
Cooking habits	
Functioning utilities	
Chipping paint	

CASE STUDY

Mr. Maxwell Cohen is an 85-year-old male who has been discharged from the acute care hospital after a fall outside of his home that was caused by a weak railing. He has multiple bruises and skin tears, as well as a left radial ulnar fracture. The cast limits his mobility but he is right-handed and does not believe this will be a problem. Mr. Cohen has been a widower for the last year and a half, and seems well-adjusted.

During the nurse's first visit, it is evident that Mr. Cohen has many friends in the neighborhood who check on him often, and several stop by during the visit. The railing has been repaired and there are no additional areas that appear to be loose. There is a non-slip mat at the front and side doors for people to wipe their shoes before entering the home. Things appear to be neat and tidy in the home with little clutter. There are two extension cords visible in the home, one of which runs under the edge of a carpet in an unused corner of the living room.

The kitchen is well-organized and clean, and the cookware is heavy but Mr. Cohen is able to lift it without difficulty with his right hand. The nurse is able to observe Mr. Cohen in the kitchen because he was making lunch at the time the nurse arrived. The client uses plastic dinnerware and drinking glasses.

Mr. Cohen states that he is healing but the progress seems to be slower than he expected. He also states that he has had difficulty changing clothes, getting in and out of the bathtub, and opening his medication bottles. His medications are lined up on the counter; none are expired and he is able to discuss his medications without difficulty.

1. What distractions limited the nurse's ability to assess and care for Mr. Cohen?

2. What safety concerns do you see in Mr. Cohen's home setting? Would these be expensive to repair?

3. What can you do to improve Mr. Cohen's safety with regard to his medication administration?

CARE PLAN CRITICAL THINKING ACTIVITY

Please use the case study above to develop a care plan listing the most important physiological, psychosocial, teaching, and safety issue.

NCLEX REVIEW QUESTIONS

1. Which factor does not affect the health of a community?
    1. Providing care in a client's home
    2. The number of extended families in a community
    3. Environmental factors such as air and water quality
    4. Access to health care
2. Community-based healthcare services allow clients to remain in the community longer. Which best describes these types of services?
    1. Services that allow clients with late stages of Alzheimer's disease to remain at home
    2. Programs that encourage physical safety, and social, nutritional, and recreation
    3. Meals on Wheels
    4. Programs that decrease the need for hospitalization days and limit costs
3. Which statement by the nurse is most accurate when discussing home health care?
    1. The purpose of home health care is to promote, maintain, or restore the level of dependence of the client.
    2. Home health care provides care for clients who need long-term daily care.
    3. The largest single source of reimbursement for home health care is Medicaid.
    4. Home health care is designed for clients who require additional assistance and education in their home.

4. A family member believes that a 43-year-old female client would benefit from home health care after a trauma. The client has no health insurance and does not think that she needs this type of care. Which is the most appropriate statement the nurse can make about home health care?
   1. Home health care is inexpensive and will help the client to return to their maximum level of wellness earlier than clients who don't have home health care support.
   2. Some home health care agencies have sliding scale or donations payment plans.
   3. Family members cannot be the person who is requesting home health care.
   4. A registered nurse can help to keep the cost lower by limiting the involvement of a physician in the client's aftercare.
5. The focus of the initial home health visit is best described as:
   1. Evaluation of client outcomes established during the acute care in-hospital stay.
   2. The time to obtain a referral and establish the nurse-client relationship.
   3. Assessment of the client, the physical environment, and support systems.
   4. The best time to determine if this client will be successful with in-home care.
6. Which statement below is the most appropriate outcome statement?
   1. Deficient knowledge related to a diagnosis of chronic obstructive pulmonary disease.
   2. Client will use oxygen.
   3. Client will demonstrate application of oxygen by the second home health visit.
   4. Apply oxygen per physician order.
7. As a coordinator of services, the home health nurse:
   1. Will discuss the client's care with the various members of the healthcare team.
   2. Will change the treatment plan at the direction of the client.
   3. Will document the client's care to meet the needs of the physician.
   4. Will fax requests to the physician's office in order to maintain the client confidentiality.
8. Which of the following can be a challenge in providing care in the client's home?
   1. The client's independence in the home
   2. Blurring of lines between nursing and the family support system
   3. Establishing a positive rapport with the client and family
   4. Caregivers who share responsibility for the client's support
9. Education is an important part of home health care. Which statement is most appropriate when it comes to client education?
   1. The nurse is the most influential source of information for the home health client.
   2. The nurse can empower the client to learn by encouraging them to listen to their own bodies and asking questions.
   3. The nurse gives the client written information about concerns he or she might have in the future.
   4. The nurse involves as many people as possible in the learning process.
10. During a home health visit, the nurse notices that the client is taking expired medications and has no heat. Which would be the most appropriate action of the nurse?
    1. Discuss the situation with social services.
    2. Ignore the situation and hope it gets better.
    3. Encourage the client to wear warmer clothing and to get the furnace fixed before winter comes.
    4. Discuss the issues with the client.

CHAPTER 4

Nursing Care of Clients Having Surgery

LEARNING OUTCOMES

After completing Chapter 4, you will be able to demonstrate the following objectives:

- Discuss the differences and similarities between outpatient and inpatient surgery.
- Describe the various classifications of surgical procedures.
- Identify diagnostic tests used in the perioperative period.
- Describe nursing implications for medications prescribed for the surgical client.
- Provide appropriate nursing care for the client in the preoperative, intraoperative, and postoperative phases of surgery.
- Identify variations in perioperative care for the older adult.
- Describe principles of pain management specific to acute postoperative pain control.
- Use the nursing process as a framework for providing individualized care for the client undergoing surgery.

CLINICAL COMPETENCIES

- Assess the physiological health status of clients for surgery to determine their ability to tolerate surgery and risks for complications.
- Assess the psychosocial health status of the client and family.
- Transfer the client safely within the operating room and throughout the postoperative stay.
- Participate in client and family teaching prior to anesthesia and prior to discharge from the facility.
- Create and maintain a sterile field in the operating room and use universal precautions to prevent infections.
- Provide equipment and supplies based on client need.
- Perform sponge, sharps, and instrument counts before discharging the client from the operating room.

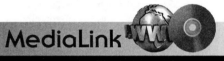

MediaLink
www.prenhall.com/lemone

Resources for this chapter can be found on the Prentice Hall Nursing MediaLink DVD accompanying this textbook, and on the Companion Website at http://www.prenhall.com/lemone. Click on Chapter 4 to select the activities for this chapter.

Prentice Hall Nursing MediaLink DVD-ROM
- Audio Glossary
- NCLEX-RN® Review

Animation/Video
- Epidural Placement

Companion Website
www.prenhall.com/lemone
- Audio Glossary
- NCLEX-RN® Review
- Care Plan Activity: Providing Postoperative Care
- Case Study: The Circulating Nurse
- MediaLink Applications
  - Anesthesia and Outpatient Surgery
  - Consent Forms
  - Joint Replacement Patient Education Program
- Links to Resources

- Physiologically monitor the client during surgery. As part of the interdisciplinary team, promote safe practice and client rehabilitation.
- Monitor and control the environment to prevent accidents or injury to the client and the healthcare team. Respect the client's rights, including privacy, at all times (AORN, 2005b).

KEY TERMS

anesthesia	informed consent
circulating nurse	interdisciplinary care
conscious sedation	intraoperative phase
dehiscence	perioperative nursing
equianalgesia	positioning
evisceration	postoperative phase
freestanding outpatient	preoperative phase
surgical facilities	regional anesthesia
general anesthesia	scrub person
independent nursing care	surgery

CHAPTER OUTLINE

   I. Settings for Surgery
  II. Legal Requirements
    A. Perioperative Risk Factors
    B. Interdisciplinary Care
       1. Diagnosis
       2. Medications
       3. Surgical Environment
       4. Client Preparation
       5. Nutrition
 III. Nursing Care
    A. Preoperative Nursing Care
    B. Preoperative Client and Family Teaching
    C. Preoperative Client Preparation
    D. Intraoperative Nursing Care
    E. Postoperative Nursing Care
       1. Immediate Postoperative Care
       2. Care When the Client Is Stable
    F. Nursing Care of Common Postoperative Complications
       1. Cardiovascular Complications
       2. Respiratory Complications
       3. Wound Complications
       4. Complications Associated with Elimination
       5. Special Considerations for Older Adults
    G. Managing Acute Postoperative Pain
    H. Using NANDA, NIC, and NOC
    I. Community-Based Care

FOCUSED STUDY TIPS

1. List and describe the three phases of the perioperative experience.

   a. _____

   b. _____

   c. _____

2. Describe the role and responsibilities of the following healthcare providers within the perioperative setting:

   a. Surgeon

   _____

   b. Circulating nurse

   _____

   c. Scrub nurse

   _____

   d. Anesthesiologist

   _____

   e. Phlebotomists

   _____

   f. X-ray technicians

   _____

   g. Transporters

   _____

3. Describe the differences between general anesthesia, regional anesthesia, and conscious sedation.

   _____

   _____

   _____

   _____

   _____

4. Describe the following postoperative complications and their appropriate nursing interventions:

   a. Hemorrhage:

   _____

   _____

   _____

   b. Deep vein thrombosis:

   _____

   _____

   _____

   c. Pneumonia:

   _____

   _____

   _____

CASE STUDY

Mrs. Elvira, a 28-year-old female, is scheduled to undergo a right radical mastectomy. Mrs. Elvira reports smoking two and a half packs of cigarettes a day and obtaining minimal exercise. She takes aspirin for frequent headaches and herbal supplements to help her lose weight. Answer the following questions based on your knowledge of client needs for undergoing surgery.

1. Mrs. Elvira's informed consent document includes the surgeon's name, the alternatives and risks of treatments, and the date and time she and her surgeon signed the consent. What is missing?

2. What postoperative complication(s) is Mrs. Elvira at most risk of developing based on her history?

3. What preoperative studies and interventions will Mrs. Elvira undergo to reduce the likelihood of intraoperative and postoperative complications?

4. Prior to discharge, Mrs. Elvira will be instructed to assess her incision site for signs of infection. What are they?

NCLEX REVIEW QUESTIONS

1. Identify the incorrect statement.
   1. Inpatient procedures decrease client, hospital, and insurance agency costs.
   2. The outpatient surgical client must cope with the need to learn a great deal of information in a short span of time.
   3. Outpatient surgery provides for less time for pain relief before discharge.
   4. Outpatient surgery provides for less interruption in the client's and family's routine.
2. Informed consent does not need to include which of the following?
   1. Description and purpose of the proposed procedure
   2. Alternative treatments or procedures available
   3. Date, time, and location of the proposed surgical procedure
   4. Right to refuse treatment or withdraw consent
3. All but which of the following interventions are appropriate nursing interventions when monitoring the client for hypothermia?
   1. Application of warm blankets upon arrival in the surgical area and after sterile drapes are removed
   2. Cool irrigation or infusion solutions as needed
   3. Humidify the airway
   4. Prevent surgical drapes from becoming wet
4. Identify the incorrect stage of general anesthesia.
   1. Induction
   2. Emergence
   3. Maintenance
   4. Deepening
5. After the client has undergone surgery with a spinal anesthetic, a postoperative spinal headache occurs. Which intervention is the appropriate one for the nurse to implement?
   1. Decrease client hydration.
   2. Raise the head of the bed 45 degrees.
   3. Prepare the client for a blood patch procedure.
   4. Restrict all caffeine products.
6. Identify the surgical team member who is responsible for documenting intraoperative nursing activities, medications, blood administration, placement of drains and catheters, and length of the procedure.
   1. Surgeon
   2. Circulating Nurse
   3. Certified Registered Nurse Anesthetist
   4. Surgical Scrub

7. An outcome of improper intraoperative surgical positioning is:
   1. Nerve damage
   2. Hyperthermia
   3. Hemorrhage
   4. Increased joint flexibility

8. The nurse knows the client understood perioperative teaching when the client demonstrates which of these behaviors?
   1. Arrives with freshly-painted nails
   2. Has eaten a full breakfast before arriving at the hospital
   3. Has completed all preoperative testing as ordered
   4. Arrives with contacts in-place

9. The client has a positive Homan's sign after surgery. Which of the following interventions is incorrect?
   1. Keep affected extremity at or below heart level.
   2. Ensure that the affected area is not rubbed or massaged.
   3. Record bilateral calf or thigh circumferences every shift.
   4. Teach and support the client and family.

10. Which is not a common assessment finding of a client who is experiencing symptoms of a pulmonary embolism?
    1. Anxiety
    2. Decreased oxygen saturation
    3. Decrease in respiratory rate
    4. Cough

CHAPTER 5

NURSING CARE OF CLIENTS EXPERIENCING LOSS, GRIEF, AND DEATH

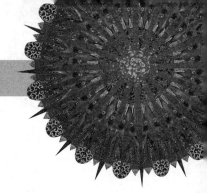

MediaLink

www.prenhall.com/lemone

Resources for this chapter can be found on the Prentice Hall Nursing MediaLink DVD accompanying this textbook, and on the Companion Website at http://www.prenhall.com/lemone. Click on Chapter 5 to select the activities for this chapter.

Prentice Hall Nursing MediaLink DVD-ROM
- Audio Glossary
- NCLEX-RN® Review

Companion Website
www.prenhall.com/lemone
- Audio Glossary
- NCLEX-RN® Review
- Care Plan Activity: Anticipatory Grieving
- Case Study: Do-Not-Resuscitate
- MediaLink Applications
  - DNR Regulations
  - Explore Your Feelings about Death
  - Grieving Process
  - Hospice: Purpose and Benefits
- Links to Resources

LEARNING OUTCOMES

After completing Chapter 5, you will be able to demonstrate the following objectives:
- Differentiate loss, grief, and mourning.
- Compare and contrast theories of loss and grief.
- Explain factors affecting responses to loss.
- Discuss legal and ethical issues in end-of-life care.
- Describe the philosophy and activities of hospice.

CLINICAL COMPETENCIES

- Identify physiological changes in the dying client.
- Provide nursing interventions to promote a comfortable death.
- Provide individualized care for clients and families experiencing loss, grief, or death.

KEY TERMS

anticipatory grieving
bereavement
chronic sorrow
death
death anxiety
do-not-resuscitate order
durable power of attorney
end-of-life nursing care
euthanasia
grief
grieving
healthcare surrogate
hospice
living will
loss
mourning
palliative care

CHAPTER OUTLINE

I. Theories of Loss and Grief
  A. Freud: Psychoanalytic Theory
  B. Bowlby: Protest, Despair, and Detachment
    1. Engel: Acute Grief, Restitution, and Long-Term Grief
  C. Lindemann: Categories of Symptoms
  D. Caplan: Stress and Loss
  E. Kübler-Ross: Stages of Coping with Loss
II. Factors Affecting Responses to Loss
  A. Age
  B. Social Support
  C. Families
  D. Cultural and Spiritual Practices
  E. Rituals of Mourning
  F. Nurses' Response to Clients' Loss
III. End-of-Life Care
  A. Nursing Considerations for End-of-Life Care
    1. Legal and Ethical Issues
  B. Settings and Services for End-of-Life Care
    1. Hospice
    2. Palliative Care
  C. Physiologic Changes in the Dying Client
    1. Pain
    2. Dyspnea
    3. Anorexia, Nausea, and Dehydration
    4. Altered Levels of Consciousness
    5. Hypotension
  D. Support for the Client and Family
  E. Death
    1. Postmortem Care
    2. Nurses' Grief
IV. Interdisciplinary Care
V. Nursing Care
  A. Health Promotion
  B. Assessment
    1. Physical Assessment
    2. Spiritual Assessment
    3. Psychosocial Assessment
  C. Nursing Diagnoses and Interventions
    1. Anticipatory Grieving
    2. Chronic Sorrow
    3. Death Anxiety
  D. Using NANDA, NIC, and NOC
  E. Community-Based Care

FOCUSED STUDY TIPS

1. List three grief theories that are included in this chapter. Based on your personal experience with grief, which theory best describes your process of handling loss?

_____

_____

_____

_____

_____

2. A client is interested in planning his funeral service and writing his obituary. He is still in the treatment phase of his disease and his family is concerned that he's just given up. They are angry that they are being so supportive and hopeful for treatment and he is morbidly planning his death.

   1. How common is this situation?

   _____

   2. Has the client given in or is he looking for control? Support your findings.

   _____

   _____

   3. The nurse caring for the client is care-focused. How will this affect the care relationship?

   _____

   _____

   _____

3. Define the following terms or concepts:

   1. Grief

   _____

   2. Hospice

   _____

   3. Euthanasia

   _____

   4. Living will

   _____

   5. Mourning

   _____

   6. Advance directive

   _____

   7. Loss

   _____

4. Cultural care is as important at the end of life as it is at any other time during the client's life. Investigate the cultural needs of a client who is from a different faith system. Discuss the challenges of meeting these needs in a medical-surgical unit.

   _____

   _____

   _____

   _____

   _____

CASE STUDY

27-year-old Alana Oberan just received a terminal diagnosis. She is a successful graduate student at a state university, and is studying medieval literature. She has a friend that she has been seeing for the last several months but has no long-term plans with this individual. Alana is an only child and both of her parents are professors of archeology at the same university that she attends.

Alana has always been an independent person but now she is confused and afraid. When she asked the doctor for a timeframe the only answer was, "Everyone responds differently, so it is very difficult to say." What the doctor didn't say was that, due to the aggressive growth of this cancer, a 12-month survival rate would be optimistic. Alana doesn't know what to tell her parents, or if she should tell them now. What if the diagnosis is wrong? Is there a treatment that this doctor doesn't know about? Why get her parents upset if the doctor is wrong? Her friend will probably leave. They've only been seeing each other for a short time and both agreed that it wasn't a serious relationship, it was just for fun. This would not be fun, not for anyone.

1. Is a hospice organization available to members of your community? What other community resources would be helpful for this client?

2. According to Kübler-Ross's stages of coping with loss, in what stage of grieving is the client? At what stage can you anticipate her parents will begin?

3. What factors will affect the parents' ability to grieve their upcoming loss?

CARE PLAN CRITICAL THINKING ACTIVITY

1. What psychological diagnosis symptoms is Mrs. Rogers demonstrating?

2. What questions could the nurse ask as part of the interview and assessment process to gain further information about Mrs. Rogers's mental health?

3. What information could the nurse gather from Mrs. Rogers's daughter that would assist in assessing the client's mental health?

NCLEX REVIEW QUESTIONS

1. The nurse enters the room and finds the client crying after the physician left the room. Which would be the best statement made by the nurse to the client?
   1. "The physician said she told you about your testing tomorrow. Is that true?"
   2. "Is there someone I can call for you?"
   3. "Tell me what is troubling you right now."
   4. "Are you upset about tomorrow's testing?"
2. A client's family has explained their important cultural ritual of taping medallions to the client's body and removing them at the time of death so that they can be given to the children. What is the best response by the nurse?
   1. "We can work with that as long as the medallions don't interfere with the client's medical care."
   2. "I'm sorry but those can pose an electrical risk to the client. I can talk to the doctor to see what what we will have to do about them."
   3. "What religious connection do these have for you?"
   4. "As long as these were approved by the physician they should be ok."
3. A client is now unresponsive after six months of aggressive treatment for pancreatic cancer. Which document would allow a designated person to make decision about the client's health care?
   1. Advanced directive
   2. Durable power of attorney
   3. Living will
   4. Client Bill of Rights

4. A client is actively dying and her husband wants to burn candles in the client's room. The hospital policy strictly forbids open flame in the facility. What would be the best response by the nurse?
   1. "I can't allow you to burn those in here because of the hospital policy."
   2. "That is alright, but please keep the door closed so no one else finds out."
   3. "Does the candle need to burn all the time or can you just light it for a few minutes at a time?"
   4. "Hospital policy does not allow for anyone to have open flame inside the building. Is there anything else you could do that would have similar meaning?"

5. The client has a do-not-resuscitate order on the chart and the family has decided to provide palliative care rather than aggressive treatment. Which nursing intervention is an appropriate nursing response to the client's moans and grimaces?
   1. Administer 2 mg IV morphine per the physician's order.
   2. Assess for pain, reposition the client, and then reassess for pain.
   3. Ask the family if this is how the client reacts to pain.
   4. Call the physician seeking a long-term pain control medication.

6. A client asks the nurse about the reputation of the physician who diagnosed his colon cancer. The client states, "I should get another opinion before I have this surgery tomorrow." In which stage of grief is this client? (Please select all that apply.)
   1. Kübler-Ross: anger
   2. Engel: acute stage
   3. Bowlby: protest
   4. Lindemann: morbid grief reaction
   5. Caplan: stress and loss

7. The client chooses palliative care for the end of his life. What would be the most appropriate action for the nurse to take in the last hours of the client's life?
   1. Hourly vital signs
   2. Repositioning the client every two hours
   3. Elevate the head of the bed and provide a fan.
   4. Encourage the client to eat to keep up his/her strength.

8. The client is complaining of being being short of breath with a respiratory rate of 38 and an oxygen saturation of 92%. Which nursing intervention would be the least appropriate?
   1. Administration of 2 mg of IV morphine
   2. Administration of oxygen 2 L/min via nasal cannula
   3. Reposition the client.
   4. Administer oxygen via 100% nonrebreather mask.

9. A client at the end of life has intractible vomiting and has refused a nasogastric tube. What other nursing interventions may aid the client's comfort?
   1. Encourage the client to drink ginger ale with ice chips.
   2. Administer morphine 1 mg IV.
   3. Administer prochlorperazine (Compazine) PO.
   4. Administer odansetron (Zofran) IV.

10. After providing care for a client, the nurse documents the care. Which is the best evaluation statement?
    1. Oral care provided, client repositioned for comfort
    2. Mucous membranes moist and intact
    3. Oxygen applied via nasal cannula
    4. Client confused, sister at bedside

CHAPTER 6

NURSING CARE OF CLIENTS WITH PROBLEMS OF SUBSTANCE ABUSE

LEARNING OUTCOMES

After completing Chapter 6, you will be able to demonstrate the following objectives:

- Explain risk factors associated with substance abuse.
- Recognize the signs and symptoms of potential substance abuse in coworkers.
- Describe common characteristics of substance abusers.
- Classify major addictive substances.
- Explain the effects of addictive substances on physiologic, cognitive, psychologic, and social well-being.
- Support interdisciplinary care for the client with substance abuse problems, including diagnostic tests, emergency care for overdose, and treatment of withdrawal.
- Develop a framework for providing individualized nursing care for clients experiencing problems with substance abuse using the nursing process.

CLINICAL COMPETENCIES

- Assess functional health status of clients with substance abuse.
- Monitor, document, and report physical manifestations of substance abuse.
- Assess for signs of withdrawal and monitor for life-threatening conditions.
- Use evidence-based research to plan and implement nursing care for clients experiencing withdrawal symptoms.
- Derive priority nursing diagnoses from assessment data.
- Formulate appropriate goals and implement individualized nursing interventions for clients with problems of substance abuse.
- Provide skilled nursing care during detoxification period.
- Collaborate with other disciplines when caring for clients with substance abuse problems.

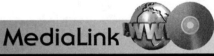

MediaLink

www.prenhall.com/lemone

Resources for this chapter can be found on the Prentice Hall Nursing MediaLink DVD accompanying this textbook, and on the Companion Website at http://www.prenhall.com/lemone. Click on Chapter 6 to select the activities for this chapter.

Prentice Hall Nursing MediaLink DVD-ROM
- Audio Glossary
- NCLEX-RN® Review

Animation
- Cocaine

Companion Website
www.prenhall.com/lemone
- Audio Glossary
- NCLEX-RN® Review
- Care Plan Activities
  - Alcohol Withdrawal
  - Tobacco Cessation
- Case Study: Alcohol Withdrawal
- MediaLink Applications
- Links to Resources

- Educate client about stress management, coping skills, nutrition, relapse prevention, and healthy lifestyle choices.
- Revise plan of care as needed to promote, maintain, or restore functional health status to clients with substance abuse problems.

KEY TERMS

alcohol
amphetamine
caffeine
cannabis sativa
central nervous system
   depressants
cocaine
co-occurring disorders
delirium tremens (DT)
dual diagnosis
dual disorder
hallucinogens
inhalants

kindling
Korsakoff's psychosis
nicotine
opiates
polysubstance abuse
psychostimulants
substance abuse
substance dependence
tolerance
Wernicke's encephalopathy
withdrawal
withdrawal symptoms

CHAPTER OUTLINE

I. Risk Factors
II. Characteristics of Abusers
III. Addictive Substances and Their Effects
   A. Caffeine
   B. Nicotine
   C. Cannabis
   D. Alcohol
   E. CNS Depressants
   F. Psychostimulants
   G. Opiates
   H. Hallucinogens
   I. Inhalants
IV. Interdisciplinary Care
   1. Diagnostic Tests
   2. Emergency Care for Overdose
   3. Treatment of Withdrawal
V. Nursing Care
   A. Health Promotion
   B. Assessment
       1. History of Past Substance Abuse
       2. Medical and Psychiatric History
       3. Psychosocial Issues
       4. Screening Tools
       5. Withdrawal Assessment Tools
   C. Nursing Diagnoses and Interventions
       1. Risk for Injury and Risk for Violence
       2. Ineffective Denial
       3. Ineffective Coping
       4. Imbalanced Nutrition: Less than Body Requirements
       5. Chronic Low or Situational Low Self-Esteem
       6. Deficient Knowledge
       7. Disturbed Sensory Perceptions
       8. Disturbed Thought Processes

      D. Using NANDA, NIC, and NOC
      E. Community-Based Care
  VI. Impaired Nurses

FOCUSED STUDY TIPS

1. Explain the following risk factors as they relate to substance abuse:

   a. Genetic factors

    _____

    _____

   b. Biological factors

    _____

    _____

   c. Psychological factors

    _____

    _____

   d. Sociocultural factors

    _____

    _____

2. Complete the following table:

Addictive Substance	Effect
Caffeine	
Nicotine	
Cannabis	
Alcohol	
CNS Depressants	
Psychostimulants	
Amphetamines	
Opiates	
Hallucinogens	
Inhalants	

3. Describe the following substance abuse screening tools:

   a. Michigan Alcohol Screening Test (MAST) brief version

   _____

   _____

   b. CAGE questionnaire

   _____

   _____

   c. Brief Drug Abuse Screening Test (B-DAST)

   _____

   _____

4. Identify community-based care options available to clients who suffer from substance abuse.

   _____

   _____

   _____

   _____

   _____

   _____

CASE STUDY

Ryan Dern is a 32-year-old male who suffers from alcoholism. He has taken the initial step of admitting to his problem and seeking medical assistance. Answer the following questions based on your knowledge of alcoholism.

1. How long does Ryan need to have had excessive drinking behaviors to be considered substance dependent?

2. What factors affect the rate of alcohol absorption?

3. What vitamin deficiency is associated with alcoholism? How will the nurse assist Ryan in meeting his nutritional needs?

4. The nurse will teach Ryan HALT. What is HALT?

CARE PLAN CRITICAL THINKING ACTIVITY

1. Describe methods used to assess Mr. Russell's motor responses.

2. Describe interventions that can be utilized to prevent Mr. Russell from experiencing a fall injury.

3. What questions can the nurse ask to assess Mr. Russell's perceptions of his alcohol intake?

4. How should the nurse respond if Mr. Russell denies an alcohol problem?

NCLEX REVIEW QUESTIONS

1. Identify the neurotransmitter that plays a pivotal role in substance abuse.
   1. Dopamine
   2. Endorphin
   3. Enkephalin
   4. Dynorphin
2. Which ethnic group reports the lowest incidence of alcohol abuse?
   1. African Americans
   2. Native Americans
   3. Hispanics
   4. Asians
3. Which is not a characteristic of substance abusers?
   1. Drug users indulge in impulsive behaviors.
   2. Abusers often have a high tolerance for frustration and pain.
   3. Drug users are rebellious against social norms.
   4. Substance abusers have an impaired social and occupational functioning.
4. Which addictive substance may be a risk factor in developing future psychotic symptoms?
   1. Cocaine
   2. Methamphetamine
   3. Cannabis
   4. OxyContin
5. The client reports using crank to the nurse. The nurse knows crank is a form of what substance?
   1. Methamphetamine
   2. Opiate
   3. Hallucinogen
   4. Alcohol
6. Which body fluid is not often tested for drug content?
   1. Saliva
   2. Tears
   3. Urine
   4. Blood
7. Which is the correct form of questioning to use when assessing a client for substance abuse?
   1. "You don't have any drug abusers in your family, do you?"
   2. "Did you ever abuse a substance in the past?"
   3. "Have you ever been treated in an alcohol or drug abuse clinic?"
   4. "Were you ever arrested for a driving while under the influence (DUI) offense?"
8. Which screening tool is most effective for the nurse to use when the client does not recognize their own substance abuse problem?
   1. Brief Drug Abuse Screening Test (B-DAST)
   2. CAGE questionnaire
   3. Michigan Alcohol Screening Test (MAST) brief version
   4. HALT Screening Assessment tool
9. The nurse caring for a client with a substance abuse addiction should employ which intervention?
   1. Assess the client's level of disorientation.
   2. Place the client alone in a private room.
   3. Accept the use of defense mechanisms.
   4. Do not encourage the client to verbalize anxieties.
10. Nurses have a higher incidence of what type of abuse?
    1. Alcohol
    2. Hallucinogen
    3. Opiate
    4. Amphetamine

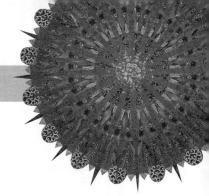

CHAPTER 7

NURSING CARE OF CLIENTS EXPERIENCING DISASTERS

LEARNING OUTCOMES

After completing Chapter 7, you will be able to demonstrate the following objectives:

- Distinguish the difference between an emergency and a disaster.
- Describe the types of injuries or symptoms that are associated with biologic, chemical, or radiologic terrorism.
- Evaluate nursing interventions for the treatment of injuries related to biological, chemical, or radiologic terrorism.
- Explain the rationale for reverse triage in disasters versus conventional triage in emergencies.
- Discuss situations requiring the need for client isolation or client decontamination.
- Discuss the role of the nurse in disaster planning, response, and mitigation.
- Identify ways that nurses are able to provide care to clients with special considerations.

CLINICAL COMPETENCIES

- Assess health status of clients who have experienced a disaster and monitor, document, and triage to the appropriate level of care.
- Use evidence-based research to plan and implement nursing care for clients with injuries suffered as a result of the disaster.
- Using assessment skills, determine priority nursing diagnoses, implement, and evaluate individualized nursing interventions for clients who are victims of disasters.
- Provide skilled nursing care to treat disaster-related injuries.
- Integrate interdisciplinary care of clients with an understanding of local, state, and federal systems of disaster response.
- Evaluate and revise plan of care and interventions based on client's condition, environmental factors, and resources to promote, maintain, or restore functional health status to clients who have sustained injuries due to a disaster.
- Provide education to promote prevention of disaster-related injuries.

KEY TERMS

bioterrorism
cold zone
conventional weapons
dirty bomb
disasters
emergency
hazardous materials
hot zone
hurricane
man-made disasters
mass casualty incidents
mitigation
multiple casualty incidents
natural disasters
nonconventional terrorist
  weapons

nuclear
personal protective
  equipment PPE)
preparedness
radiation sickness
radiologic dispersion bomb
reconstruction
recovery
response
reverse triage
surge capacity
surveillance
terrorism
triage
tsunami
warm zone

CHAPTER OUTLINE

FOCUSED STUDY TIPS

1. Describe and give examples of natural and manmade disasters.

   _____

   _____

   _____

   _____

   _____

2. Describe and give examples of conventional and nonconventional weapons.

   _____

   _____

   _____

   _____

   _____

3. What agencies are involved in the following levels of disasters?

   a. Level I

   _____

   b. Level II

   _____

   c. Level III

   _____

4. Describe triage. Develop your own triage system.

   _____

   _____

   _____

   _____

   _____

   _____

   _____

   _____

   _____

CASE STUDY

Mrs. Deckman, a 72-year-old female, has been trapped in her home as a result of a hurricane with flooding. She is a diabetic who controls her blood sugar with oral hypoglycemics. She has no other significant past medical history. Answer the following questions based on your knowledge of the care of patients experiencing disasters.

1. What is a hurricane?

2. What physical effects of a hurricane is Mrs. Deckman at risk for, regardless of her past medical history?

3. Mrs. Deckman was given a triage level of red after she was taken to a local shelter. What does this mean?

4. Mrs. Deckman asks the nurse for assistance in developing a disaster box to be used in case of another disaster. What items should the nurse suggest to be kept in the box?

CARE PLAN CRITICAL THINKING ACTIVITY

1. How should the nurse respond if Mr. Jones refused to speak about his feelings of loss and grief?

2. What role could Mr. Jones's daughter play in assisting him with expressing his feelings of loss and grief?

3. What community-based resources could be accessed to assist Mr. Jones in dealing with his emotional and financial losses?

NCLEX REVIEW QUESTIONS

1. Identify the nonconventional terrorist weapon.
   1. Incendiary bomb
   2. Shoulder-fired missiles
   3. Anthrax
   4. Hand grenade
2. Identify the correct statement about thunderstorm-related injuries.
   1. A person who has been struck by lightning carries an electrical charge.
   2. The immediate flashover of current around the body usually results in skin breakdown and tissue burns.
   3. The body's low electrolyte and water content conducts the greatest electrical current.
   4. High resistors to electric current are bone, tendon, and fat.
3. Which is not a source of ionizing radiation?
   1. Stars
   2. Sun
   3. X-ray machines
   4. Cell phones
4. A disaster that requires mutual aid from surrounding communities and regional efforts is what level of disaster?
   1. Level I
   2. Level II
   3. Level III
   4. Level IV
5. The pre-disaster preparedness stage involves which activity?
   1. Planning and preparation
   2. Warning, preimpact mobilization, and evacuation if appropriate
   3. The community experiences the immediate effects
   4. The immediate response to the effects of the disaster
6. The nurse color-codes a client as yellow during the triage process. The yellow code identifies the client as:
   1. Requiring the most support and immediate emergency care.
   2. Being less critical but still in need of transport to emergency centers for care.
   3. Having minor injuries and do not warrant transport to an emergency center.
   4. Being least likely to survive or are already deceased.
7. The site of the disaster where a weapon was released or where the contamination occurred is called the _____ zone.
   1. Cold
   2. Warm
   3. Hot
   4. Safe

8. Identify the nursing diagnosis that does not apply during a disaster.
    1. Feeling of powerfulness
    2. Risk for injury
    3. Impaired communication
    4. Anxiety
9. Identify the incorrect statement concerning the disaster preparation needs of immunocompromised clients.
    1. Clients should carry treatment calendars with them at all times.
    2. Clients should plan a back-up location to visit for chemotherapy if their usual office is inaccessible.
    3. Clients must avoid raw seafood or possibly contaminated water.
    4. Bone marrow transplant clients are instructed to eat raw fruits and vegetables to maintain their increased nutritional needs.
10. Overexertion and exhaustion are major problems during what type of disaster?
    1. Blast
    2. Snow
    3. Earthquake
    4. Tornado

CHAPTER 8

GENETIC IMPLICATIONS OF ADULT HEALTH NURSING

LEARNING OUTCOMES

After completing Chapter 8, you will be able to demonstrate the following objectives:

- Discuss the role of genetic concepts in health promotion and health maintenance.
- Apply knowledge of the principles of genetic transmission and risk factors for genetic disorders.
- Describe the significance of delivering genetic education and counseling follow-up in a professional manner.
- Identify the implications of genetic advances on the role of nurses with particular attention to spiritual, cultural, ethical, legal, and social issues.
- Identify the significance of recent advances in human genetics and the impact on healthcare delivery.

CLINICAL COMPETENCIES

- Integrate genetic physical assessment and the use of a pedigree family history into delivery of nursing care.
- Identify clients or families with actual or potential genetic conditions and initiate referrals to a genetics professional.
- Prepare clients and their families for a genetic evaluation and facilitate the genetic counseling process.
- Integrate basic genetic concepts into client and family education and the reinforcement of information provided to clients by genetic professionals.

KEY TERMS

alleles
autosomes
carriers
chromosomes

MediaLink

www.prenhall.com/lemone

Resources for this chapter can be found on the Prentice Hall Nursing MediaLink DVD accompanying this textbook, and on the Companion Website at http://www.prenhall.com/lemone. Click on Chapter 8 to select the activities for this chapter.

Prentice Hall Nursing MediaLink DVD-ROM
- Audio Glossary
- NCLEX-RN® Review

Animation
- Human Genome Project

Companion Website
www.prenhall.com/lemone
- Audio Glossary
- NCLEX-RN® Review
- Care Plan Activity: Genetic Implications of Adult Health Nursing Care
- Case Study: Genetic Implications
- MediaLink Application: Create and Analyze a Family Pedigree
- Links to Resources

DNA-based tests
gene
gene expression
genetic locus
genotype
heterozygous
homologous chromosomes
homozygous
human genome
meiosis
mitochondria
mitosis
monosomy
multifactorial conditions

nondisjunction
penetrance
phenotype
polymorphisms
sex chromosomes
somatic cell
test sensitivity
test specificity
translocation
trisomy 21
wild-type gene
x-linked dominant
x-linked recessive

CHAPTER OUTLINE

  I. Integrating Genetics into Nursing Practice
 II. Genetic Basics
      A. Cell Division
      B. Chromosomal Alterations
           1. Alterations in Chromosome Number
           2. Alterations in Chromosome Structure
      C. Genes
           1. Function and Distribution of Genes
           2. Mitochondrial Genes
           3. Gene Alterations and Disease
           4. Gene Alterations That Decrease Risk of Disease
           5. Single Nucleotide Polymorphisms
III. Principles of Inheritance
      A. Mendelian Pattern of Inheritance
           1. Recessive vs. Dominant Disorders
           2. Autosomal Dominant
           3. Autosomal Recessive
           4. X-Linked Recessive
           5. X-Linked Dominant
      B. Variability in Classic Mendelian Patterns of Inheritance
           1. Penetrance
           2. New Mutation
           3. Anticipation
           4. Variable Expressivity
      C. Multifactorial (Polygenic or Complex) Disorders
 IV. Interdisciplinary Care
      A. Genetic Testing
  V. Nursing Care
      A. The Role of the Nurse in Genetic Testing
           1. Ensuring Confidentiality and Privacy for Genetic Testing
           2. Psychosocial Issues
           3. Economic Issues
      B. Assessment
           1. Health Promotion and Health Maintenance
           2. Client Intake and History
           3. Pedigrees
           4. Genetic Physical Assessment

      C. Nursing Diagnosis and Interventions
         1. Genetic Referrals and Counseling
         2. Client Teaching
         3. Psychosocial Care
      D. Evaluation
  VI. Visions for the Future

FOCUSED STUDY TIPS

1. Discuss the difference between mitosis and meiosis cell division. What role do they play in chromosomal alteration?

2. Explain the principles of inheritance and how nurses can apply these principles when performing genetic counseling.

3. List several examples of genetic testing and what condition, disease, or trait the test screens.

4. Discuss the importance of performing a thorough client genetic intake and history. List items that must be included in a comprehensive genetic intake and history.

CASE STUDIES

Case Study 1

Janine Steinman, a 27-year-old married female, is being seen for her first prenatal visit by Dr. Williams. Mrs. Steinman reports that her relatives have a history of Tay Sachs disease and she is concerned about her child's potential for developing the disease. Dr. Williams orders a carrier test followed by genetic counseling.

1. Why did the physician order carrier testing for Mrs. Steinman?

2. What type of genetic disorder is Tay Sachs classified as?

3. How can the Steinmans be assured of the accuracy of their genetic testing results?

4. Who may obtain the results of the Steinmans' genetic testing?

Case Study 2

Dianne Simmons, a 42-year-old female, is considering having an elective bilateral mastectomy. Ms. Simmons has a strong family history of breast cancer. Ms. Simmons's mother, sister, maternal aunt, and great-grandmother have all been diagnosed and treated for breast cancer. Ms. Simmons is consulting with Dr. Powers and his team to determine if elective bilateral mastectomies will lessen the likelihood of her developing a form of breast cancer.

1. Describe the predictive genetic testing that Ms. Simmons will have performed.

2. Why is it important to discuss and map Ms. Simmons's family tree in relation to breast cancer?

3. What type of nursing diagnoses will the nurse include in Ms. Simmons's genetic counseling care plan?

4. How can the testing information obtained by Ms. Simmons be used in the care of her extended family members?

NCLEX REVIEW QUESTIONS

1. A nurse is reviewing the client's chromosomal report. The nurse recognizes that the correct number of chromosomes per nucleus is:
   1. 23.
   2. 33.
   3. 46.
   4. 52.
2. DNA molecules consist of long sequences of nucleotides or bases represented by the letters:
   1. A, G, T, and C.
   2. A, H, P, and S.
   3. T, O, D, and P.
   4. A, D, S, and M.
3. Down syndrome is better known as:
   1. Trisomy 5
   2. Duosomy 19
   3. Trisomy 21
   4. Monosomic 16

4. A nurse is counseling a client known to be homozygous for the CCR5 mutation. The nurse explains to the client that they will be resistant to what virus?
   1. Hepatitis B
   2. HIV I
   3. Hepatitis C
   4. Human papilloma virus
5. The nurse is providing inheritance risk assessment and teaching to a client. Which of the following statements is incorrect?
   1. Autosomal recessive disorders are more severe and have an earlier onset than conditions with other patterns of inheritance.
   2. The sex chromosome, X, is evenly distributed to males and females.
   3. An individual with a recessive condition has inherited one altered gene from their mother and one from their father.
   4. Homozygous dominant conditions are generally more severe than heterozygous dominant conditions and are often lethal.
6. A newborn undergoes what type of genetic newborn testing for phenylketonuria (PKU)?
   1. Predictive genetic testing
   2. Pharmacogenetic testing
   3. Carrier testing
   4. Newborn screening
7. Prior to genetic testing, the nurse discusses all but which of the following with the client?
   1. Risks and benefits of the testing
   2. Emotional stress caused by the testing and results
   3. Cost of the procedure to be performed and its impact on family resources
   4. Verbal consent is the preferred method of consent to avoid disclosing the client's identity on a written consent.
8. Evaluation of successful genetic counseling with a client who has a strong family history for the BRCA1 and BRCA2 tumor suppressor genes would observe whether the client:
   1. Undergoes her first mammogram by age 50.
   2. Keeps the counseling session information private.
   3. Begins early clinical breast screenings at a young age.
   4. Does not perform self breast exams due to unlikelihood of feeling these tumors.
9. Mitochondrial genes and any diseases due to DNA alterations on those genes are transmitted by what means?
   1. Through the mother in a matrilineal pattern
   2. Through the father in a patrilineal pattern
   3. By either parent
   4. Mitochondrial diseases are not transmitted based on a sex link.
10. A genetic counselor has just informed a female client that carrier testing has confirmed that she, her husband, and infant daughter are positive for the sickle cell trait. You would expect the client to express all but which of the following emotions?
    1. Survivor guilt
    2. Fear
    3. Shame
    4. Self-image disturbance

CHAPTER 9

NURSING CARE OF CLIENTS EXPERIENCING PAIN

LEARNING OUTCOMES

After completing Chapter 9, you will be able to demonstrate the following objectives:

- Describe the neurophysiology of pain.
- Compare and contrast definitions and characteristics of acute, chronic, central, phantom, and psychogenic pain.
- Discuss factors affecting individualized responses to pain.
- Clarify myths and misconceptions about pain.
- Discuss interdisciplinary care for the client in pain, including medications, surgery, transcutaneous electrical nerve stimulation, and complementary therapies.
- Use the nursing process as a framework for providing individualized nursing care for clients experiencing pain.

CLINICAL COMPETENCIES

- Assess client's pain intensity; quality; location; pattern; intensifiers; nullifiers; side effects of analgesics; effect on physical, psychologic, and social function, mood, and support for managing pain.
- Determine client's desire and preference for pain management.
- Intervene with client-approved pharmacologic and nonpharmacologic methodologies. Administer medications knowledgeably and safely.
- Utilize equianalgesia tables for transitioning among opioid analgesics. Match continuous pain with around-the-clock, long-acting dosing and intermittent pain with short-acting medications.
- Provide client and family teaching about effective pain control.
- Evaluate effectiveness of interventions to relieve pain; retreat or adjust doses of medication and interventions as necessary.
- Revise plan of care according to client's response to interventions and need for control.

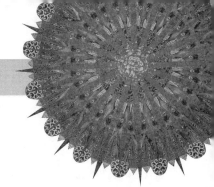

MediaLink

www.prenhall.com/lemone

Resources for this chapter can be found on the Prentice Hall Nursing MediaLink DVD accompanying this textbook, and on the Companion Website at http://www.prenhall.com/lemone. Click on Chapter 9 to select the activities for this chapter.

Prentice Hall Nursing MediaLink DVD-ROM
- Audio Glossary
- NCLEX-RN® Review

Animation/Video
- Epidural Placement
- Morphine
- Naproxen
- Reflex Arc

Companion Website
www.prenhall.com/lemone
- Audio Glossary
- NCLEX-RN® Review
- Care Plan Activity: The Client in Pain
- Case Study: Assessing the Client in Pain
- MediaLink Applications
- Links to Resources

KEY TERMS

acute pain

addiction

analgesic

breakthrough pain

central pain

chronic pain

incident pain

malignant pain

nociception

nociceptors

pain

pain tolerance

phantom pain

psychogenic pain

titrate

transdermal

CHAPTER OUTLINE

I. Neurophysiology and Theories of Pain
   A. Neurophysiology
   B. Pain Pathway
   C. Inhibitory Mechanisms
   D. Pain Theories
II. Types and Characteristics of Pain
   A. Acute Pain
   B. Chronic Pain
   C. Breakthrough Pain
   D. Central Pain
   E. Phantom Pain
   F. Psychogenic Pain
III. Factors Affecting Responses to Pain
   A. Age
   B. Sociocultural Influences
   C. Emotional Status
   D. Past Experiences with Pain
   E. Source and Meaning
   F. Knowledge
IV. Myths and Misconceptions about Pain
V. Interdisciplinary Care
   1. Medications
   2. Surgery
   3. Transcutaneous Electrical Nerve Stimulation
   4. Complementary Therapies
VI. Nursing Care
   A. Assessment
      1. Client Perceptions
      2. Physiologic Responses
      3. Behavioral Responses
      4. Self-Management of Pain
   B. Nursing Diagnoses and Interventions
      1. Acute Pain or Chronic Pain
   C. Using NANDA, NIC, and NOC
   D. Community-Based Care

FOCUSED STUDY TIPS

1. Discuss the unique characteristics of acute vs. chronic pain.

   _____

   _____

   _____

   _____

2. List factors that influence the client's response to pain.

   _____

   _____

   _____

   _____

   _____

3. Describe the different routes of medication administration.

   _____

   _____

   _____

   _____

   _____

4. What are the nurse's responsibilities in teaching clients about pain and pain control strategies?

   _____

   _____

   _____

   _____

   _____

CASE STUDY

Case Study 1

J.S. Browning was brought into the emergency room after suffering a traumatic amputation of his right lower leg. An emergency above-knee amputation was performed soon after his arrival.

1. What nerve fibers will be involved in sensing pain from J.S. Browning's injury site?

2. What form of acute pain will J.S. experience immediately after the injury?

3. What form of chronic pain may J.S. experience for several months after the amputation?

4. What strategies will the nurse employ to assess J.S. Browning's pain tolerance?

Case Study 2

Bailey Bowen is a 32-year-old male who suffers with recurrent lower back pains from an impinged nerve. Mr. Bowen has come to your family practice center for pain relief.

1. What factors will influence Mr. Bowen's perceived level of pain?

2. What strategies other than medication administration can be used to lessen Mr. Bowen's perceived level of pain?

3. What types of medications would you expect this client to be placed on for pain control at home?

4. Mr. Bowen's doctor has discussed placing a TENS unit on the client. Explain the unit and its benefit to a client with chronic pain.

CARE PLAN CRITICAL THINKING ACTIVITY

1. What side effects of nonnarcotic analgesics must Susan be made aware of?

2. What types of relaxation exercises can Susan use to reduce pain while in the work environment?

3. What environmental factors will impact Susan's perceived level of pain?

NCLEX REVIEW QUESTIONS

1. Which of the following statements about pain is accurate?
    1. Pain is always real.
    2. Pain affects the whole body, usually positively.
    3. Pain has no sociocultural dimension.
    4. Pain does not serve as a warning of potential trauma.
2. The client is complaining of dull and poorly-localized cramping and intermittent pain. The nurse notes that the client is experiencing accompanying nausea, vomiting, hypotension, and restlessness. The client is experiencing what type of pain?
    1. Somatic pain
    2. Visceral pain
    3. Referred pain
    4. Hyperesthesias pain
3. The client is experiencing breakthrough pain. What intervention can the nurse use to alleviate and prevent further episodes of this type of pain?
    1. Provide medication on an as-needed basis.
    2. Reposition the client frequently.
    3. Time repeated doses in relation to patterns of breakthrough.
    4. Suggest that the baseline medication dosage be decreased and subsequent doses be increased.
4. In caring for a geriatric client, the nurse is aware that:
    1. The perception of pain decreases with age.
    2. Opioids cause excessive respiratory depression in older adults.
    3. Older adult clients fear narcotic addiction.
    4. Pain is a part of growing older.
5. Identify the correct misconception about pain control.
    1. Pain is a cause, not a result.
    2. Narcotic medication is widely used in chronic pain.
    3. Clients do not lie about the existence or severity of their pain.
    4. Pain relief interferes with diagnosis.

6. The client has been diagnosed with herpes zoster. The nurse is aware that initial pain control will be from which class of medications?
   1. Local anesthetic
   2. Anticonvulsants
   3. Narcotics
   4. Nonsteroidal anti-inflammatory drugs (NSAIDs)
7. The nurse understands the advantage to administering analgesics before the pain occurs is that:
   1. The client may spend less time in pain.
   2. Frequent administration allows for larger doses.
   3. The client's fear and anxiety about the return of pain will increase.
   4. The client will be less physically active.
8. The client has been ordered a transdermal analgesic patch. Which of the following statements demonstrate the client understands the use and application of the patch?
   1. The patch must be changed every 24 hours.
   2. The patch must be applied to the same site each time.
   3. The application of a heating pad over the site will accelerate absorption.
   4. The therapeutic level is reached within 12 hours of initial application.
9. The client is scheduled to undergo a cordotomy. How will the nurse explain this procedure to the client?
   1. "During the procedure a nerve will be removed."
   2. "A needle will be placed in the lower back and the bundle of sympathetic nerves will be injected with medication."
   3. "A surgical severing of the dorsal spinal roots will be performed."
   4. "An incision will be made into the anterolateral tracts of the spinal cord to interrupt the transmission of pain."
10. Physical manifestations of pain include all but which of the following?
    1. Shallow rapid breathing
    2. Increased blood pressure
    3. Increased pulse rate
    4. Constricted pupils

NURSING CARE OF CLIENTS WITH ALTERED FLUID, ELECTROLYTE, AND ACID–BASE BALANCE

MediaLink

www.prenhall.com/lemone

Resources for this chapter can be found on the Prentice Hall Nursing MediaLink DVD accompanying this textbook, and on the Companion Website at http://www.prenhall.com/lemone. Click on Chapter 10 to select the activities for this chapter.

Prentice Hall Nursing MediaLink DVD-ROM
- Audio Glossary
- NCLEX-RN® Review

Animations
- Acid–Base Balance
- Fluid Balance
- Furosemide
- Membrane Transport

Companion Website
www.prenhall.com/lemone
- Audio Glossary
- NCLEX-RN® Review
- Care Plan Activities
  - Fluid Volume Deficit
  - Hypocalcemia
- Case Studies
  - Third Spacing
  - Hypernatremia
- MediaLink Applications
  - Metabolic Acidosis and Type 1 Diabetes
  - Alterations in Electrolytes, Medications, Fluid Volumes
- Links to Resources

LEARNING OUTCOMES

After completing Chapter 10, you will be able to demonstrate the following objectives:
- Describe the functions and regulatory mechanisms that maintain water and electrolyte balance in the body.
- Compare and contrast the causes, effects, and care of the client with fluid volume or electrolyte imbalance.
- Explain the pathophysiology and manifestations of imbalances of sodium, potassium, calcium, magnesium, and phosphorus.
- Describe the causes and effects of acid–base imbalances.

CLINICAL COMPETENCIES

- Assess and monitor fluid, electrolyte, and acid–base balance for assigned clients.
- Administer fluids and medications knowledgeably and safely.
- Determine priority nursing diagnoses, based on assessment data, to select and implement individualized nursing interventions.
- Provide client and family teaching about diet and medications used to restore, promote, and maintain fluid, electrolyte, and acid–base balance.
- Integrate interdisciplinary care into care of clients with altered fluid, electrolyte, and acid–base balance.

KEY TERMS

acidosis	electrolytes
acids	filtration
active transport	fluid volume deficit (FVD)
alkalis	fluid volume excess
alkalosis	glomerular filtration rate
anasarca	homeostasis
anion gap	Kussmaul's respirations
arterial blood gases (ABGs)	orthopnea
ascites	osmosis
atrial natriuretic peptide (ANP)	$Paco_2$
base excess (BE)	Pao_2
bases	polyuria
buffers	serum bicarbonate
dehydration	stridor
diffusion	tetany
dyspnea	third spacing
edema	volatile acids

CHAPTER OUTLINE

I. Overview of Normal Fluid and Electrolyte Balance
  A. Body Fluid Composition
    1. Water
    2. Electrolytes
  B. Body Fluid Distribution
    1. Body Fluid Movement
  C. Body Fluid Regulation
    1. Thirst
    2. Kidneys
    3. Renin–Angiotensin–Aldosterone System
    4. Antidiuretic Hormone
    5. Atrial Natriuretic Peptide
II. Changes in the Older Adult
III. Fluid Imbalance
  A. The Client with Fluid Volume Deficit
    1. Pathophysiology
    2. Manifestations
  B. Interdisciplinary Care
    1. Diagnosis
    2. Fluid Management
  C. Nursing Care
    1. Health Promotion
    2. Assessment
    3. Nursing Diagnoses and Interventions
      i. Deficient Fluid Volume
      ii. Ineffective Tissue Perfusion
      iii. Risk for Injury
    4. Using NANDA, NIC, and NOC
    5. Community-Based Care
  B. The Client with Fluid Volume Excess
    1. Pathophysiology
    2. Manifestations and Complications

3. Interdisciplinary Care
   a. Diagnosis
   b. Medications
   c. Treatments
4. Nursing Care
   a. Health Promotion
   b. Assessment
   c. Nursing Diagnoses and Interventions
      i. Excess Fluid Volume
      ii. Risk for Impaired Skin Integrity
      iii. Risk for Impaired Gas Exchange
   d. Community-Based Care
IV. Sodium Imbalance
   A. Overview of Normal Sodium Balance
   B. The Client with Hyponatremia
      1. Pathophysiology
      2. Manifestations
      3. Interdisciplinary Care
         a. Diagnosis
         b. Medications
         c. Fluid and Dietary Management
      4. Nursing Care
      5. Health Promotion
         a. Assessment
         b. Nursing Diagnoses and Interventions
            i. Risk for Imbalanced Fluid Volume
            ii. Risk for Ineffective Cerebral Tissue Perfusion
         c. Community-Based Care
   C. The Client with Hypernatremia
      1. Pathophysiology
      2. Manifestations
      3. Interdisciplinary Care
         a. Diagnosis
         b. Medications
      4. Nursing Care
         a. Health Promotion
         b. Assessment
         c. Nursing Diagnoses and Interventions
            i. Risk for Injury
         d. Community-Based Care
V. Potassium Imbalance
   A. Overview of Normal Potassium Balance
   B. The Client with Hypokalemia
      1. Pathophysiology
      2. Manifestations
      3. Interdisciplinary Care
         a. Diagnosis
         b. Medications
         c. Nutrition
      4. Nursing Care
         a. Health Promotion
         b. Assessment
         c. Nursing Diagnoses and Interventions
            i. Decreased Cardiac Output
            ii. Activity Intolerance

iii. Risk for Imbalanced Fluid Volume

iv. Acute Pain

d. Using NANDA, NIC, and NOC

e. Community-Based Care

C. The Client with Hyperkalemia

1. Pathophysiology

2. Manifestations

3. Interdisciplinary Care

a. Diagnosis

b. Medications

c. Dialysis

4. Nursing Care

a. Health Promotion

b. Assessment

c. Nursing Diagnoses and Interventions

i. Risk for Decreased Cardiac Output

ii. Risk for Activity Intolerance

iii. Risk for Imbalanced Fluid Volume

d. Community-Based Care

VI. Calcium Imbalance

A. Overview of Normal Calcium Balance

B. The Client with Hypocalcemia

1. Risk Factors

2. Pathophysiology

3. Manifestations and Complications

4. Interdisciplinary Care

a. Diagnosis

b. Medications

c. Nutrition

5. Nursing Care

a. Health Promotion

b. Assessment

c. Nursing Diagnoses and Interventions

i. Risk for Injury

d. Community-Based Care

C. The Client with Hypercalcemia

1. Pathophysiology

2. Manifestations and Complications

3. Interdisciplinary Care

a. Diagnosis

b. Medications

c. Fluid Management

4. Nursing Care

5. Health Promotion

a. Assessment

b. Nursing Diagnoses and Interventions

i. Risk for Injury

ii. Risk for Excess Fluid Volume

c. Community-Based Care

VII. Magnesium Imbalance

A. Overview of Normal Magnesium Balance

B. The Client with Hypomagnesemia

1. Risk Factors

2. Pathophysiology

3. Manifestations and Complications

5. Nursing Care
   a. Health Promotion
   b. Assessment
   c. Nursing Diagnoses and Interventions
      i. Risk for Impaired Gas Exchange
      ii. Deficient Fluid Volume
   d. Community-Based Care
D. The Client with Respiratory Acidosis
   1. Risk Factors
   2. Pathophysiology
   3. Manifestations
   4. Interdisciplinary Care
      a. Diagnosis
      b. Medications
      c. Respiratory Support
   5. Nursing Care
      a. Health Promotion
      b. Assessment
      c. Nursing Diagnoses and Interventions
         i. Impaired Gas Exchange
         ii. Ineffective Airway Clearance
      d. Using NANDA, NIC, and NOC
      e. Community-Based Care
E. The Client with Respiratory Alkalosis
   1. Risk Factors
   2. Pathophysiology
   3. Manifestations
   4. Interdisciplinary Care
      a. Diagnosis
      b. Medications
      c. Respiratory Therapy
   5. Nursing Care
      a. Health Promotion
      b. Assessment, Diagnoses, and Interventions
         i. Ineffective Breathing Pattern
      c. Community-Based Care

FOCUSED STUDY TIPS

1. Describe the difference between intracellular and extracellular fluid.

_____

_____

_____

_____

2. Describe the following body fluid movements:

   a. Osmosis

_____

_____

   b. Diffusion

_____

_____

c. Filtration

_____

_____

d. Active transport

_____

_____

3. Fill in the following table:

Condition	Definition	Manifestations	Medications
Hypernatremia			
Hyponatremia			
Hypokalemia			
Hyperkalemia			
Hypocalcemia			
Hypercalcemia			
Hypomagnesemia			
Hypermagnesemia			
Hypophosphatemia			
Hyperphosphatemia			

4. Describe the differences between:

a. Metabolic acidosis and alkalosis

_____

_____

_____

b. Respiratory acidosis and alkalosis

_____

_____

_____

CASE STUDY

Mr. Sweeney has been admitted with a diagnosis of metabolic acidosis. Answer the following questions based on his diagnosis.

1. What is normal pH? What would the nurse expect Mr. Johnson's pH to be?

2. The nurse would expect Mr. Johnson's respirations to be of what quality and depth?

3. What are the early manifestations of metabolic acidosis?

4. What are vital teaching areas for Mr. Johnson?

NCLEX REVIEW QUESTIONS

1. Of the following, which can be immediately replaced intravascularly?
   1. Plasma
   2. Urine
   3. Synovial fluid
   4. Perspiration

2. Identify the primary process that controls body fluid movement between the intracellular fluid (ICF) and extracellular fluid (ECF) compartments.
   1. Osmosis
   2. Diffusion
   3. Active transport
   4. Filtration

3. A poor indicator of fluid volume deficit in the older adult is monitoring which of the following?
   1. Skin turgor
   2. Tongue turgor
   3. Blood pressure
   4. Weight

4. Your client is diagnosed with a fluid volume deficit due to a severe burn injury. Which laboratory finding is incorrect?
   1. Decrease in potassium
   2. Elevated hemoglobin
   3. Increase in urine specific gravity
   4. Decreased hematocrit

5. Your client is ordered to undergo a fluid challenge. The nurse knows to administer the challenge at what volume and rate?
   1. Administer by IV an initial fluid volume of 100 to 200 mL over two to five minutes.
   2. Administer by IV an initial fluid volume of 200 to 300 mL over five to ten minutes.
   3. Administer by IV infusion an initial fluid volume of 300 to 400 mL over three to five minutes.
   4. Administer by IV infusion an initial fluid volume of 400 to 500 mL over 15 to 20 minutes.

6. Which of the following is not an appropriate nursing action when caring for a client with fluid volume excess?
   1. Assess for lower extremity edema.
   2. Provide oral hygiene at least every two hours.
   3. Teach the client about sodium restricted diets.
   4. Obtain weights at varying times during the day.

7. Which of the following is the initial manifestation of hypernatremia?
   1. Lethargy
   2. Weakness
   3. Thirst
   4. Irritability

8. Identify the early manifestation of hypokalemia.
   1. Ileus
   2. Flattened T waves
   3. Vomiting
   4. Muscle cramping

9. A buffer prevents major changes in pH by releasing _____ ions.
   1. Hydrogen
   2. Calcium
   3. Sodium
   4. Magnesium

10. Your client is experiencing metabolic acidosis. You will document their respirations as _____ respirations.
    1. Stridor
    2. Paradoxical
    3. Trousseau's
    4. Kussmaul's

CHAPTER 11

NURSING CARE OF CLIENTS EXPERIENCING TRAUMA AND SHOCK

LEARNING OUTCOMES

After completing Chapter 11, you will be able to demonstrate the following objectives:

- Describe the components and types of trauma.
- Discuss causes, effects, and initial management of trauma.
- Describe steps of the primary survey to diagnose and manage life-threatening injuries.
- Discuss diagnostic tests used in assessing clients experiencing trauma and shock.
- Describe collaborative interventions for clients experiencing trauma and shock, including medications, blood transfusion, and intravenous fluids.
- Explain organ donation and forensic implications of traumatic injury or death.
- Discuss the risk factors, etiologies, and pathophysiologies of hypovolemic shock, cardiogenic shock, obstructive shock, and distributive shock.
- Use the nursing process as a framework for providing individualized care to clients experiencing trauma and shock.
- Describe the role of the nurse in trauma prevention education and evaluate a plan of care to restore the functional health status of trauma clients.
- Understand and comply with guidelines related to Uniform Anatomical Gift Act.

MediaLink

www.prenhall.com/lemone

Resources for this chapter can be found on the Prentice Hall Nursing MediaLink DVD accompanying this textbook, and on the Companion Website at http://www.prenhall.com/lemone. Click on Chapter 11 to select the activities for this chapter.

Prentice Hall Nursing MediaLink DVD-ROM
- Audio Glossary
- NCLEX-RN® Review

Animation/Video
- Administering Blood
- Hypovolemic Shock
- Trauma Injuries

Companion Website
www.prenhall.com/lemone
- Audio Glossary
- NCLEX-RN® Review
- Care Plan Activity: Clients Experiencing Trauma and Shock
- Case Studies
  - A Client Experiencing Trauma
  - Identifying Types of Shock
- MediaLink Applications
  - Injury Prevention
  - Organ Donation
  - Shock
- Links to Resources

CLINICAL COMPETENCIES

- Obtain initial data about the trauma client to include history taking, assessment, review of past medical history, and communication with prehospital and other healthcare providers and family members.
- Evaluate client response to medical and surgical interventions for clients sustaining multiple trauma and shock.
- Communicate significant data and changes in the condition of a client who has sustained trauma.
- Formulate nursing diagnoses based on manifestations during the nursing assessment.
- Develop a plan of care for the trauma client based on scientific knowledge and client diversity.
- Advocate for clients' rights as indicated by documents that address end-of-life issues.

KEY TERMS

abrasions
anaphylactic shock
blunt trauma
brain death criteria
cardiac output (CO)
cardiogenic shock
contusions
distributive shock
full-thickness avulsion
    injuries
hypovolemic shock
lacerations
mean arterial pressure (MAP)
minor trauma

multiple trauma
neurogenic shock
obstructive shock
penetrating trauma
pnuemothorax
puncture wounds
septic shock
shock
stroke volume (SV)
tension pneumothorax
transfusion
trauma
vasogenic shock

CHAPTER OUTLINE

I. The Client Experiencing Trauma
  A. Components of Trauma
  B. Types of Trauma
  C. Effects of Traumatic Injury
    1. Airway Obstruction
    2. Tension Pneumothorax
    3. Hemorrhage
    4. Integumentary Effects
    5. Abdominal Effects
    6. Musculoskeletal Effects
    7. Neurologic Effects
    8. Multiple Organ Dysfunction Syndrome
    9. Effects on the Family
    10. Interdisciplinary Care
      a. Prehospital Care
      b. Emergency Department Care
      c. Emergency Surgery
      d. Organ Donation
      e. Forensic Considerations
    11. Nursing Care
      a. Health Promotion
      b. Assessment
      c. Nursing Diagnoses and Interventions

          i. Ineffective Airway Clearance
          ii. Risk for Infection
          iii. Impaired Physical Mobility
          iv. Spiritual Distress
          v. Post-Trauma Syndrome
        d. Using NANDA, NIC, and NOC
        e. Community-Based Care

II. The Client Experiencing Shock
    A. Overview of Cellular Homeostasis and Hemodynamics
    B. Pathophysiology
       1. Stage I: Early, Reversible, and Compensatory Shock
       2. Stage II: Intermediate or Progressive Shock
       3. Stage III: Refractory or Irreversible Shock
       4. Effects of Shock on Body Systems
    C. Types of Shock
       1. Hypovolemic Shock
       2. Cardiogenic Shock
       3. Obstructive Shock
       4. Distributive Shock
       5. Septic Shock
       6. Neurogenic Shock
       7. Anaphylactic Shock
    D. Interdisciplinary Care
       1. Diagnosis
       2. Medications
       3. Oxygen Therapy
       4. Fluid Replacement
    E. Nursing Care
       1. Health Promotion and Assessment
       2. Nursing Diagnoses and Interventions
         a. Decreased Cardiac Output
         b. Ineffective Tissue Perfusion
         c. Anxiety
       3. Using NANDA, NIC, and NOC
       4. Community-Based Care

FOCUSED STUDY TIPS

1. Define pneumothorax and describe its treatment.

_____

_____

_____

_____

_____

2. Describe the five types of integumentary injuries and their common causes.

_____

_____

_____

_____

_____

3. Which blood type is the universal receiver?

_____

4. Which blood type is the universal donor?

_____

5. Discuss the Uniform Anatomical Gift Act.

_____

_____

_____

_____

_____

CASE STUDY

Richard Key, a 26-year-old male was involved in a motorcycle accident along a single-lane country road. He was found by a passing motorist on the side of the road with his bike twisted against a tree. Answer the following questions based on knowledge of caring for clients experiencing trauma.

1. What type(s) of trauma could Richard potentially experience?

2. What method of transportation will most likely be used to transport Richard to the hospital? What trauma level hospital should he be transported to?

3. What is the highest priority of need in caring for a trauma victim?

4. What diagnostic studies may be performed on Richard once he reaches the trauma center?

CARE PLAN CRITICAL THINKING ACTIVITY

1. What types of injuries will Jane likely experience?

2. What forces of energy did Jane experience?

3. The hospital that Jane was taken to was a level 3 trauma center. Can this center meet her needs? If not, what is the appropriate course of action to care for Jane's needs?

NCLEX REVIEW QUESTIONS

1. What type of energy is the most common type of energy that is transferred to a host in trauma?
   1. Mechanical
   2. Gravitational
   3. Thermal
   4. Electrical
2. You received a report that your incoming client has suffered a minor trauma. Which of the following injuries would you expect your client to present with?
   1. Gun shot wound
   2. Compression injury
   3. Stab wound
   4. Fractured clavicle

3. Which of the following indicates that a C-spine injury is unlikely?
    1. Midline cervical spine tenderness
    2. Normal alertness
    3. Intoxication
    4. Painful distracting injury
4. Identify the organ system that is not involved in Multiple Organ Dysfunction Syndrome.
    1. Reproductive
    2. Pulmonary
    3. Hepatic
    4. Cardiovascular
5. The nurse will not administer which medication to the client who has experienced trauma?
    1. Opioids
    2. Vasodilators
    3. Inotropic drugs
    4. Crystalloids
6. Identify the incorrect statement about blood compatibility.
    1. The person with blood type B has A antibodies.
    2. The person with type A blood has B antibodies.
    3. The person with type O blood has both types of antibodies.
    4. The person with blood type AB has O antibodies.
7. Your client is experiencing shock. Which symptom would the nurse find on assessment?
    1. Tachycardia
    2. Increased carbon dioxide levels
    3. Increased gastric motility
    4. Cerebral hypoxia
8. What type of shock is the leading cause of death for clients in intensive care units?
    1. Hypovolemic shock
    2. Septic shock
    3. Distributive shock
    4. Neurogenic shock
9. The goal of blood administration is to keep the hematocrit at what level?
    1. Between 20-25%
    2. Between 30-35%
    3. Between 40-45%
    4. Between 50-55%
10. Which finding would not be appropriate in a client suspected of having decreased tissue perfusion to the lower leg?
    1. Dry skin
    2. Pale skin
    3. Cool skin
    4. Cyanosis

CHAPTER 12

NURSING CARE OF CLIENTS WITH INFECTION

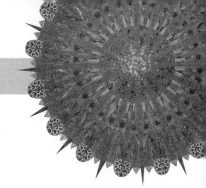

LEARNING OUTCOMES

After completing Chapter 12, you will be able to demonstrate the following objectives:

- Discuss the components and functions of the immune system and the immune response.
- Compare antibody-mediated and cell-mediated immune responses.
- Describe the pathophysiology of wound healing, inflammation, and infection.
- Identify factors responsible for nosocomial infections.
- Use the nursing process as a framework to provide individualized care to clients with inflammation and infection.

CLINICAL COMPETENCIES

- Apply universal precautions, particularly hand washing, to prevent spread of infection within the client, to other clients in the facility, and to members of the interdisciplinary team and visitors.
- Assess for signs and symptoms of inflammation and infection.
- Determine priority nursing diagnosis, based on assessment data, to select and implement individualized nursing interventions for clients with infections.
- Integrate interdisciplinary care into care of clients with infection.
- Promote therapeutic levels of anti-inflammatory and anti-infective medication through prompt administration and client and family teaching.
- Be alert for hypersensitivities to anti-infectives prior to administering and during administration.
- Provide teaching for clients with inflammation or an infection and their families.
- Revise plan of care as needed to provide effective care to promote, maintain, or restore functional health patterns to clients with infections.

MediaLink

www.prenhall.com/lemone

Resources for this chapter can be found on the Prentice Hall Nursing MediaLink DVD accompanying this textbook, and on the Companion Website at http://www.prenhall.com/lemone. Click on Chapter 12 to select the activities for this chapter.

Prentice Hall Nursing MediaLink DVD-ROM
- Audio Glossary
- NCLEX-RN® Review

Animations/Video
- Inflammatory Response
- Penicillin
- White Blood Cells

Companion Website
www.prenhall.com/lemone
- Audio Glossary
- NCLEX-RN® Review
- Care Plan Activity: Postoperative Infection
- Case Study: The Client with an Infection
- MediaLink Applications
  - Antibiotic-Resistant Organisms
  - Hospital-Acquired Infections
- Links to Resources

KEY TERMS

acquired immunity
active immunity
anergy
antibodies
antibody-mediated (humoral)
   immune response
antigen
B lymphocytes (B cells)
bactericidal agent
bacteriostatic agent
cell-mediated (cellular)
   immune response
cytokines
endotoxins
exotoxins
immunity
immunocompetent

immunoglobulin (Ig)
infection
inflammation
leukocytes
leukocytosis
leukopenia
lymphocytes
macrophages
natural killer cells (NK cells,
   null cells)
nosocomial infections
passive immunity
pathogens
phagocytosis
T lymphocytes (T cells)
vaccines

CHAPTER OUTLINE

  I. Overview of the Immune System
    A. Immune System Components
      1. Leukocytes
      2. Lymphoid System
    B. Nonspecific Inflammatory Response
      1. Vascular Response
      2. Cellular Response
      3. Phagocytosis
      4. Healing
    C. Specific Immune Response
      1. Antibody-Mediated Immune Response
      2. Cell-Mediated Immune Response
    D. The Client with Natural or Acquired Immunity
      1. Pathophysiology
      2. Interdisciplinary Care
        a. Diagnosis
        b. Immunizations
      3. Nursing Care
        a. Health Promotion
        b. Assessment
        c. Nursing Diagnoses and Interventions
          i. Health-Seeking Behaviors: Immunization
        d. Community-based Care
 II. Normal Immune Responses
    A. The Client with Tissue Inflammation
    B. Pathophysiology of Tissue Inflammation
      1. Acute Inflammation
      2. Chronic Inflammation
      3. Complications
      4. Interdisciplinary Care
        a. Diagnosis
        b. Medications
        c. Nutrition

5. Nursing Care
   a. Health Promotion
   b. Assessment
   c. Nursing Diagnoses and Interventions
      i. Pain
      ii. Impaired Tissue Integrity
      iii. Risk for Infection
   d. Community-Based Care
C. The Client with an Infection
   1. Pathophysiology
   2. Stages of the Infectious Process
   3. Complications
   4. Nosocomial Infections
   5. Antibiotic-Resistant Microorganisms
   6. Biological Threat Infections
   7. Infectious Process in Older Adults
   8. Interdisciplinary Care
      a. Diagnosis
      b. Medications
      c. Isolation Techniques
      d. Standard Precautions
      e. Transmission-Based Precautions
   9. Nursing Care
      a. Health Promotion
      b. Assessment
      c. Nursing Diagnoses and Interventions
         i. Risk for Infection
         ii. Anxiety
         iii. Hyperthermia
         iv. Pain, Acute
      d. Using NANDA, NIC, and NOC
      e. Community-Based Care

FOCUSED STUDY TIPS

1. Describe the function of the following lymphoid tissues:

   a. Spleen

   _____

   _____

   b. Thymus gland

   _____

   _____

   c. Bone marrow

   _____

   _____

2. Explain the difference between acquired immunity and passive immunity:

   a. Acquired immunity

   _____

   _____

b. Passive immunity

_____

_____

3. Identify the cardinal signs of inflammation.

_____

_____

4. Explain why antibiotics are not effective on virus pathogens.

_____

_____

CASE STUDY

Sally Chase, a 12-year-old client, is being seen in the clinic this morning. She is complaining about a sore throat and headache. Upon examination, her throat is found to be reddened with pustules developing on each tonsil. Answer the following questions based on knowledge of the care of clients with infections.

1. What questions should the nurse ask Sally about her symptoms?

2. What testing may be performed to identify the infecting organism?

3. What are the key nursing diagnoses the nurse should create for Sally?

4. Sally has been placed on antibiotics. What symptoms should she report to her healthcare provider?

CARE PLAN CRITICAL THINKING ACTIVITY

1. What potential adverse reactions would you instruct Mr. Adams to report immediately?

2. How would you respond if Mr. Adams refuses the immunizations ordered?

3. Mr. Adams reports that he does not drive and has no family in the area. How can you assist him in obtaining his required typhoid vaccine in one week?

NCLEX REVIEW QUESTIONS

1. Identify the largest leukocyte.
    1. Basophil
    2. Neutrophil
    3. Monocyte
    4. Eosinophils
2. Which is not a peripheral lymphoid organ?
    1. Spleen
    2. Bone marrow
    3. Tonsils
    4. Lymph nodes
3. Identify the function of the vascular response.
    1. Leukocytes marginate and emigrate into the damaged tissue.
    2. It is a process by which a foreign agent or target cell is engulfed, destroyed, and digested.
    3. It involves the introduction of antigens into the body.
    4. It localizes invading bacteria and keeps them from spreading.

4. Identify the correct statement about vaccines.
   1. Vaccines are suspensions of whole or fractionated bacteria or viruses that have been treated to make them pathogenic.
   2. Vaccines are administered to reduce an immune response.
   3. All vaccines are completely effective and entirely safe.
   4. Vaccines stimulate active immunity by inducing the production of antibodies and antitoxins.
5. Identify the incorrect nursing responsibility when administering a vaccine.
   1. Administration of active immunologic products in the presence of an upper respiratory infection (URI), or other infection, is not a concern.
   2. Do not administer oral polio vaccine (OPV); measles, mumps, and rubella (MMR); or any live virus vaccine to immunosuppressed clients.
   3. Prior to administering a prescribed vaccine, check the expiration date and manufacturer's instructions.
   4. Keep epinephrine 1:1000 readily available for subcutaneous injection when administering immunizations.
6. Which statement demonstrates that the client understands how to care for their infectious process?
   1. "I must restrict my intake of water."
   2. "I must keep active."
   3. "I must eat a well-balanced diet."
   4. "I must take an anti-inflammatory at the first sign of swelling."
7. Which nursing intervention to promote tissue integrity is inappropriate?
   1. Clean inflamed tissue gently.
   2. Keep the inflamed area moist and prevent exposure to air as much as possible.
   3. Balance rest with the tolerable degree of mobility.
   4. Provide protection and support for inflamed tissue.
8. Identify the most common nosocomial infection.
   1. Urinary tract infection
   2. Pneumonia
   3. Bacteremia
   4. *Clostridium difficile*
9. The hospital is undergoing a biological weapon drill. Which pathogen will the nurses not need to protect themselves against?
   1. Anthrax
   2. Smallpox
   3. Botulism
   4. Hepatitis
10. The nurse is assessing the client for an opportunistic infection. Which sign will not be found?
    1. Foul-smelling hard, compact stools
    2. Fuzzy growth on the tongue
    3. Vaginal discharge
    4. Blood in the urine

CHAPTER 13

NURSING CARE OF CLIENTS WITH ALTERED IMMUNITY

LEARNING OUTCOMES

After completing Chapter 13, you will be able to demonstrate the following objectives:

- Review normal anatomy and physiology of the immune system.
- Describe the four types of hypersensitivity reactions.
- Discuss the pathophysiology of autoimmune disorders and tissue transplant rejection.
- Discuss the characteristics of immunodeficiencies.
- Identify laboratory and diagnostic tests used to diagnose and monitor immune response.
- Describe pharmacologic and other collaborative therapies used in treating clients with altered immunity.
- Correlate the pathophysiological alterations with the manifestations of HIV/AIDS infection.
- Use the nursing process as a framework to provide individualized care to clients with altered immune responses.

CLINICAL COMPETENCIES

- Assess functional health status of clients with altered immunity and monitor, document, and report abnormal manifestations.
- Use evidence-based practice to plan and implement nursing care for clients with AIDS.
- Assess for hypersensitivities and anticipate treatment if signs and symptoms develop.
- Provide client teaching about hypersensitivities, avoidance of sensitizing agents, and prophylactic treatment.
- Determine priority nursing diagnoses, based on assessment data, to select and implement individualized nursing interventions and teaching for clients with altered immunity.

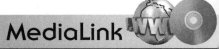

MediaLink

www.prenhall.com/lemone

Resources for this chapter can be found on the Prentice Hall Nursing MediaLink DVD accompanying this textbook, and on the Companion Website at http://www.prenhall.com/lemone. Click on Chapter 13 to select the activities for this chapter.

Prentice Hall Nursing MediaLink DVD-ROM
- Audio Glossary
- NCLEX-RN® Review
- Crossword Puzzle: The Immune System

Animation/Video
- Histamine
- Immune System
- Immune System in the Older Adult

Companion Website
www.prenhall.com/lemone
- Audio Glossary
- NCLEX-RN® Review
- Care Plan Activity: A Client with AIDS
- Case Study: HIV Prevention
- MediaLink Application: At Risk for HIV/AIDS
- Links to Resources

- Protect clients who are immune suppressed.
- Recognize manifestations of developing anaphylaxis.
- Recognize manifestations of infection and minimize nosocomial exposure.
- Utilize universal precautions to protect self and clients from HIV exposure.
- Recognize the burden and benefit of HAART for the client with HIV infection.
- Integrate interdisciplinary care into care of the client with altered immunity.
- Revise plan of care as needed to provide effective interventions to promote, maintain, or restore functional health status to clients with altered immunity.

KEY TERMS

acquired immunodeficiency
  syndrome (AIDS)
allergy
allograft
anaphylaxis
autograft
autoimmune disorder
histocompatibility
human immunodeficiency
  virus (HIV)
hypersensitivity
immunosuppression
isograft
Kaposi's sarcoma (KS)
seroconversion
xenograft

CHAPTER OUTLINE

VII. The Client with a Tissue Transplant
    A. Pathophysiology
    B. Interdisciplinary Care
       1. Diagnosis
       2. Medications
    C. Nursing Care
       1. Health Promotion
       2. Assessment
       3. Nursing Diagnoses and Interventions
          a. Ineffective Protection
          b. Risk for Impaired Tissue Integrity: Allograft
          c. Anxiety
       4. Community-Based Care
VIII. Impaired Immune Responses
  IX. The Client with HIV Infection
    A. Incidence and Prevalence
    B. Pathophysiology and Manifestations
       1. AIDS Dementia Complex and Neurologic Effects
       2. Opportunistic Infections
       3. Secondary Cancers
    C. Interdisciplinary Care
       1. Diagnosis
       2. Medications
    D. Nursing Care
       1. Prevention
       2. Assessment
       3. Nursing Diagnoses and Interventions
          a. Ineffective Coping
          b. Impaired Skin Integrity
          c. Imbalanced Nutrition: Less than Body Requirements
          d. Ineffective Sexuality Patterns
       4. Using NANDA, NIC, and NOC
       5. Community-Based Care

FOCUSED STUDY TIPS

1. Describe the difference between antibody-mediated immune response and cell-mediated immunity.

    _____

    _____

    _____

    _____

2. Describe the following hypersensitivity reactions and their triggering mechanisms.

    a. Type I IgE-mediated hypersensitivity

    _____

    _____

    b. Type II cytotoxic hypersensitivity

    _____

    _____

c. Type III immune complex

_____

_____

d. Type IV delayed hypersensitivity

_____

_____

3. Describe interventions to be taken for clients with a nursing diagnosis of ineffective airway clearance.

_____

_____

_____

_____

_____

4. Explain the differences between the following grafts:

a. Autograft

_____

b. Isograft

_____

c. Allograft

_____

d. Xenograft

_____

CASE STUDY

Gary Jones is a 25-year-old African-American homosexual who was diagnosed with AIDS. Answer the following questions based on knowledge of HIV and AIDS.

1. What are the risk factors for HIV that are specific to this client?

2. How long after exposure would the nurse expect seroconversion to occur in Gary?

3. What acute symptomology can the nurse expect Gary to experience after seroconversion?

4. How long of an asymptomatic period may Gary experience after an acute phase?

5. What opportunistic infections are most common in the AIDS client?

NCLEX REVIEW QUESTIONS

1. Identify the assessment finding that is inconsistent with an altered immune system function.
   1. Fatigue and weakness
   2. Unexplained weight gain
   3. Pale or jaundiced skin
   4. Boggy nasal mucosa

2. The client is being screened for a hypersensitivity reaction. Which laboratory test is not an effective screening tool for the identification of allergens or hypersensitivity reactions?
   1. Red blood cell (RBC) count
   2. Blood type and crossmatch
   3. Direct Coombs'
   4. Complement assay
3. Which of the following statements indicates the client's understanding of managing their hypersensitivity to bee venom?
   1. "If I take an antihistamine daily, it will prevent a reaction if I am stung."
   2. "If I use Nasalirom immediately after I am stung, it will stop a reaction."
   3. "I should carry a bee sting kit at all times."
   4. "If I get daily steroid injections, it will prevent a hypersensitivity reaction."
4. The client is undergoing a blood transfusion. Identify the incorrect protocol to follow.
   1. Monitor the client for complaints of back pain or chest pain.
   2. If signs or symptoms of a reaction occur, keep running the transfusion and call the physician for treatment.
   3. Infuse the blood through a separate site than any other IV.
   4. Two healthcare professionals must identify the blood product prior to transfusion.
5. Cadaver tissue is known as what type of graft?
   1. Autograft
   2. Isograft
   3. Allograft
   4. Xenograft
6. Graft-versus-host disease occurs within what timeframe after transplantation?
   1. Within two to three days
   2. Between four days to three months
   3. Between four months to years after transplantation
   4. Within the first 100 days following transplantation
7. The client has undergone a tissue transplantation. Which nursing intervention is incorrect?
   1. Monitor lab values closely and report changes to the physician.
   2. Change IV bags and tubing every 72 hours.
   3. Monitor client for signs of an adverse reaction to medications.
   4. Offer supplemental feeding.
8. Identify the malignancy that is not classified by the CDC as a cancer associated with AIDS.
   1. Hodgkin's lymphoma
   2. Kaposi's sarcoma
   3. Primary lymphoma of the brain
   4. Invasive cervical cancer
9. The client is being screened for HIV. Which study will provide the most specific diagnosis?
   1. ELISA
   2. CD4 cell count
   3. Western Blot antibody testing
   4. Blood culture for HIV
10. The client with HIV has a pressure blister on the right heel. Identify the appropriate nursing intervention.
    1. Rub the skin directly over the blister to enhance circulation.
    2. Open and drain the blister.
    3. Apply heat three times daily to the area until healed.
    4. Encourage ambulation to increase circulation and maintain muscle tone.

CHAPTER 14

NURSING CARE OF CLIENTS WITH CANCER

LEARNING OUTCOMES

After completing Chapter 14, you will be able to demonstrate the following objectives:

- Define cancer and differentiate benign from malignant neoplasms.
- Describe the theories of carcinogenesis.
- Explain and discuss known carcinogens and identify risk factors for cancer.
- Compare the mechanisms and characteristics of normal cells with those of malignant cells.
- Describe physical and psychologic effects of cancer.
- Describe and compare laboratory and diagnostic tests for cancer.
- Discuss the role of chemotherapy in cancer treatment and classify chemotherapeutic agents.
- Discuss the role of surgery, radiation therapy, and biotherapy in the treatment of cancer.
- Identify causes and discuss the nursing interventions for common oncologic emergencies.
- Design an appropriate care plan for clients with cancer and their families regarding cancer diagnosis, treatment, and coping strategies.

CLINICAL COMPETENCIES

- Assess functional health status of clients with cancer, and monitor, document, and report abnormal manifestations.
- Incorporate evidence-based research into the plan of nursing care for clients with cancer.
- Prioritize nursing diagnosis based on assessment data and implement appropriate nursing interventions for clients with cancer during cancer diagnosis, treatment, and rehabilitation.
- Administer chemotherapeutic medications and other medications for pain, nausea, and vomiting, mucositis, or anemia knowledgeably and safely.

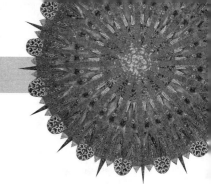

MediaLink

www.prenhall.com/lemone

Resources for this chapter can be found on the Prentice Hall Nursing MediaLink DVD accompanying this textbook, and on the Companion Website at http://www.prenhall.com/lemone. Click on Chapter 14 to select the activities for this chapter.

Prentice Hall Nursing MediaLink DVD-ROM
- Audio Glossary
- NCLEX-RN® Review

Animation/Video
- Cancer
- Cell Division
- Mini-infusion Pumps

Companion Website
www.prenhall.com/lemone
- Audio Glossary
- NCLEX-RN® Review
- Care Plan Activity: Weight Loss and Chemotherapy
- Case Studies
  - Cancer Therapies
  - Pain Management
- MediaLink Applications
  - Cancer Research
  - Interpreting Lab Results
- Links to Resources

- Use the nursing process as a framework for planning and providing individualized care and integrating interdisciplinary care for clients with cancer to meet their healthcare needs.
- Include cultural variation and diverse values in designing and implementing individualized plans of care for clients with cancer.
- Design and provide individualized client and family teaching to restore, promote, and maintain clients' functional status.
- Revise plan of care as needed to provide effective interventions for clients with cancer and their families.

KEY TERMS

anaplasia
biotherapy
cachexia
cancer
carcinogenesis
carcinogens
cell cycle
chemotherapy
differentiation
dysplasia
hospice

hyperplasia
metaplasia
metastasis
neoplasms
oncogene
oncologic emergencies
oncology
radiation therapy
tumor marker
xerostomia

CHAPTER OUTLINE

I. Incidence and Mortality
    A. Risk Factors
        1. Heredity
        2. Age
        3. Gender
        4. Poverty
        5. Stress
        6. Diet
        7. Occupation
        8. Infection
        9. Tobacco Use
        10. Alcohol Use
        11. Recreational Drug Use
        12. Obesity
        13. Sun Exposure
II. Pathophysiology
    A. Normal Cell Growth
    B. The Cell Cycle
    C. Differentiation
III. Etiology
    A. Theories of Carcinogenesis
        1. Cellular Mutation
        2. Oncogenes
        3. Tumor Suppressor Genes
    B. Known Carcinogens
        1. Viruses
        2. Drugs and Hormones
        3. Chemical Agents
        4. Physical Agents

C. Types of Neoplasms
1. Benign Neoplasms
2. Malignant Neoplasms
D. Characteristics of Malignant Cells
E. Tumor Invasion and Metastasis
1. Invasion
2. Metastasis
IV. Physiologic and Psychologic Effects of Cancer
A. Disruption of Function
B. Hematologic Alterations
C. Infection
D. Hemorrhage
E. Anorexia-Cachexia Syndrome
F. Paraneoplastic Syndromes
G. Pain
1. Types of Cancer Pain
2. Causes of Cancer Pain
H. Physical Stress
I. Psychologic Stress
J. Interdisciplinary Care
1. Diagnosis
2. Cancer Treatment
3. Pain Management
K. Nursing Care
1. Health Promotion
2. Assessment
a. Focused Interview
b. Physical Assessment
3. Nursing Diagnoses and Interventions
a. Anxiety
b. Disturbed Body Image
c. Anticipatory Grieving
d. Risk for Infection
e. Risk for Injury
f. Imbalanced Nutrition: Less than Body Requirements
g. Impaired Tissue Integrity
4. Nursing Interventions for Oncologic Emergencies
a. Pericardial Effusions and Neoplastic Cardiac Tamponade
b. Superior Vena Cava Syndrome
c. Sepsis and Septic Shock
d. Spinal Cord Compression
e. Obstructive Uropathy
f. Hypercalcemia
g. Hyperuricemia
h. Syndrome of Inappropriate Antidiuretic Hormone Secretion
i. Tumor Lysis Syndrome
5. Using NANDA, NIC, and NOC
6. Health Education for the Client and Family
a. Prevention
b. Rehabilitation and Survival
7. Community-Based Care
a. Hospice Care

FOCUSED STUDY TIPS

1. Identify the following cancer risk factors as controllable or uncontrollable. If controllable, indicate how they can be modified.

   a. Heredity

   _____

   _____

   b. Age

   _____

   _____

   c. Gender

   _____

   _____

   d. Poverty

   _____

   _____

   e. Stress

   _____

   _____

   f. Diet

   _____

   _____

   g. Occupation

   _____

   _____

   h. Infection

   _____

   _____

   i. Tobacco

   _____

   _____

   j. Alcohol/Recreational drug use

   _____

   _____

   k. Obesity

   _____

   _____

   l. Sun exposure

   _____

   _____

2. What role do viruses play in the development of cancer?

_____

_____

_____

3. Explain the difference between a benign and malignant neoplasm.

_____

_____

_____

_____

4. Explain the following cancer treatments:

   a. Surgery

   _____

   _____

   b. Chemotherapy

   _____

   _____

   c. Radiation

   _____

   _____

   d. Biotherapy

   _____

   _____

   e. Photodynamic therapy

   _____

   _____

CASE STUDY

Donna Lee is a 54-year-old female who has been diagnosed with carcinoma of her right breast. She is scheduled to undergo a right modified radical mastectomy. Her current medication includes an estrogen supplement. She has experienced menopause. Answer the following questions based on knowledge of caring for a client with cancer.

1. What race experiences a higher prevalence of breast cancer?

2. What role does Donna's age play in her cancer?

3. What role does estrogen play in breast cancer?

4. During the surgical procedure, the axillary lymph nodes are removed for examination. Why is this done?

5. How can the nurse assist the client in adjusting to her new body image post-mastectomy?

CARE PLAN CRITICAL THINKING ACTIVITY

1. What strategies could Mr. Casey use to increase his nutritional intake, even though he reports a lack of appetite?

2. How can Mr. Casey maintain his muscle tone and flexibility given his decreased stamina for exercise?

3. What community-based services could assist Mr. Casey and his daughter to meet his care needs now and in the future?

NCLEX REVIEW QUESTIONS

1. Which type of cancer would the nurse screen for more closely in men than in women clients?
   1. Skin
   2. Bladder
   3. Lung
   4. Thyroid
2. The correct definition of dysplasia is:
   1. An increase in the number or density of normal cells.
   2. A change in the normal pattern of differentiation.
   3. A loss of DNA control over the differentiation that occurs in response to adverse conditions.
   4. Regression of a cell to an immature or undifferentiated cell type.
3. Identify the false statement about malignant cells.
   1. Malignant cells undergo rapid cell division.
   2. Malignant cells perform typical cellular functions.
   3. Malignant cells do not respect other cellular boundaries.
   4. Transformation of a malignant cell is irreversible.
4. Identify the incorrect statement about tumor markers.
   1. Decreased enzyme levels in the blood indicate a tumor.
   2. Proteins narrow down the type of tissue that may be malignant.
   3. Increased hormone levels may signify a hormone-secreting malignancy.
   4. The presence of a large amount of antigens reflects tumor cells.
5. The client has a diagnosis of lung cancer. Which imaging technique will provide the greatest accuracy in tumor diagnosis?
   1. Ultrasonography
   2. Magnetic resonance imaging
   3. Computed tomography
   4. Nuclear imaging
6. The client has been newly diagnosed with cancer and is undergoing their first chemotherapy treatment. Which statement indicates that the client understands pre-chemotherapy education?
   1. "I will not lose my hair."
   2. "My body will respond quicker to an infection."
   3. "I may develop a loss of taste."
   4. "I will become pregnant easily while undergoing chemotherapy."
7. The client has been diagnosed with an anxiety disorder. Which behavioral sign would the client not display.
   1. Using direct eye contact
   2. Hyperactivity
   3. Trembling
   4. Withdrawal
8. The client has recently undergone a right radical mastectomy. Which behavior indicates that the client has maintained a positive body image after surgery?
   1. The client denies a change in physical body appearance.
   2. The client is willing to look at their wound.
   3. The client requests no visitors.
   4. The client prefers that only nursing staff perform care to the affected area.

9. Mr. Packer has recently been diagnosed with cancer. Which oral hygiene practice must be avoided?
    1. Use of a soft-tipped toothbrush.
    2. Use of an alcohol-based mouthwash.
    3. Soaking dentures in hydrogen peroxide.
    4. The use of waxed dental floss.
10. The client is suspected to be undergoing tumor lysis syndrome. Which signs and symptoms of the disorder would the nurse expect to find during assessment?
    1. Hypouricemia
    2. Hyperphosphatemia
    3. Hypokalemia
    4. Hyponatremia

CHAPTER 15

ASSESSING CLIENTS WITH INTEGUMENTARY DISORDERS

LEARNING OUTCOMES

After completing Chapter 15, you will be able to demonstrate the following objectives:

- Describe the anatomy, physiology, and functions of the skin, hair, and nails.
- Discuss factors that influence skin color.
- Identify specific topics for a health history interview of the client with problems involving the skin, hair, and nails.
- Explain techniques for assessing the skin, hair, and nails.
- Compare and contrast normal and abnormal findings when conducting an assessment of the integumentary system.
- Describe normal variations in assessment findings for the older client.
- Identify abnormal findings that may indicate impairment of the integumentary system.

CLINICAL COMPETENCIES

- Conduct and document a health history for clients who have or are at risk for alterations in the skin, hair, or nails.
- Conduct and document a physical assessment of the integumentary system.
- Monitor the results of diagnostic tests and report findings.

EQUIPMENT NEEDED

- Disposable gloves
- Ruler
- Flashlight

MediaLink

www.prenhall.com/lemone

Resources for this chapter can be found on the Prentice Hall Nursing MediaLink DVD accompanying this textbook, and on the Companion Website at http://www.prenhall.com/lemone. Click on Chapter 15 to select the activities for this chapter.

Prentice Hall Nursing MediaLink DVD-ROM
- Audio Glossary
- NCLEX-RN® Review

Companion Website www.prenhall.com/lemone
- Audio Glossary
- NCLEX-RN® Review
- Care Plan Activity: Integumentary Disorders
- Case Studies
  - Assessing a Rash
  - Skin Assessment for a Client with a Bacterial Infection
- MediaLink Applications
  - Moles
  - Skin Cancer
- Links to Resources

KEY TERMS

alopecia

cyanosis

ecchymosis

edema

erythema

hirsutism

jaundice

keratin

melanin

pallor

sebum

urticaria

vitiligo

CHAPTER OUTLINE

I. Anatomy, Physiology, and Functions of the Integumentary System
   A. The Skin
      1. The Epidermis
      2. The Dermis
      3. Superficial Fascia
      4. Glands of the Skin
      5. Skin Color
   B. The Hair
   C. The Nails
II. Assessing the Integumentary System
   A. Diagnosis
   B. Genetic Considerations
   C. Health Assessment Interview
   D. Physical Assessment
III. Integumentary Assessments

CASE STUDY

42-year-old Cassandra Messersmith was admitted to a medical surgical unit with a diagnosis of bradycardia and hypotension. Her vital signs are as follows: heart rate 28, blood pressure 89/56, and respiratory rate 24. She denies pain at this time. Her past medical history is significant for a small basal cell carcinoma on the side of her nose. The lesion was surgically excised without complication one year ago.

During the morning assessment, the nurse observes a red scaly area on the back of the client's scalp at the base of the hairline with papules. When the nurse questions the client about the area, the client states that it just appeared about a week ago, and it bleeds occasionally when she brushes her hair. The nurse measures the area (which is 3 mm), completes the assessment, and makes certain the client is comfortable. The nurse then documents the findings and calls the physician with the morning lab results.

1. Is the area on the back of the client's scalp a recurrence of her basal cell carcinoma? Why or why not?

   _____

   _____

2. What risk factors increase the client's risk of developing this type of skin disorder?

   _____

   _____

   _____

3. The lesion is located on the back of the client's head and she noticed it a week ago. The lesion is 3 mm in size now. Based on knowledge of this type of lesion, has the client waited too long to seek treatment?

_____

4. Is there a connection between the reason for the client's admission and the lesion found on the back of her head?

_____

_____

_____

NCLEX REVEW QUESTIONS

1. A frail elderly client has been ordered to bedrest after placement of a pacemaker defibrillator. What precautions should the nurse institute to prevent the development of pressure ulcers?
   1. Reposition the client every half hour.
   2. Change the client's diet to increase protein and vitamin B intake.
   3. Develop a written turning schedule.
   4. Ambulate the client in the room.
2. During a blood pressure screening, the nurse notices that the client is scratching her abdomen. When the nurse asks about scratching, the client states that she has a red itchy rash under her breast. What is the most appropriate response from the nurse?
   1. "That happens in hot weather. It is probably just dry skin from bathing too much."
   2. "Scratching will only make it worse."
   3. "I think it is your new detergent. You should go back to what you were using before."
   4. "How long ago did the itching start?"
3. While assessing a client, the nurse sees that the client's ankles and feet are swollen to the point that her shoes are too tight. However, the skin slowly returns to normal when depressed by the nurse's thumb. This finding is most accurately documented as:
   1. 1+
   2. 2+
   3. 3+
   4. 4+
4. A client has a significantly receding hairline and a dark suntan. The nurse notices that he has a bandage on top of his head. When asked about it he states that it is an odd mole that bleeds sometimes. Which of the following factors would increase the client's risk of skin cancer?
   1. Smoking one pack of cigarettes a day for 15 years
   2. Construction worker for ten years
   3. High-fat diet
   4. Hypothyroidism
5. A nurse has been asked to speak to a community group about the risks factors associated with skin cancers. Which statement by the nurse would be the most accurate?
   1. "A tendency to sunburn, even with sunscreen, increases your risk."
   2. "Family history is the strongest indicator of your risk."
   3. "Women have twice the risk of skin cancer as do men."
   4. "Your risk of skin cancer is less if you have a mild tan to the skin from a tanning bed."
6. When assessing a client with dark skin color for jaundice, the best place to look is the:
   1. Nail beds.
   2. Eyes.
   3. Forearm.
   4. Mucous membranes.

7. The nurse notices that a client is scratching her head. The nurse assesses the area and finds pustules and some hair loss. The nurse knows that these symptoms are associated with:
   1. Ringworm.
   2. Head lice.
   3. Seborrhea.
   4. Boils.
8. When assessing a client's nails, the nurse notices that they are thick and yellow in color. The nurse knows that this is associated with:
   (Select all that Apply.)
   1. Fungal infection.
   2. Trauma to the nail.
   3. Pseudomonas infection.
   4. Psoriasis.
9. A client is schedule for a Tzanct test. Which statement is the most accurate when discussing this test with the client?
   1. "This test will differentiate herpes simplex from herpes zoster."
   2. "This test is simply a small skin biopsy and should not be painful."
   3. "The fluid will be examined under a microscope and will tell us if you have a herpes infection."
   4. "This test will tell us which antibiotic will be effective in treating your infection."
10. When assessing the skin of a client, the nurse notices that it is coarse. The nurse knows that coarse, dry skin is associated with:
    1. Hypothyroidism.
    2. Acne vulgaris.
    3. Fever.
    4. Seborrhea.

CHAPTER 16

NURSING CARE OF CLIENTS WITH INTEGUMENTARY DISORDERS

LEARNING OUTCOMES

After completing Chapter 16, you will be able to demonstrate the following objectives:

- Describe the manifestations and nursing care of common skin problems and lesions.
- Compare and contrast the etiology, pathophysiology, interdisciplinary care, and nursing care of clients with infections and infestations, inflammatory disorders, and malignancies of the skin.
- Explain the risk factors for, pathophysiology of, and nursing interventions to prevent and care for pressure ulcers.
- Discuss surgical options for excision of neoplasms, reconstruction of facial or body structures, and cosmetic procedures.
- Explain the pathophysiology of selected disorders of the hair and nails.
- Discuss the effects and nursing implications of medications and treatments used to treat disorders of the integument.

CLINICAL COMPETENCIES

- Assess functional health status of clients with integumentary disorders, and monitor, document, and report abnormal manifestations.
- Use evidence-based research to plan and implement nursing care for clients with pressure ulcers.
- Determine priority nursing diagnoses, based on assessed data, to select and implement individualized nursing interventions for clients with integumentary disorders.
- Administer topical, oral, and injectable medications used to treat integumentary disorders knowledgeably and safely.
- Integrate interdisciplinary care into care of clients with integumentary disorders.
- Provide teaching appropriate for prevention and self-care of disorders of the integumentary system.
- Revise plan of care as needed to provide effective interventions to promote, maintain, or restore functional health status to clients with disorders of the integument.

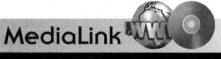

MediaLink

www.prenhall.com/lemone

Resources for this chapter can be found on the Prentice Hall Nursing MediaLink DVD accompanying this textbook, and on the Companion Website at http://www.prenhall.com/lemone. Click on Chapter 16 to select the activities for this chapter.

Prentice Hall Nursing MediaLink DVD-ROM
- Audio Glossary
- NCLEX Review

Animation/Video
- Pressure Ulcers

Companion Website
www.prenhall.com/lemone
- Audio Glossary
- NCLEX-RN® Review
- Care Plan Activity: Pressure Ulcers
- Case Study: Lesions and Pruritis
- MediaLink Applications
- Links to Resources

KEY TERMS

acne
actinic keratosis
angioma
basal cell cancer
candidiasis
carbuncle
cellulitis
comedones
cyst
dermatitis
dermatophytoses
erysipelas
folliculitis
frostbite
furuncle
herpes simplex
herpes zoster
keloids

keratosis
lichen planus
malignant melanoma
nevi
paronychia
pediculosis
pemphigus vulgaris
pressure ulcer
pruritus
psoriasis
scabies
skin graft
squamous cell cancer
toxic epidermal necrolysis
    (TEN)
warts
xerosis

CHAPTER OUTLINE

CASE STUDY

Chrissy Green is a 30-year-old attorney with blonde hair and green eyes. She is very tan and reports a lot of sun exposure since childhood. She has been seen in the physician's office for a large, dark, pigmented area on her right shoulder. The lesion is irregular in shape and has grown in size over the past year. Answer the following questions based on knowledge of malignant melanoma.

1. What factors place Chrissy at risk for developing malignant melanoma?

_____

_____

_____

2. What is Chrissy's prognosis?

_____

_____

3. What treatments are available to Chrissy?

_____

_____

4. How often must Chrissy be seen for a checkup after removal of the lesion?

_____

_____

NCLEX REVIEW QUESTIONS

1. Upon assessment, the nurse finds a skin lesion that looks like a flat or raised macule or papule with a rounded, well-defined border. The nurse suspects what type of diagnosis?
   1. Cyst
   2. Nevi
   3. Keloid
   4. Skin tag
2. Which is not an appropriate instruction to teach a client about the care for psoriasis?
   1. Avoid exposure to the sun.
   2. Avoid exposure to contagious illnesses.
   3. Avoid trauma to the skin.
   4. Indomethacin (Indocin), lithium, and beta-adrenergic blocking agents are known to precipitate exacerbations of psoriasis.
3. Which of the following is an infection of the skin most often caused by group A streptococci?
   1. Cellulitis
   2. Carbuncle
   3. Furuncle
   4. Erysipelas
4. Which behavior demonstrates the client's understanding of the nurse's teaching about a vaginal _candida albicans_ infection?
   1. The client wears tight clothing such as jeans and pantyhose.
   2. The client wears silk or silk-lined underwear.
   3. The client reports bathing more frequently.
   4. The client reports not discussing the infection with their sexual partner.
5. Which form of dermatitis is a chronic inflammatory disorder of the skin that involves the scalp, eyebrows, eyelids, ear canals, nasolabial folds, axillae, and trunk?
   1. Contact dermatitis
   2. Atopic dermatitis
   3. Seborrheic dermatitis
   4. Exfoliative dermatitis
6. Which is not a risk factor for nonmelanoma skin cancer?
   1. Blonde hair, and blue or green eyes
   2. A family history of skin cancer
   3. Protected exposure to UV radiation
   4. Occupational exposures to coal tar

7. At what temperature does skin freeze?
    1. 0-10 degrees Fahrenheit
    2. 14-24.8 degrees Fahrenheit
    3. 32-50 degrees Fahrenheit
    4. 55-72 degrees Fahrenheit
8. The client has a port wine stain. What treatment will be used to reduce the lesion?
    1. Chemical destruction
    2. Sclerotherapy
    3. Curettage
    4. Laser surgery
9. Identify the correct statement about skin grafts.
    1. A split-thickness graft contains both epidermis and dermis.
    2. A common donor site for a skin graft is the posterior thigh.
    3. Skin grafting is an effective way to cover wounds that are infected.
    4. A full-thickness graft is best able to withstand trauma.
10. Which is not a cause of hirsutism?
    1. Polycystic ovary syndrome
    2. Uterine tumors
    3. Cushing's syndrome
    4. Central nervous system disorders

CHAPTER 17

NURSING CARE OF CLIENTS WITH BURNS

LEARNING OUTCOMES

After completing Chapter 17, you will be able to demonstrate the following objectives:

- Discuss the types and causative agents of burns.
- Explain burn classification by depth and extent of injury.
- Describe the pathophysiology, interdisciplinary care, and nursing care for the client with a minor burn.
- Discuss the systemic pathophysiologic effects of a major burn and the stages of burn wound healing.
- Explain the interdisciplinary care and nursing implications necessary during the emergent/resuscitative stage, the acute stage, and the rehabilitative stage of a major burn.

CLINICAL COMPETENCIES

- Assess functional health status of clients with burns, and monitor, document, and report abnormal manifestations.
- Use evidence-based research to plan and implement nursing care for clients with burns.
- Determine priority nursing diagnoses, based on assessed data, to select and implement individualized nursing interventions for client with burns.
- Administer medications knowledgeably and safely to clients with burns.
- Integrate interdisciplinary care into care of clients with burns.
- Provide teaching appropriate for prevention of burns.
- Revise plan of care as needed to provide effective interventions to promote, maintain, or restore functional health status to clients with burns.

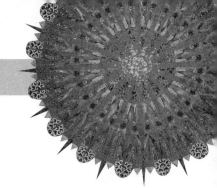

MediaLink

www.prenhall.com/lemone

Resources for this chapter can be found on the Prentice Hall Nursing MediaLink DVD accompanying this textbook, and on the Companion Website at http://www.prenhall.com/lemone. Click on Chapter 17 to select the activities for this chapter.

Prentice Hall Nursing MediaLink DVD-ROM
- Audio Glossary
- NCLEX-RN® Review

Companion Website
www.prenhall.com/lemone
- Audio Glossary
- NCLEX-RN® Review
- Care Plan Activities
  - A Client Having a Skin Graft
  - A Client with Burns
  - Inhalation Injury
- Case Studies
- MediaLink Applications
- Links to Resources

KEY TERMS

allograft
autografting
burn
burn shock
compartment syndrome
contractures
Curling's ulcers
debridement
eschar
escharotomy
fascial excision

fasciectomy
fluid resuscitation
full-thickness burn
heterograft
homograft
hypertrophic scar
keloid
partial-thickness burn
superficial burn
surgical debridement
xenograft

CHAPTER OUTLINE

   I. Types of Burn Injury
      A. Thermal Burns
      B. Chemical Burns
      C. Electrical Burns
      D. Radiation Burns
  II. Factors Affecting Burn Classification
      A. Depth of the Burn
         1. Superficial Burns
         2. Partial-Thickness Burns
         3. Full-Thickness Burns
      B. Extent of the Burn
 III. Burn Wound Healing
  IV. The Client with a Minor Burn
      A. Pathophysiology
         1. Sunburn
         2. Scald Burn
      B. Interdisciplinary Care
      C. Nursing Care
         1. Community-Based Care
   V. The Client with a Major Burn
      A. Pathophysiology
         1. Integumentary System
         2. Cardiovascular System
         3. Respiratory System
         4. Gastrointestinal System
         5. Urinary System
         6. Immune System
         7. Metabolism
      B. Interdisciplinary Care
         1. Stages of Interdisciplinary Care
         2. Prehospital Client Management
         3. Emergency and Acute Care
         4. Diagnosis
         5. Medications
         6. Treatments
      C. Nursing Care
         1. Health Promotion
         2. Assessment
         3. Nursing Diagnoses and Interventions

a. Impaired Skin Integrity
b. Deficient Fluid Volume
c. Acute Pain
d. Risk for Infection
e. Impaired Physical Mobility
f. Imbalanced Nutrition: Less than Body Requirements
g. Powerlessness
4. Using NANDA, NIC, and NOC
5. Community-Based Care

FOCUSED STUDY TIPS

1. Label the burn diagram. Note the difference in depth with each degree of burn.

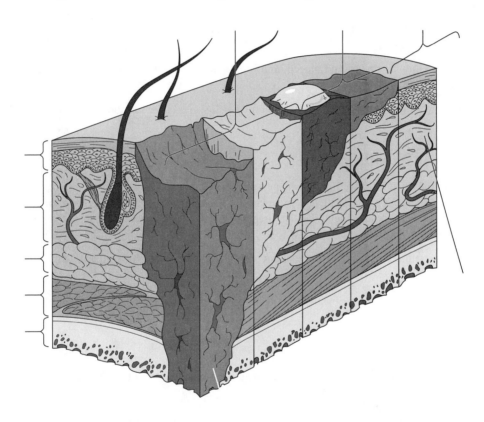

2. Using the Lund & Bowder burn assessment chart, determine the total body surface area affected by the burns described below.

Description	Percentage of Burn Area
24-year-old with second-degree burns to right hand	
57-year-old with second- and third-degree burns to both legs, upper and lower, and groin	
85-year-old with second-degree burns to chest, arms, right hand, neck, and face	

CASE STUDY

74-year-old Viola Baker arrives in the emergency department following a fire in her apartment. She has first- and second-degree burns over 50% of her body including her face, chest, and arms. Viola was cooking when grease caught fire, catching her clothing on fire as well. There are soot marks around her nostrils and her eyebrows are singed. She is using a 100% nonrebreather mask, and has a pulse oximetry reading of 89%. She is being given normal saline solution by IV in addition to the 5 mg morphine sulfate for pain that she was given in the ambulance. Her vital signs are as follows: heart rate 116, blood pressure 104/76, and respiratory rate 35. She opens her eyes to verbal stimuli, and her conversation is confused but she answers some simple questions and withdraws from pain. The client's past medical history is significant for osteoporosis, bilateral cataract surgery, and type II diabetes mellitus that is controlled with diet and exercise. The client's family was notified by the apartment manager and they are on the way to the emergency department.

1. What changes need to be made immediately in the client's care?

2. To what setting will this client likely be transferred when she is stable?

3. Why would the client be intubated and placed on a ventilator?

4. Based on the client's injuries, from what type of immediate surgical intervention might she benefit?

CARE PLAN CRITICAL THINKING ACTIVITY

Please answer the following question in light of the previous case study.

The client's son arrives in the emergency department with the client's advanced directive granting him power of attorney. Her son is confused because the advanced directive states that she does not want life support if she is determined to be in an irrecoverable state. The client was intubated and is receiving ventilatory support.

1. Develop an impromptu teaching plan for the client's son and power of attorney regarding the client condition.

2. Develop a care map including any interventions from which she might benefit.

NCLEX REVIEW QUESTIONS

1. The client who weighs 68 kg has sustained second-degree burns over 40% of his body. Which fluid resuscitation is correct according to the Parkland calculation?
   1. 10.88 liters of lactated Ringer's solution in 24 hours
   2. 5.44 liters of lactated Ringer's solution in eight hours and 5.44 liters of LR over the next 16 hours
   3. 5.44 liters of lactated Ringer's solution in eight hours and 5.44 liters of D5W over the next 16 hours
   4. 10.88 liters of D5W in 24 hours
2. Which nursing intervention holds the highest priority for a client with burns to her face and upper respiratory tract?
   1. Elevate the head of the bed to at least 30 degrees.
   2. Administer six liters of oxygen via nasal cannula.
   3. Medicate the client prior to repositioning the client in bed.
   4. Prevent moving the skin around the burn site.
3. When caring for a client with chemical burns, which task could the registered nurse assign to unlicensed nursing personnel?
   1. Documentation about the dressing change and wound bed.
   2. First ambulation of hospital stay.
   3. Encouraging the client to use patient-controlled analgesia for pain and the incentive spirometer hourly.
   4. Checking urinary output for adequacy of fluid resuscitation.

4. When teaching a community group about radiation burns, which statement best reflects the goals of treatment?
    1. Radiation burns are usually mild, and involve only the surface of the skin.
    2. Severe radiation burns are usually caused by industrial accidents.
    3. Radiation burns are much less common than thermal burns.
    4. Promoting wound and body healing are the most important goals of treatment.
5. Which is an appropriate order when caring for a client with a burn?
    1. Provide 4000 Kcal per 24 hours.
    2. Administer four liters of lactated Ringer's solution for a 105 lb client with a 10% total body surface area.
    3. Administer six liters of oxygen via nasal cannula without humidification with a pulse oximetry reading of 99%.
    4. Apply support garments beginning on the fourth day postburn.
6. Which is the highest priority for the nurse when caring for a client with an electrical burn?
    1. Disconnect the client from the electrical source.
    2. Ensure that clients have a cervical collar and be placed on a back board prior to care.
    3. Monitor for cardiac dysrhythmia.
    4. Clients may require changes in fluid resuscitation as compared to clients with other types of burns.
7. Which client will require skin grafting for wound closure?
    1. The client with a 31.5% heavy superficial chemical burn.
    2. The client with a 12mm full-thickness thermal burn.
    3. The client with a moderate partial-thickness burn.
    4. The client with an 18% partial-thickness burn to the lower limbs.
8. A major burn is defined as:
    1. 20% total body surface area in adults less than 40 years of age.
    2. 5% total body surface area full-thickness burn in adults greater than 40 years of age.
    3. A household electrical burn with a cervical spine injury.
    4. A burn that caused the oxygen saturation rate to drop below 95%.
9. Please document on the diagram below a burn that involves 22.5% of the client's body surface area.

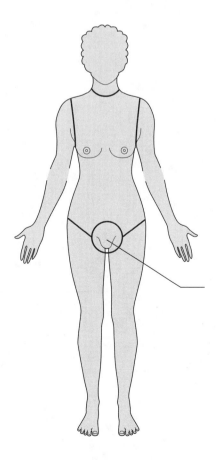

10. Clients with major burns are at risk for many system issues. Which is the highest priority for the nurse caring for a client with a major burn?
    1. Compartment syndrome
    2. Hypovolemia
    3. Thermal burn and dysrrhythmia
    4. Acute renal failure

CHAPTER 18

ASSESSING CLIENTS WITH ENDOCRINE DISORDERS

LEARNING OUTCOMES

After completing Chapter 18, you will be able to demonstrate the following objectives:

- Describe the anatomy and physiology of the endocrine glands.
- Explain the functions of the hormones secreted by the endocrine glands.
- Identify specific topics to consider during a health history interview of the client with health problems involving endocrine function.
- Describe techniques for assessing the thyroid gland and the effects of altered endocrine function.
- Describe normal variations in assessment findings for the older adult.
- Identify abnormal findings that may indicate malfunction of the glands of the endocrine system.

CLINICAL COMPETENCIES

- Conduct and document a health history for clients who have or are at risk for alterations in the structure or function of the endocrine glands.
- Monitor the results of diagnostic tests and report abnormal findings.
- Conduct and document a physical assessment of the structure of the thyroid gland and the effects of altered endocrine function on other body structures and functions.

EQUIPMENT NEEDED

- Reflex hammer
- Safety pin, cotton ball, containers with hot and cold water, tuning fork
- Blood pressure cuff
- Stethoscope

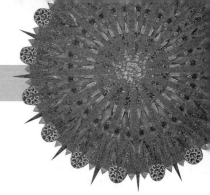

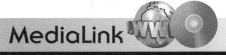

MediaLink

www.prenhall.com/lemone

Resources for this chapter can be found on the Prentice Hall Nursing MediaLink DVD accompanying this textbook, and on the Companion Website at http://www.prenhall.com/lemone. Click on Chapter 18 to select the activities for this chapter.

Prentice Hall Nursing MediaLink DVD-ROM
- Audio Glossary
- NCLEX-RN® Review

Companion Website www.prenhall.com/lemone
- Audio Glossary
- NCLEX-RN® Review
- Care Plan Activity: Type 2 Diabetes
- Case Studies
  - Assessing a Client for Hypocalcemia
  - Endocrine Assessment
- MediaLink Application: Endocrine Hormones
- Links to Resources

KEY TERMS

acromegaly   exophthalmos
carpal spasm   goiter
Chvostek's sign   tetany
dwarfism   Trousseau's sign

CHAPTER OUTLINE

I. Anatomy, Physiology, and Functions of the
    Endocrine System
    A. Pituitary Gland
        1. Anterior Pituitary
        2. Posterior Pituitary
    B. Thyroid Gland
    C. Parathyroid Glands
    D. Adrenal Glands
    E. Pancreas
    F. Gonads

II. An Overview of Hormones
III. Assessing Endocrine Function
     A. Diagnostic Tests
     B. Genetic Considerations
     C. Health Assessment Interview
     D. Physical Assessment
IV. Endocrine Assessments

FOCUSED STUDY TIPS

- Practice completing a health history interview and physical assessment with a peer or family member. Provide
  your partner with a list of symptoms or various endocrine disorders and try to identify the abnormal descriptions
  or findings.

  _____

  _____

  _____

  _____

  _____

- Fill in the diagram below identifying both the hormone produced and the target cells.

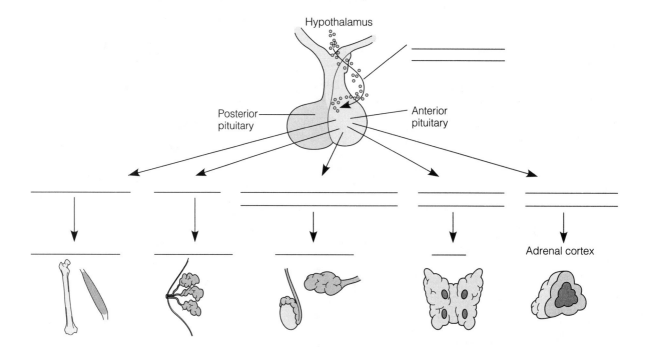

- Complete the chart below with normal and abnormal findings for an endocrine health history interview or physical assessment.

Endocrine Organ	Normal Findings	Abnormal Findings
Pituitary gland		
Thyroid gland		
Parathyroid glands		
Adrenal glands		
Pancreas		
Reproductive glands		

CASE STUDY

Karmen Aummert is a 42-year-old female that has been admitted complaining of a severe decrease in her energy level and feeling sluggish. Her vital signs are stable now, heart rate 39, blood pressure 98/62, respiratory rate 14. Karmen has one child, age three, and works full-time as a department assistant for a small credit agency. She began to notice these changes six months prior to her admission: increase in weight, cold intolerance, and lack of energy. She blamed her symptoms on working so many hours, being a single parent, and her divorce, but became concerned when she fell at work today and lost consciousness for a reported 25 seconds. She is very worried about this hospital admission because this means her 66-year-old parents are taking care of her daughter.

1. What questions should be included in the client's health history inventory related to her current endocrine issues?

2. What endocrine-specific diagnostic tests might be used to correctly diagnose Ms. Aummert's health problem?

3. List the top two physiologic and psychosocial nursing diagnoses for this client.

4. What possible impediments might the nurse encounter while trying to develop a plan of care for Ms. Aummert?

NCLEX REVIEW QUESTIONS

1. Pituitary hormones control:
   1. Emotional growth and development.
   2. Red blood cell production.
   3. The release of thyroid hormones.
   4. Production of calcium.
2. When assessing a client who is concerned about weight gain, hair loss, and generalized weakness, how should the nurse adapt physical assessment to focus on the client's concern?
   1. Perform a focused abdominal assessment.
   2. Assess the neck and swallowing.
   3. Test the balance and gait.
   4. Assess height and weight.
3. The nurse understands carbohydrate metabolism occurs in which gland?
   1. Pancreas
   2. Pituitary
   3. Thyroid
   4. Parathyroid

4. Epinephrine is produced by which gland?
   1. Pancreas
   2. Thyroid
   3. Adrenal medulla
   4. Adrenal cortex

5. The nurse knows that a problem with this gland would affect corticosteroid production.
   1. Pituitary
   2. Parathyroid
   3. Adrenal cortex
   4. Adrenal medulla

6. The gland located in the abdomen behind the stomach is the:
   1. Pancreas.
   2. Duodenum.
   3. Thyroid.
   4. Adrenal cortex.

7. The hormone responsible for development of secondary female sexual characteristics is:
   1. Oxytocin.
   2. Vasopressin.
   3. Follicle-stimulating hormone (FSH).
   4. Luteinizing hormone (LH).

8. Which of the following is not considered to be a genetic consideration of endocrine disorders?
   1. Age of symptom onset
   2. Length of time the client experiences symptoms
   3. Gender
   4. Immediate family blood connection

9. What is the role of the nurse in caring for a client experiencing diagnostic testing of a possible endocrine disorder?
   1. Identify the client's specific disorder.
   2. Obtain consent for the diagnostic testing.
   3. Provide the client and family with the results of the diagnostic testing.
   4. Assess the client's medication list for anything that may affect the outcome of the testing.

10. Chvostek's sign is a diagnostic tool that is used to assess for:
    1. Hypocalcemic tetany.
    2. Hypercalcemic tetany.
    3. Hyperkalemic tetany.
    4. Hyperinsulinism.

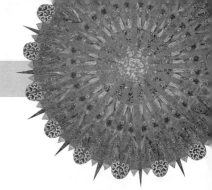

CHAPTER 19

NURSING CARE OF CLIENTS WITH ENDOCRINE DISORDERS

LEARNING OUTCOMES

After completing Chapter 19, you will be able to demonstrate the following objectives:

- Apply knowledge of normal anatomy, physiology, and assessments of the thyroid, parathyroid, adrenal, and pituitary glands when providing nursing care for clients with endocrine disorders.
- Compare and contrast the manifestations of disorders that result from hyperfunction and hypofunction of the thyroid, parathyroid, adrenal, and pituitary glands.
- Explain the nursing implications for medications prescribed to treat disorders of the thyroid and adrenal glands.
- Provide appropriate nursing care for the client before and after a subtotal thyroidectomy and an adrenalectomy.
- Use the nursing process as a framework for providing individualized care to clients with disorders of the thyroid, parathyroid, adrenal, and pituitary glands.

CLINICAL COMPETENCIES

- Assess functional health status of clients with endocrine disorders and monitor, document, and report abnormal manifestations.
- Use evidence-based research to provide appropriate teaching for self-medicating with thyroid hormone.
- Determine priority nursing diagnoses, based on assessed data, to select and implement individualized nursing interventions for clients with endocrine disorders.
- Teach clients that hormone replacement is lifelong, and how to take medications efficiently and effectively.
- Monitor respiratory function after thyroidectomy.
- Monitor for latent tetany following parathyroid removal, planned or inadvertent.
- Anticipate and recognize the effects of adrenal hormones.
- Revise plan of care as needed to provide effective interventions to promote, maintain, or restore functional health status to clients with endocrine disorders.

KEY TERMS

acromegaly
Addisonian crisis
Addison's disease
Cushing's syndrome
diabetes insipidus
euthyroid
exophthalmos
gigantism
goiter
Graves' disease
Hashimoto's thyroiditis
hyperparathyroidism
hyperthyroidism
hypoparathyroidism

hypothyroidism
myxedema
myxedema coma
pheochromocytoma
pretibial myxedema
proptosis
syndrome of inappropriate
    ADH secretion (SIADH)
tetany
thyroid storm or crisis
thyroidectomy
thyroiditis
thyrotoxicosis
toxic multinodular goiter

CHAPTER OUTLINE

XIV. The Client with Disorders of the Posterior Pituitary Gland
   A. Pathophysiology and Manifestations
      1. Syndrome of Inappropriate ADH Secretion
      2. Diabetes Insipidus
   B. Interdisciplinary Care
   C. Nursing Care

FOCUSED STUDY TIPS

1. Discuss the incidence, manifestations, and treatment for Graves' disease:

   a. Incidence

   _____

   _____

   b. Manifestations

   _____

   _____

   c. Treatment

   _____

   _____

2. Discuss the incidence, manifestations, and treatment of hypothyroidism:

   a. Incidence

   _____

   _____

   b. Manifestations

   _____

   _____

   c. Treatment

   _____

   _____

3. Describe Cushing's syndrome as well as its signs and symptoms and treatment.

   _____

   _____

   _____

   _____

   _____

4. Compare and contrast gigantism and acromegaly.

   _____

   _____

   _____

   _____

CASE STUDY

Judy Moss is a 43-year-old white female who has been recently diagnosed with Addison's disease. Answer the following questions based on knowledge of caring for clients with endocrine disorders.

1. How should the nurse explain Addison's disease to Ms. Moss?

2. What manifestations should the nurse look for during the assessment of Ms. Moss?

3. What skin changes should the nurse expect Ms. Moss to experience?

4. What diagnostic testing procedures may have been used to diagnose Ms. Moss's condition?

CARE PLAN CRITICAL THINKING ACTIVITY: CLIENT WITH HYPOTHYROIDISM

1. What metabolic processes are occurring in the body that cause constipation to occur in hypothyroid clients?

2. Mrs. Lee states that she hates her appearance and does not want to go out into public anymore. How should the nurse respond?

3. What strategies could Mrs. Lee employ to help her to communicate easier?

NCLEX REVIEW QUESTIONS

1. Which would not be found on the nurse's assessment for a client with the diagnosis of hyperthyroidism?
    1. Increased appetite
    2. Insomnia
    3. Increased sweating
    4. Constipation
2. Identify the inappropriate nursing intervention to use with a client in thyroid storm.
    1. Replace fluids.
    2. Reduce body temperature by administering aspirin.
    3. Apply oxygen.
    4. Replace electrolytes.
3. Which behavior demonstrates that the client understands the care for hyperthyroidism?
    1. The client participates in continuous activity.
    2. The client practices stress-reduction techniques.
    3. The client weighs self weekly.
    4. The client restricts carbohydrates and protein in their diet.
4. The nurse will administer which medication to increases thyroid function?
    1. Anabolic steroids
    2. Estrogen
    3. Lithium
    4. Propranolol
5. Which statement about Hashimoto's thyroiditis is incorrect?
    1. It is more common in men.
    2. It is an autoimmune disorder.
    3. It causes a goiter to form.
    4. It has a familial link.

6. Which nursing intervention is contraindicated in a client with hyperthyroidism?
   1. Avoid mobility.
   2. Avoid thiazide diuretics.
   3. Infuse IV saline.
   4. Administer large doses of vitamins A and D.
7. The nurse understands which client population is less likely to develop hypercortisolism?
   1. Women between the ages of 30 and 50.
   2. Teen males.
   3. Clients on long-term steroids.
   4. Clients undergoing chemotherapy.
8. Identify the behavior that demonstrates the client understands health teaching about Cushing's syndrome.
   1. The client refuses to discuss their body changes with professionals.
   2. The client decreases their intake of vitamins A and C in their diet.
   3. The client restricts fluids.
   4. The client uses dim lighting to induce a relaxing environment.
9. Clients experience symptoms of Addison's disease after what percent of adrenal gland function is lost?
   1. 40%
   2. 50%
   3. 70%
   4. 90%
10. Which is not a manifestation of diabetes insipidus?
    1. Polyuria
    2. Polydipsia
    3. Hypoosmolality
    4. Low urine specific gravity

CHAPTER 20

NURSING CARE OF CLIENTS WITH DIABETES MELLITUS

LEARNING OUTCOMES

After completing Chapter 20, you will be able to demonstrate the following objectives:

- Apply knowledge of normal endocrine anatomy, physiology, and assessments when providing nursing care for clients with diabetes mellitus.
- Describe the prevalence and incidence of diabetes mellitus.
- Explain the pathophysiology, risk factors, manifestations, and complications of type 1 and type 2 diabetes mellitus.
- Compare and contrast the manifestations and interdisciplinary care of hypoglycemia, diabetic ketoacidosis, and hyperosmolar hyperglycemic state.
- Identify the diagnostic tests used for screening, diagnosis, and monitoring of diabetes mellitus.
- Discuss the nursing implications for insulin and oral hypoglycemic agents used to treat clients with diabetes mellitus.
- Provide accurate information to clients with diabetes mellitus to facilitate self-management of medications, diet planning, exercise, and self-assessment, including foot care.
- Use the nursing process as a framework for providing individualized care to clients with diabetes mellitus.

CLINICAL COMPETENCIES

- Assess blood glucose levels and patterns of hyper- and hypoglycemia in clients with diabetes mellitus.
- Recognize the importance of early diagnosis and control of blood glucose to prevent complications.
- Determine priority nursing diagnoses, based on assessed data, to select and implement individualized nursing interventions for clients with type I and type II diabetes mellitus.
- Administer oral and injectable medications used to treat type I and type II diabetes mellitus knowledgeably and safely.

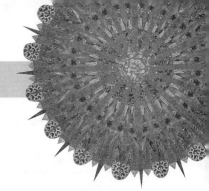

MediaLink

www.prenhall.com/lemone

Resources for this chapter can be found on the Prentice Hall Nursing MediaLink DVD accompanying this textbook, and on the Companion Website at http://www.prenhall.com/lemone. Click on Chapter 20 to select the activities for this chapter.

Prentice Hall Nursing MediaLink DVD-ROM
- Audio Glossary
- NCLEX-RN® Review

Animations
- Glipizide
- Responding to Hypoglycemia

Companion Website www.prenhall.com/lemone
- Audio Glossary
- NCLEX-RN® Review
- Care Plan Activity: Diabetes Mellitus Type 2
- Case Studies
  - Compare and Contrast SIADH and DI
  - Diabetes Mellitus Type 1
- MediaLink Applications
  - Diabetes and Nutrition
  - Diabetes Foot Care
  - Diabetic Neuropathy
- Links to Resources

- Provide skilled care to clients with diabetic ketoacidosis and hyperosmolar hyperglycemic states.
- Integrate interdisciplinary care into care of clients with type I and type II diabetes mellitus, especially foot and eye care.
- Provide appropriate teaching to facilitate blood glucose monitoring, administration of oral and injectable hypoglycemic medications, diabetic diet, appropriate exercise, and foot care.
- Revise plan of care as needed to provide effective interventions to promote, maintain, or restore normal glucose levels.
- Teach the relationship of hygiene, neuropathy, and impaired microcirculation to infection; teach the principles and procedures of effective foot care.
- Assess clients' ability to read markings on syringes and to identify correct insulin and hypoglycemics.
- Relate insulin (endogenous and exogenous), dietary intake, and exercise to control of blood glucose.

KEY TERMS

dawn phenomenon
diabetes mellitus (DM)
diabetic ketoacidosis (DKA)
diabetic nephropathy
diabetic neuropathies
diabetic retinopathy
endogenous insulin
exogenous insulin
gluconeogenesis
glucosuria
glycogenolysis
hyperglycemia
hyperosmolar hyperglycemic
   state (HHS)

hypoglycemia
insulin
insulin reaction
ketonuria
ketosis
lipoatrophy
lipodystrophy
microalbuminuria
polydipsia
polyphagia
polyuria
Somogyi phenomenon
type 1 DM
type 2 DM

CHAPTER OUTLINE

   I. Incidence and Prevalence
  II. Overview of Endocrine Pancreatic Hormones and Glucose Homeostasis
     A. Hormones
     B. Blood Glucose Homeostasis
 III. Pathophysiology of Diabetes
     A. Type 1 Diabetes
        1. Risk Factors
        2. Manifestations
     B. Type 2 Diabetes
        1. Risk Factors
        2. Manifestations
     C. Diabetes in the Older Adult
     D. Interdisciplinary Care
        1. Diagnosis
        2. Monitoring Blood Glucose
        3. Medications
        4. Nutrition
        5. Exercise
        6. Treatments
 IV. Complications of Diabetes
     A. Acute Complications: Alterations in Blood Glucose Levels
        1. Hyperglycemia
        2. Hypoglycemia

B. Chronic Complications
1. Alterations in the Cardiovascular System
2. Alterations in the Peripheral and Autonomic Nervous Systems
3. Mood Alterations
4. Increased Susceptibility to Infection
5. Periodontal Disease
6. Complications Involving the Feet
C. Nursing Care
1. Health Promotion
2. Assessment
3. Nursing Diagnoses and Interventions
   a. Risk for Impaired Skin Integrity
   b. Risk for Infection
   c. Risk for Injury
   d. Sexual Dysfunction
   e. Ineffective Coping
4. Using NANDA, NIC, and NOC
5. Community-Based Care

FOCUSED STUDY TIPS

1. Describe the differences between type I and type II diabetes.

_____

_____

_____

_____

_____

2. What diagnostic tests are used to monitor diabetes management?

_____

_____

_____

_____

_____

3. Describe the different types of insulin preparations.

_____

_____

_____

_____

_____

4. Explain the cause of diabetic ketoacidosis (DKA) and its treatment.

_____

_____

_____

_____

_____

CASE STUDY

Jack Brown is a 56-year-old male who was just recently diagnosed with diabetes. He has spent the past three days on the unit with a diagnosis of hypoglycemia secondary to diabetes. He is being discharged with prescriptions for an oral hypoglycemic. Answer the following questions based on knowledge of caring for clients with diabetes.

1. What type of diabetes would Mr. Brown be diagnosed with and why?

2. How do oral hypoglycemics regulate blood sugar?

3. What modifications will Mr. Brown need to make to his diet?

4. How should Mr. Brown be taught to manage an episode of hypoglycemia?

CARE PLAN CRITICAL THINKING ACTIVITY

1. What information should the nurse reinforce to Mr. Meligrito about his insulin administration?

2. What roles, both positive and negative, does Mr. Meligrito's father play in his management of his diabetes?

3. What resources can Mr. Meligrito use to assist his diet planning?

NCLEX REVIEW QUESTIONS

1. The nurse understands which statement to be true about type 2 diabetes mellitus.
    1. Its onset begins most often in childhood.
    2. It is the nonketonic form of diabetes.
    3. It can be triggered by a viral infection.
    4. An exogenous source of insulin is required.
2. When performing the client assessment with a diagnosis of type 2 diabetes mellitus (DM), the nurse expects which of the following findings to be present?
    1. Polydipsia
    2. Polyuria
    3. Paresthesias
    4. Polyphagia
3. The normal fasting glucose level is:
    1. 40 mg/dL.
    2. 60mg/dL.
    3. 100 mg/dL.
    4. 200 mg/dL.
4. Which syringe is not available for administering insulin?
    1. 0.3 mL (30 U) syringe
    2. 0.5 mL (50 U) syringe
    3. 1.0 mL (100 U) syringe
    4. 1.5 mL (150 U) syringe
5. Identify the incorrect method of insulin injection.
    1. Inject the needle at a 90-degree angle.
    2. Massage the site after administering the injection.
    3. Rotate sites of injection.
    4. Insulin should not be injected into an area that will be exercised.

6. How should the nurse explain the use of alcohol to the client?
   1. Alcohol places you at increased risk for an insulin reaction.
   2. Your oral hypoglycemic will not interact with alcohol.
   3. Light beer should be avoided; only regular beer should be ingested.
   4. Alcohol should be consumed between meals.
7. The dawn phenomenon is a rise in blood glucose between what hours?
   1. 12:00 a.m. – 2:00 a.m.
   2. 3:00 a.m. – 8:00 a.m.
   3. 4:00 a.m. – 8:00 a.m.
   4. 6:00 a.m. – 9:00 a.m.
8. Which is not a characteristic of diabetic nephropathy?
   1. Albumin in the urine
   2. Hypotension
   3. Edema
   4. Progressive renal insufficiency
9. Which is not an alteration in the peripheral and autonomic nervous systems of diabetic clients?
   1. Palsy of the third cranial nerve
   2. Loss of cutaneous sensation, most often located in the chest
   3. Pain, weakness, and areflexia in the anterior thigh and medial calf
   4. Compression of the radial nerve at the wrist
10. Which behavior indicates the client is following proper foot care?
    1. The client inspects the feet monthly for changes.
    2. The client wears tight-fitting shoes to facilitate circulation.
    3. The client keeps the feet in a dependent position the majority of the day.
    4. After bathing the feet, the client pats the foot dry and dries the areas between the toes well.

CHAPTER 21

ASSESSING CLIENTS WITH NUTRITIONAL AND GASTROINTESTINAL DISORDERS

MediaLink

www.prenhall.com/lemone

Resources for this chapter can be found on the Prentice Hall Nursing MediaLink DVD accompanying this textbook, and on the Companion Website at http://www.prenhall.com/lemone. Click on Chapter 21 to select the activities for this chapter.

Prentice Hall Nursing MediaLink DVD-ROM
- Audio Glossary
- NCLEX-RN® Review

Animation
- GI A&P

Companion Website
www.prenhall.com/lemone
- Audio Glossary
- NCLEX-RN® Review
- Care Plan Activity: Gallstones
- Case Studies
  - Assessing Dietary Intake
  - Counseling a College Student about Vitamins
- Teaching Plan: Regular Dental Check-Ups and Older Adults
- MediaLink Application: Nursing Tools for Assessing the Nutritional Status of Clients
- Links to Resources

LEARNING OUTCOMES

After completing Chapter 21, you will be able to demonstrate the following objectives:
- Describe the sources of nutrients, and their functions in the human body.
- Describe the anatomy, physiology, and functions of the gastrointestinal system.
- Explain the processes of carbohydrate, fat, and protein metabolism.
- Identify specific topics to consider during a health history assessment interview of the client with nutritional and gastrointestinal disorders.
- Explain techniques used for assessing nutritional and gastrointestinal status.
- Describe normal variations in assessment findings for the older adult.
- Identify abnormal findings that may indicate alterations in gastrointestinal function.

CLINICAL COMPETENCIES

- Conduct and document a health history for clients who have or are at risk for alterations in nutrition and gastrointestinal function.
- Conduct and document a physical assessment of nutritional status and the gastrointestinal system.
- Monitor the results of diagnostic tests and report abnormal findings.

EQUIPMENT NEEDED

- Stethoscope
- Balance scale with height measuring attachment
- Tape measure
- Skin fold calipers

KEY TERMS

bile	leukoplakia
borborygmus	metabolism
bruit	nutrition
cheilosis	peristalsis
gingivitis	striae
glossitis	

CHAPTER OUTLINE

I. Nutrients
   A. Carbohydrates
   B. Proteins
   C. Fats (Lipids)
   D. Vitamins
   E. Minerals
II. Anatomy, Physiology, and Functions of the Gastrointestinal System
   A. The Mouth
   B. The Pharynx
   C. The Esophagus
   D. The Stomach
   E. The Small Intestine
   F. The Accessory Digestive Organs
     1. The Liver and Gallbladder
III. The Exocrine Pancreas
IV. Metabolism
V. Assessing Nutritional Status and Gastrointestinal Function
   A. Diagnostic Tests
   B. Genetic Considerations
   C. The Health Assessment Interview
   D. Physical Assessment
VI. Nutritional and Gastrointestinal Assessments

FOCUSED STUDY TIPS

1. Locate and label the major digestive organs in the diagram below. Draw quadrants over the diagram to orient yourself to organ location.

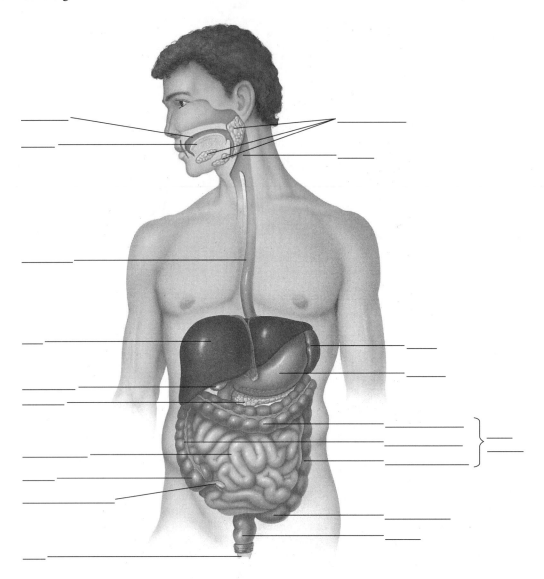

2. Assess four peers, friends, or family members for the following: height-to-weight ratio, waist-to-hip ratio, triceps skin folds, and midarm circumference. Compare your findings to the tables.

3. Track your dietary intake over the course of 24 hours. How does your diet compare to the current dietary guidelines? Where could you improve your diet to reduce your health risk?

_____

_____

_____

_____

_____

4. Practice auscultating abdominal gastric and vascular sounds. Remember to use the diaphragm for gastric sounds and the bell for vascular sounds.

CASE STUDY

During a community health screening, a 36-year-old client states that he has epigastric pain three to five times per week. He describes the discomfort as burning and says that he often feels nausea with the discomfort. When questioned about the discomfort and diet, the client states that he tries to eat two or three balanced meals daily, he drinks coffee several times throughout the day, and usually stops to have a single beer with his coworkers on the way home each evening. He is a non-smoker and feels that aside from this discomfort and newly-identified hypertension he is healthy. He takes no medications (one was prescribed for his hypertension but he has not filled the prescription yet). He has no immediate family history of gastric disease.

1. What additional questions should the nurse ask this client?

2. Epigastric pain of this type is often associated with what disorders? If the client's pain is more intense between meals and less intense after eating, it is more likely to be what disorder?

3. What diagnostic studies might be ordered to further assess the client's epigastric pain?

4. What type of teaching needs does this client have?

NCLEX REVIEW QUESTIONS

1. When teaching a client about diet, which statement is most important to include?
    1. Protein is the most important nutrient and should comprise the majority of the daily caloric intake.
    2. Daily intake of carbohydrates should be about 150 grams.
    3. Milk is an excellent source of vitamins C and D.
    4. Vitamin E is water-soluble and must be replenished every day.
2. When obtaining a medical history from a client, the nurse learns that he had several feet of his small bowel, including his duodenum, removed because of a trauma. What concerns should the nurse have regarding this client's nutritional status related to the location of the removal?
    1. Malabsorption
    2. Loose stools and potential for dehydration.
    3. Poor production of vitamin D.
    4. Inadequate bile production and a need to decrease dietary fat.
3. When teaching a client who is a vegan about stable, inexpensive sources of protein, what is the best response?
    1. A salad with 4 ounces of salmon.
    2. Steamed broccoli with heavy cream sauce.
    3. Peanut butter.
    4. Italian wedding soup.
4. During a client assessment, which finding is indicative of a client with severe malnutrition?
    1. Triceps skin fold thickness 10% below standard.
    2. Midarm muscle circumference less than 60% of standard.
    3. Greater than 10% ideal body weight (IBW).
    4. Decreased midarm circumference (MAC).
5. When percussing the liver of a client, the dullness ends at the costal margin. The nurse know that this finding is:
    1. Indicative of cirrhosis.
    2. Venous congestion of the liver.
    3. A normal finding.
    4. Ascites.
6. Which statement regarding bowel sound assessment is accurate? Bowel sounds:
    1. Are most active in the upper left quadrant.
    2. Should take no longer than 4 minutes.
    3. Are present in all or no quadrants.
    4. Could take up to 20 minutes to assess.

7. A client describes painful vertical fissures on the tongue. These are:
   1. Cheliosis.
   2. Associated with dehydration.
   3. Associated with an acute infection.
   4. Candidiasis.
8. During an abdominal assessment, the client stops breathing in during palpation due to sharp pain. This is often associated with:
   1. Gastric ulcers.
   2. Pancreatitis.
   3. Appendicitis.
   4. Cholecystitis.
9. Which finding during an abdominal assessment is a normal finding?
   1. Plaque on the teeth.
   2. Bowel sounds every 15 seconds.
   3. Borborygmus.
   4. Venous hum.
10. The first step of assessing the abdomen is to:
    1. Auscultate.
    2. Inspect.
    3. Percuss.
    4. Palpate.

CHAPTER 22

NURSING CARE OF CLIENTS WITH NUTRITIONAL DISORDERS

LEARNING OUTCOMES

After completing Chapter 22, you will be able to demonstrate the following objectives:
- Compare and contrast the pathophysiology and manifestations of nutritional disorders.
- Identify causes and predict effects of nutritional disorders on client health status.
- Explain interdisciplinary care for clients with nutritional disorders.
- Develop strategies to promote nutrition for client populations.

CLINICAL COMPETENCIES

- Assess the functional health status of clients with nutritional disorders.
- Monitor nutritional status and responses to care; document and report abnormal or unexpected responses.
- Use assessed data to determine priority nursing diagnoses, and select and implement nursing interventions.
- Administer medications and enteral and parenteral nutrition knowledgeably and safely.
- Integrate interdisciplinary care in the plan of care.
- Adapt cultural values and variations into the plan of care for clients with nutritional disorders.
- Plan and provide client and family teaching to restore, promote, and maintain functional health status.
- Evaluate responses to care and use data to revise plan of care as needed.

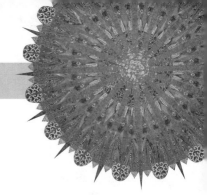

MediaLink

www.prenhall.com/lemone

Resources for this chapter can be found on the Prentice Hall Nursing MediaLink DVD accompanying this textbook, and on the Companion Website at http://www.prenhall.com/lemone. Click on Chapter 22 to select the activities for this chapter.

Prentice Hall Nursing MediaLink DVD-ROM
- Audio Glossary
- NCLEX-RN® Review

Companion Website
www.prenhall.com/lemone
- Audio Glossary
- NCLEX-RN® Review
- Care Plan Activity: Malnutrition
- Case Studies
  - Enteral Feeding Complications
  - Obesity
- MediaLink Applications
  - Anorexia Nervosa
  - Establishing a Balanced Diet
  - Adapting Diet Plans to Individualize Care

KEY TERMS

anorexia nervosa

basal metabolic rate (BMR)

binge-eating disorder

body mass index (BMI)

bulimia nervosa

catabolism

enteral nutrition

lower body obesity

malnutrition

morbid obesity

nutrients

obesity

protein-calorie malnutrition

  (PCM)

starvation

total parenteral nutrition (TPN)

triglycerides

upper body obesity

very low calorie diets

  (VLCD)

CHAPTER OUTLINE

  I. The Client with Obesity

    A. Incidence and Prevalence

    B. Risk Factors

    C. Overview of Normal Physiology

    D. Pathophysiology

      1. Complications of Obesity

    E. Interdisciplinary Care

      1. Diagnosis

      2. Medications

      3. Treatments

      4. Maintaining Weight Loss

    F. Nursing Care

      1. Health Promotion

      2. Assessment

      3. Nursing Diagnoses and Interventions

        a. Imbalanced Nutrition: More than Body Requirements

        b. Activity Intolerance

        c. Ineffective Therapeutic Regimen Management

        d. Chronic Low Self-Esteem

      4. Using NANDA, NIC, and NOC

      5. Community-Based Care

  II. The Client with Malnutrition

    A. Incidence and Prevalence

      1. Risk Factors

    B. Pathophysiology

      1. Manifestations

    C. Interdisciplinary Care

      1. Diagnosis

      2. Medications

      3. Nutrition

    D. Nursing Care

      1. Health Promotion

      2. Assessment

      3. Nursing Diagnoses and Interventions

        a. Imbalanced Nutrition: Less than Body Requirements

        b. Risk for Infection

        c. Risk for Deficient Fluid Volume

        d. Risk for Impaired Skin Integrity

      4. Using NANDA, NIC, and NOC

      5. Community-Based Care

III. The Client with an Eating Disorder
   A. Anorexia Nervosa
   B. Bulimia Nervosa
   C. Binge-Eating Disorder
   D. Interdisciplinary Care
      1. Diagnosis
      2. Treatment
   E. Nursing Care

FOCUSED STUDY TIPS

1. Define obesity and explain its health concerns.

   _____

2. Describe the forms of bariatric procedures performed in the United States.

   _____

   _____

   _____

   _____

   _____

3. Describe the manifestations that clients with malnutrition will experience.

   _____

   _____

   _____

   _____

   _____

4. Explain the difference between anorexia nervosa and bulimia nervosa.

   _____

   _____

   _____

   _____

CASE STUDY

Barbara Spencer is a 50-year-old woman who has been diagnosed with binge-eating disorder. She has been referred to the mental health unit for counseling. Answer the following questions based on knowledge of caring for clients with a binge-eating disorder.

1. What psychosocial factors may have contributed to Ms. Spencer's eating disorder?

2. What diagnostic studies may be ordered to assess Ms. Spencer's nutritional status?

3. What treatments are instituted for clients with a binge-eating disorder?

4. What role can Ms. Spencer's family play in assisting her to be successful with her treatment regimen?

CARE PLAN CRITICAL THINKING ACTIVITY: A CLIENT WITH OBESITY

1. What psychological factors may contribute to Mr. Elliot's weight gain?

2. How can Mr. Elliot's family assist him in reaching his goal weight?

3. What role does Mr. Elliot's culture have in his weight loss success?

NCLEX REVIEW QUESTIONS

1. The nurse understands a client with a BMI of _____ kg/m2 indicates obesity.
   1. 20
   2. 23
   3. 27
   4. 30
2. The most important factor that contributes to obesity is:
   1. Physical inactivity
   2. Genetics
   3. Ethnicity
   4. Low self-esteem
3. Which is not a manifestation of metabolic syndrome?
   1. Increased waist circumference
   2. High HDL cholesterol
   3. Hypertension
   4. Increase in fasting blood glucose
4. The client reports fecal urgency. The nurse recognizes this as a side effect of which medication?
   1. Dexatrim
   2. Acutrim
   3. Meridia (Sibutramine)
   4. Xenical (Orlistat)
5. The client reports a history of stomach reduction surgery that consisted of the creation of a small sac for a stomach. The nurse knows that the client underwent which of the following procedures?
   1. Biliopancreatic diversion
   2. Roux-en-Y gastric bypass
   3. Adjustable gastric banding
   4. Vertical banded gastroplasty
6. Which nursing intervention is not appropriate for a client who needs to reduce their weight?
   1. Assist the client to identify their cues to eating.
   2. Establish a weight loss goal of 3–4 pounds per week.
   3. Assist the client to develop a well-balanced food menu.
   4. Monitor laboratory values.
7. The client presents with malnutrition. The nurse should assess the client for what manifestations?
   1. Recent acute infection
   2. Weight loss of greater than 10% of usual weight
   3. Inability to eat for more than two days
   4. Affluent lifestyle

8. Which finding requires an immediate intervention when monitoring the client's parental nutrition?
   1. The nurse finds that the nutrition is being infused through a central line.
   2. The solution is being administered by gravity.
   3. The client is afebrile.
   4. The parental solution is found to be mixed with intralipids.
9. The client is a 12-year-old female who was recently diagnosed with anorexia nervosa. Identify the incorrect home-based intervention.
   1. The mother reports feeding her daughter three large meals a day.
   2. The daughter weighs herself at the same time weekly with adult supervision.
   3. The mother administers vitamin supplements daily.
   4. Family members do not allow the daughter to use the bathroom unattended after meals.
10. Dumping syndrome occurs with diets that are high in what nutrient?
    1. Fiber
    2. Protein
    3. Simple carbohydrates
    4. Fat

CHAPTER 23

NURSING CARE OF CLIENTS WITH UPPER GASTROINTESTINAL DISORDERS

LEARNING OUTCOMES

After completing Chapter 23, you will be able to demonstrate the following objectives:

- Describe the pathophysiology of common disorders of the mouth, esophagus, and stomach.
- Relate manifestations and diagnostic test results to the pathophysiologic processes involved in upper gastrointestinal disorders.
- Explain interdisciplinary care for clients with upper gastrointestinal disorders.
- Describe the role of the nurse in interdisciplinary care of clients with upper gastrointestinal disorders.

CLINICAL COMPETENCIES

- Assess the functional health status of clients with upper gastrointestinal disorders.
- Monitor, document, and, as needed, report manifestations of upper gastrointestinal disorders and their complications.
- Plan nursing care using evidence-based research.
- Determine priority nursing diagnoses and interventions based on assessed data.
- Administer medications and prescribed care knowledgeably and safely.
- Coordinate and integrate interdisciplinary care into plan of care.
- Construct and revise individualized plans of care considering the culture and values of the client.
- Plan and provide client and family teaching to promote, maintain, and restore functional health.

KEY TERMS

achalasia

acute gastritis

anorexia

cachectic

chronic gastritis

Curling's ulcers

Cushing's ulcers

diffuse esophageal spasm

dumping syndrome

duodenal ulcers

dysphagia

erosive (stress-induced)
  gastritis

esophagojejunostomy

gastric lavage

gastric mucosal barrier

gastric outlet obstruction

gastric ulcers

gastritis

gastroduodenostomy
  (Billroth I)

gastroesophageal reflux

gastroesophageal reflux
  disease (GERD)

gastrojejunostomy
  (Billroth II)

hematemesis

hematochezia

hemmorrhage

hiatal hernia

melena

nausea

occult bleeding

partial gastrectomy

peptic ulcer disease (PUD)

peptic ulcers

perforation

steatorrhea

stomatitis

total gastrectomy

ulcer

vomiting

Zollinger-Ellison syndrome

CHAPTER OUTLINE

I. Disorders of the Mouth

II. The Client With Stomatitis

   A. Pathophysiology and Manifestations

   B. Interdisciplinary Care

      1. Medications

   C. Nursing Care

      1. Health Promotion

      2. Assessment

      3. Nursing Diagnoses and Interventions

         a. Impaired Oral Mucous Membrane

         b. Imbalanced Nutrition: Less than Body Requirements

      4. Using NANDA, NIC, and NOC

      5. Community-Based Care

III. The Client with Oral Cancer

   A. Pathophysiology and Manifestations

   B. Interdisciplinary Care

   C. Nursing Care

      1. Health Promotion

      2. Assessment

      3. Nursing Diagnoses and Interventions

         a. Risk for Ineffective Airway Clearance

         b. Imbalanced Nutrition: Less than Body Requirements

         c. Impaired Verbal Communication

         d. Disturbed Body Image

      4. Community-Based Care

IV. Disorders of the Esophagus

XIII. The Client with Gastritis
    A. Pathophysiology
       1. Acute Gastritis
       2. Erosive Gastritis
       3. Chronic Gastritis
    B. Interdisciplinary Care
       1. Diagnosis
       2. Medications
       3. Treatments
    C. Nursing Care
       1. Health Promotion
       2. Assessment
       3. Nursing Diagnoses and Interventions
         a. Deficient Fluid Volume
         b. Imbalanced Nutrition: Less than Body Requirements
       4. Community-Based Care
XIV. The Client with Peptic Ulcer Disease
    A. Risk Factors
    B. Pathophysiology
    C. Manifestations
    D. Complications
    E. Zollinger-Ellison Syndrome
    F. Interdisciplinary Care
       1. Diagnosis
       2. Medications
       3. Treatments
       4. Treatment of Complications
    G. Nursing Care
       1. Health Promotion
       2. Assessment
       3. Nursing Diagnoses and Interventions
         a. Pain
         b. Disturbed Sleep Pattern
         c. Imbalanced Nutrition: Less than Body Requirements
         d. Deficient Fluid Volume
       4. Using NANDA, NIC, and NOC
       5. Community-Based Care
    H. The Client with Cancer of the Stomach
    I. Risk Factors
    J. Pathophysiology
    K. Manifestations
    L. Interdisciplinary Care
       1. Diagnosis
       2. Surgery
    M. Complications
       1. Other Therapies
    N. Nursing Care
       1. Health Promotion
       2. Assessment
       3. Nursing Diagnoses and Interventions
         a. Imbalanced Nutrition: Less than Body Requirements
         b. Anticipatory Grieving
       4. Using NANDA, NIC, and NOC
       5. Community-Based Care

FOCUSED STUDY TIPS

1. Who is at risk for developing stomatitis? Describe the manifestations and nursing care.

_____

_____

_____

_____

_____

2. Discuss the nursing diagnoses and their interventions for clients with oral cancer.

_____

_____

_____

_____

_____

3. Explain a hiatal hernia. Describe its causes, manifestations, and treatment.

_____

_____

_____

_____

_____

4. Describe the difference between acute and chronic gastritis.

_____

_____

_____

_____

_____

CASE STUDY

Kevin Hess is a 40-year-old male who has been diagnosed with a duodenal ulcer. Kevin has a 2-pack-per-day smoking history since age 15. He also admits to using Excedrin in large amounts to ease pain in his right knee. Answer the following questions based on knowledge of caring for clients with peptic ulcer disease.

1. What role does Mr. Hess's age, smoking history, and Excedrin use play in his peptic ulcer disease?

2. Why might Mr. Hess be screened for _H. pylori_ infection?

3. What symptoms of peptic ulcer disease must the nurse assess Mr. Hess for?

4. Describe the most lethal complication of peptic ulcer disease and its symptomology.

CARE PLAN CRITICAL THINKING ACTIVITY: A CLIENT WITH ORAL CANCER

1. Mr. Chavez states that he quit smoking but the nurse sees a pack of cigarettes in his shirt pocket and he smells of smoke. What should the nurse do?

2. What techniques can be used to assist Mr. Chavez to communicate during the immediate postoperative period?

3. What behaviors will demonstrate that Mr. Chavez's anxiety has lessened about his speech?

NCLEX REVIEW QUESTIONS

1. Which of the following behaviors indicate the client's understanding of stomatitis prevention?
   1. The client brushes and flosses the teeth every 48 hours to avoid trauma to oral mucosa.
   2. The client uses an alcohol-based mouthwash to quickly dry the oral mucosa.
   3. The client wears loose-fitting dentures to avoid the rubbing of dentures against the sensitive oral mucosa.
   4. The client limits their intake of highly spiced, acidic foods.
2. The nurse would not expect an oral cancer to form in what location?
   1. Tongue
   2. Upper lip
   3. Lower lip
   4. Floor of the mouth
3. The client has undergone surgery for cancer of the mouth. What nursing interventions should not be used to maintain an open airway?
   1. Turn the client every 2 hours.
   2. Have the client practice deep breathing.
   3. Place the client in Fowler's position.
   4. Place the client in Trendelenberg position.
4. The nurse expects that the client will not be able to communicate verbally after oral surgery. What communication planning should be done?
   1. Have the client record all questions preoperatively on a tape recorder.
   2. Require that a spokesperson be available at the client's bedside at all times.
   3. Place a tablet and pens next to the bed for the client to write on.
   4. Provide the client with the nursing staff's unit cell phone numbers.
5. Which diagnostic study would not be routinely performed for a client with gastroesophageal reflux disease (GERD)?
   1. Barium enema
   2. 24-hour ambulatory pH monitoring
   3. Barium swallow
   4. Upper endoscopy
6. Adenocarcinoma is one of two forms of esophageal cancer. Identify the other common form.
   1. Squamous cell
   2. Basal cell
   3. Epithelial cell
   4. Stratus cell
7. Which is not a complication of vomiting?
   1. Hyperkalemia
   2. Metabolic acidosis
   3. Aspiration
   4. Tears of the esophagus
8. To help relieve nausea and vomiting, the nurse could suggest using which aromatic root?
   1. Anise
   2. Catmint
   3. Sage
   4. Ginger

9. Hematochezia is defined as:
    1. Vomiting blood.
    2. Black and tarry stools.
    3. Frankly bloody stools.
    4. Frothy white vomitus.
10. Which client statement reflects their understanding of preventing dumping syndrome?
    1. "I eat three large meals a day."
    2. "I do not drink liquids with my meal."
    3. "I have decreased the amount of protein in my diet."
    4. "I have increased the amount of sugars in my diet."

CHAPTER 24

NURSING CARE OF CLIENTS WITH GALLBLADDER, LIVER, AND PANCREATIC DISORDERS

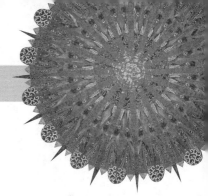

LEARNING OUTCOMES

After completing Chapter 24, you will be able to demonstrate the following objectives:

- Describe the pathophysiology of commonly occurring disorders of the gallbladder, liver, and exocrine pancreas.
- Use knowledge of normal anatomy and physiology to understand the manifestations and effects of biliary, hepatic, and pancreatic disorders.
- Relate changes in normal assessment data to the pathophysiology and manifestations of gallbladder, liver, and exocrine pancreatic disorders.

CLINICAL COMPETENCIES

- Assess functional health status of clients with gallbladder, liver, or pancreatic disease.
- Monitor for, document, and report expected and unexpected manifestations in clients with gallbladder, liver, or pancreatic disease.
- Prepare clients for and understand the purpose and significance of diagnostic tests for gallbladder, liver, and pancreatic disorders.
- Integrate appropriate dietary, pharmacologic, and other interdisciplinary measures into nursing care and teaching of the client with a gallbladder, liver, or pancreatic disorder.
- Provide appropriate nursing care for the client who has surgery of the gallbladder, liver, or pancreas.
- Integrate psychosocial, cultural, and spiritual considerations into the plan of care for a client with a gallbladder, liver, or pancreatic disorder.

MediaLink

www.prenhall.com/lemone

Resources for this chapter can be found on the Prentice Hall Nursing MediaLink DVD accompanying this textbook, and on the Companion Website at http://www.prenhall.com/lemone. Click on Chapter 24 to select the activities for this chapter.

DVD-ROM
- Audio Glossary
- NCLEX-RN® Review

Animation/Video
- Cirrhosis

Companion Website
www.prenhall.com/lemone
- Audio Glossary
- NCLEX-RN® Review
- Care Plan Activity: A Client with Hepatitis A
- Case Studies
  - Hepatitis B
  - Traditional Native American Diet and Gallbladder Disease
- MediaLink Applications
  - GI Disorders and Gall Bladder Disease
  - Treatment of Liver Cancer
- Links to Resources

- Use evidence-based practice to develop, implement, evaluate, and, as needed, revise the plan of care for clients with disorders of the gallbladder, liver, or pancreas.
- Provide appropriate client and family teaching to promote, maintain, and restore functional health status for clients with gallbladder, liver, and pancreatic disorders.

KEY TERMS

alcoholic cirrhosis
ascites
balloon tamponade
biliary colic
cholecystitis
cholelithiasis
chronic hepatitis
cirrhosis
esophageal varices
fulminant hepatitis
gastric lavage
hematochezia
hepatitis

hepatorenal syndrome
jaundice
laparoscopic
   cholecystectomy
liver transplantation
pancreatitis
paracentesis
portal hypertension
portal systemic
   encephalopathy
steatorrhea
transjugular intrahepatic
   portosystemic shunt (TIPS)

CHAPTER OUTLINE

I. Gallbladder Disorders
II. The Client with Gallstones
  A. Physiology Review
  B. Pathophysiology and Manifestations
    1. Cholelithiasis
    2. Cholecystitis
  C. Interdisciplinary Care
    1. Diagnosis
    2. Medications
    3. Treatments
  D. Nursing Care
    1. Health Promotion
    2. Assessment
    3. Nursing Diagnoses and Interventions
      a. Pain
      b. Imbalanced Nutrition: Less than Body Requirements
      c. Risk for Infection
    4. Community-Based Care
III. The Client with Cancer of the Gallbladder
IV. Liver Disorders
  A. Physiology Review
  B. Common Manifestations of Liver Disorders
    1. Hepatocellular Failure
    2. Jaundice
    3. Portal Hypertension
V. The Client with Hepatitis
  A. Pathophysiology and Manifestations
    1. Viral Hepatitis
    2. Chronic Hepatitis

IX. The Client with Liver Abscess
  A. Pathophysiology and Manifestation
  B. Interdisciplinary Care
  C. Nursing Care
 X. Exocrine Pancreas Disorders
XI. The Client with Pancreatitis
  A. Physiology Review
  B. Pathophysiology
    1. Acute Pancreatitis
    2. Chronic Pancreatitis
  C. Interdisciplinary Care
    1. Diagnosis
    2. Medications
    3. Treatments
  D. Nursing Care
    1. Health Promotion
    2. Assessment
    3. Nursing Diagnoses and Interventions
      a. Pain
      b. Imbalanced Nutrition: Less than Body Requirements
      c. Risk for Deficient Fluid Volume
    4. Using NANDA, NIC, and NOC
    5. Community-Based Care
XII. Client with Pancreatic Cancer
  A. Pathophysiology and Manifestations
  B. Interdisciplinary Care

FOCUSED STUDY TIPS

1. Describe the manifestations, diagnosis, treatment, and nursing interventions for clients with cholecystitis.

_____

_____

_____

_____

_____

2. Explain the physiologic process of jaundice.

_____

_____

_____

_____

_____

3. Define the various forms of hepatitis.

_____

_____

_____

_____

_____

4. Identify causes of liver trauma, resulting manifestations, and required nursing care.

_____

_____

_____

_____

_____

CASE STUDY

Joseph Wales, a 62-year-old male has been admitted with a diagnosis of chronic hepatitis. Mr. Wales has a past medical history that includes acute pancreatitis and alcohol abuse. Answer the following questions based on knowledge of caring for clients with chronic pancreatitis.

1. What role does Mr. Wales's past medical history play in his current episode of chronic pancreatitis?

2. What symptoms will Mr. Wales experience?

3. What complications from chronic pancreatitis must be assessed by the nurse?

4. Describe discharge teaching that must occur with Mr. Wales.

CARE PLAN CRITICAL THINKING ACTIVITY: A CLIENT WITH CHOLELITHIASIS

1. What role did Mrs. Red Wing's diet play in the development of cholelithiasis?

2. How can tribal medicine complement traditional medical therapies for Mrs. Red Wing?

3. What strategies can Mrs. Red Wing's family utilize to decrease the likelihood of another family member developing cholelithiasis?

NCLEX REVIEW QUESTIONS

1. The nurse knows the majority of gallstones consist of what element?
   1. Cholesterol
   2. Bile salts
   3. Calcium
   4. Lecithin
2. The nurse understands the client with acute cholecystitis will not experience which symptom?
   1. Nausea
   2. Fever
   3. Right upper quadrant pain
   4. Diarrhea
3. Teaching to reduce the risk of cholelithiasis includes:
   1. Avoiding cholesterol lowering medications.
   2. Instructing the client to follow a low-fat, low-cholesterol diet.
   3. Instructing the client to decrease their activity level.
   4. Instructing the client to increase carbohydrates in their diet.

4. Jaundice is first noticeable in what tissue?
   1. Nailbeds
   2. Skin
   3. Sclera
   4. Oral mucosa

5. The client presents with abnormal liver function studies and impaired consciousness. The nurse knows the client is experiencing what effect?
   1. Portal systemic encephalopathy
   2. Ascites
   3. Hepatorenal syndrome
   4. Splenomegaly

6. A vaccine is available for which form of viral hepatitis?
   1. Hepatitis A
   2. Hepatitis C
   3. Hepatitis Delta
   4. Hepatitis E

7. Which statement indicates client understanding of hepatitis C transmission and care?
   1. "I can share needles because hepatitis B is not present in blood."
   2. "I will get very sick suddenly when I am infected with the hepatitis C virus."
   3. "I must use a condom during sex."
   4. "Once I am exposed to the infection, I will become immune."

8. Which body part is not affected by asterixis?
   1. Tongue
   2. Feet
   3. Arms
   4. Eyes

9. Identify the incorrect nursing diagnosis for a client with liver trauma.
   1. Deficient fluid volume related to hemorrhage
   2. Risk for infection related to wound or abdominal contamination
   3. Ineffective protection related to impaired coagulation
   4. Altered body image related to bruising

10. Which is not a risk factor for pancreatic cancer?
    1. Exposure to industrial chemicals
    2. Following a low-fat diet
    3. Diabetes mellitus
    4. Smoking

CHAPTER 25

ASSESSING CLIENTS WITH BOWEL ELIMINATION DISORDERS

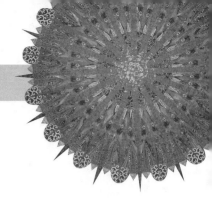

LEARNING OUTCOMES

After completing Chapter 25, you will be able to demonstrate the following objectives:

- Describe the anatomy, physiology, and functions of the intestines.
- Explain the physiologic processes involved in bowel elimination.
- Identify specific topics to consider during a health history assessment interview of the client with problems of bowel elimination.
- Describe techniques used to assess bowel integrity and function.
- Describe normal variations in assessment findings for the older adult.
- Identify manifestations of altered intestinal function.

CLINICAL COMPETENCIES

- Conduct and document a health history for clients who have or are at risk for alterations in bowel elimination.
- Conduct and document a physical assessment of the intestinal system.
- Monitor the results of diagnostic tests and report abnormal findings.

EQUIPMENT NEEDED

- Water-soluble lubricant
- Occult blood test kit, such as Occultest or Hemoccult II
- Disposable gloves
- Stethoscope

KEY TERMS

borborygmus
bruits
constipation
diarrhea
flatus
hernia
melena

occult blood
ostomy
peristalsis
steatorrhea
striae
Valsalva's maneuver

CHAPTER OUTLINE

   I. Anatomy, Physiology and Functions of the Intestines
     A. The Small Intestine
     B. The Large Intestine
  II. Assessing Bowel Function
     A. Diagnostic Tests
     B. Genetic Considerations
     C. Health Assessment Interview
     D. Physical Assessment
 III. Bowel Assessment

FOCUSED STUDY TIPS

1. Discuss the differences in function between the small and large intestine.

_____

_____

_____

_____

2. What radiologic modalities are used to assess bowel function?

_____

_____

_____

3. Describe the difference between borborygmus and bruits.

_____

_____

_____

_____

4. Identify three abnormal findings of a perianal assessment.

_____

_____

_____

CASE STUDY

Jerry Parsons is being seen in the office complaining of constipation. He describes episodes of feeling as if he is going to pass out while bearing down during a bowel movement. Answer the following based on knowledge of the digestive system.

1. What is the condition Mr. Parsons is describing when he mentions feeling as if he will pass out while bearing down during a bowel movement?

2. What could result from frequent bouts of constipation?

3. What radiographic study may be performed to assess Mr. Parsons's large bowel function?

4. Would you screen a client who describes bouts of constipation for depression or an anxiety disorder?

NCLEX REVIEW QUESTIONS

1. Which structure is not found in the large bowel?
    1. Ileum
    2. Cecum
    3. Colon
    4. Rectum
2. Which of the following enzymatic processes is not performed in the small intestine?
    1. Pancreatic amylase acts on starches.
    2. Pancreatic enzymes break down proteins.
    3. Triglycerides break down dextrin.
    4. Triglycerides are coated by bile salts and emulsified.
3. Identify the product of digestion that is left to enter the large intestine.
    1. Electrolytes
    2. Indigestible fibers
    3. Vitamins
    4. Nutrients
4. Stool specimen examination does not include which component of assessment?
    1. Odor
    2. Water
    3. Color
    4. WBC
5. Which is not a part of a bowel function assessment?
    1. Ask the client if they have traveled to a foreign country.
    2. Question the client about allergies.
    3. Ask the client to describe their sexual history.
    4. Question the client about stressors in their lifestyle.
6. To effectively perform an abdominal examination, the client should be placed in what position?
    1. Lithotomy
    2. Supine
    3. Standing
    4. Sims'
7. Identify the abnormal abdominal assessment finding.
    1. A concave abdomen
    2. Gurgling or clicking sound heard upon auscultation
    3. Tympany heard over gas-filled bowels upon palpation
    4. Dullness heard over the abdomen during palpation

8. Rebound tenderness located in the right lower quadrant is an indicator of what disease process?
   1. Acute appendicitis
   2. Acute cholecystitis
   3. Acute pancreatitis
   4. Acute diverticulitis
9. Which of the following is not a cause of anal fissures?
   1. Hemorrhoids
   2. Large stools
   3. Hard stools
   4. Diarrhea
10. When assessing the anus, slowly insert a gloved finger and point it toward:
    1. The rectal floor.
    2. The umbilicus.
    3. The right lung.
    4. The heart.

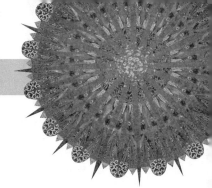

CHAPTER 26

NURSING CARE OF CLIENTS WITH BOWEL DISORDERS

LEARNING OUTCOMES

After completing Chapter 26, you will be able to demonstrate the following objectives:

- Compare and contrast the causes, pathophysiology, manifestations, interdisciplinary care and nursing care of clients with diarrhea, constipation, irritable bowel syndrome, and fecal incontinence.
- Explain the pathophysiology, manifestations, complications, interdisciplinary care, and nursing care of clients with acute inflammatory and infectious bowel disorders, chronic inflammatory bowel disorders, malabsorption syndromes, neoplastic disorders, structural and obstructive bowel disorders, and anorectal disorders.
- Discuss the purposes, nursing implications, and health education for the client and family of medications used to treat bowel disorders.
- Explain the rationale for using selected diets, including those for diarrhea and constipation and low-residue, gluten-free, and high-fiber diets.
- Describe the surgical procedures of the bowel, including colectomy, colostomy, ileostomy, and perianal surgery.

CLINICAL COMPETENCIES

- Assess the functional status of clients with bowel disorders, and monitor, document, and report abnormal manifestations.
- Use evidence-based research to prevent aspiration in critically ill clients with enteral feedings, and to make accurate assessments of fecal incontinence in older adults.
- Determine priority nursing diagnoses, based on assessed data, to select and implement individualized nursing interventions for clients with bowel disorders.
- Administer medications used to treat bowel disorders knowledgeably and safely.

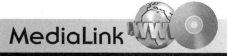

MediaLink

www.prenhall.com/lemone

Resources for this chapter can be found on the Prentice Hall Nursing MediaLink DVD accompanying this textbook, and on the Companion Website at http://www.prenhall.com/lemone. Click on Chapter 26 to select the activities for this chapter.

Prentice Hall Nursing MediaLink DVD-ROM
- Audio Glossary
- NCLEX-RN® Review

Companion Website
www.prenhall.com/lemone
- Audio Glossary
- NCLEX-RN® Review
- Care Plan Activity: Irritable Bowel Syndrome
- Case Studies
  - Enteral Tube Complications
  - Irritable Bowel Syndrome
- Teaching Plan: Colon Cancer
- MediaLink Applications
  - Crohn's Disease and Ulcerative Colitis
  - Crohn's Disease Teaching Sheet

133

- Provide skilled care to clients having an ileostomy, colostomy, or perianal surgery.
- Integrate interdisciplinary care into care of clients with bowel disorders.
- Provide appropriate teaching to promote nutrition, prevent infectious and helminthic infestations, encourage preventive screening for colon cancer, and facilitate community-based care for healthcare needs resulting from bowel disorders.
- Revise plan of care as needed to provide effective interventions to promote, maintain, or restore functional health status to clients with bowel disorders.

KEY TERMS

appendicitis
borborygmi
Crohn's disease
colectomy
colostomy
constipation
diarrhea
diverticulosis
fecal impaction
gastroenteritis
hematochezia
hemorrhoids
hernia

ileostomy
inflammatory bowel disease
   (IBD)
irritable bowel syndrome
   (IBS)
lactose intolerance
malabsorption
paralytic ileus
peritonitis
sprue
steatorrhea
stoma
ulcerative colitis

CHAPTER OUTLINE

   I. Disorders of Intestinal Motility
  II. The Client with Diarrhea
     A. Pathophysiology
     B. Manifestations
     C. Complications
     D. Interdisciplinary Care
       1. Diagnosis
       2. Medications
       3. Nutrition
       4. Complementary and Alternative Therapies
     E. Nursing Care
       1. Health Promotion
       2. Assessment
       3. Nursing Diagnoses and Interventions
         a. Diarrrhea
         b. Risk for Deficient Fluid Volume
         c. Risk for Impaired Skin Integrity
       4. Using NANDA, NIC, and NOC
       5. Community-Based Care
  III. The Client with Constipation
     A. Pathophysiology
     B. Manifestations
     C. Interdisciplinary Care
       1. Diagnosis
       2. Medications
       3. Nutrition
       4. Enemas
       5. Complementary and Alternative Therapies

D. Nursing Care
   1. Health Promotion
   2. Assessment
   3. Nursing Diagnoses and Interventions
      a. Constipation
   4. Community-Based Care

IV. The Client with Irritable Bowel Syndrome
   A. Pathophysiology
   B. Manifestations
   C. Interdisciplinary Care
      1. Diagnosis
      2. Medications
      3. Nutrition
      4. Complementary and Alternative Therapies
   D. Nursing Care
      1. Assessment
      2. Nursing Diagnoses and Interventions
      3. Community-Based Care

V. The Client with Fecal Incontinence
   A. Pathophysiology
   B. Interdisciplinary Care
   C. Nursing Care
      1. Health Promotion
      2. Assessment
      3. Nursing Diagnoses and Interventions
         a. Bowel Incontinence
         b. Risk for Impaired Skin Integrity
      4. Community-Based Care

VI. Acute Inflammatory and Infectious Bowel Disorders

VII. The Client with Appendicitis
   A. Pathophysiology
   B. Manifestations
   C. Complications
   D. Interdisciplinary Care
      1. Diagnosis
      2. Medications
      3. Surgery
   E. Nursing Care
      1. Assessment
      2. Nursing Diagnoses and Interventions
         a. Risk for Infection
         b. Acute Pain
      3. Using NANDA, NIC, and NOC
      4. Community-Based Care

VIII. The Client with Peritonitis
   A. Pathophysiology
   B. Manifestations
   C. Complications
   D. Interdisciplinary Care
      1. Diagnosis
      2. Medications
      3. Surgery
      4. Nutrition

E. Nursing Care
   1. Assessment
   2. Nursing Diagnoses and Interventions
      a. Acute Pain
      b. Deficient Fluid Volume
      c. Ineffective Protection
      d. Anxiety
   3. Using NANDA, NIC, and NOC
   4. Community-Based Care

IX. The Client with Gastroenteritis
  A. Pathophysiology
  B. Manifestations
  C. Complications
    1. Specific Types of Gastrointestinal Infections
  D. Interdisciplinary Care
    1. Diagnosis
    2. Medications
    3. Nutrition and Fluids
    4. Gastric Lavage
    5. Plasmapheresis
    6. Dialysis
  E. Nursing Care
    1. Health Promotion
    2. Assessment
    3. Nursing Diagnoses and Interventions
    4. Community-Based Care

X. The Client with a Protozoal Bowel Infection
  A. Pathophysiology and Manifestations
    1. Giardiasis
    2. Amebiasis
    3. Cryptosporidiosis (Coccidiosis)
  B. Interdisciplinary Care
    1. Diagnosis
    2. Medications
  C. Nursing Care

XI. The Client with a Helminthic Disorder
  A. Pathophysiology
  B. Interdisciplinary Care
    1. Diagnosis
    2. Medications
  C. Nursing Care

XII. Chronic Inflammatory Bowel Disorders

XIII. The Client with Inflammatory Bowel Disease
  A. Ulcerative Colitis
    1. Pathophysiology
    2. Manifestations
    3. Complications
  B. Crohn's Disease
    1. Pathophysiology
    2. Manifestations
    3. Compications
  C. Interdisciplinary Care
    1. Diagnosis
    2. Medications

FOCUSED STUDY TIPS

1. Discuss the impact that diarrhea has on a client's physiological well-being. Include nursing interventions that need to be instituted to maintain physiological well-being.

_____

_____

_____

_____

_____

2. Describe the pathophysiology, treatment, and nursing interventions for clients diagnosed with peritonitis.

_____

_____

_____

_____

_____

3. Describe the similarities and differences between ulcerative colitis and Crohn's disease.

_____

_____

_____

_____

4. Define polyps, their location, manifestations, and how they are treated.

_____

_____

_____

CASE STUDY

Lynn Bowman is a 16-year-old female who comes into the emergency room with complaints of lower right lower quadrant pain, nausea, vomiting, and a fever of 101°F. She exhibits a positive McBurney's sign, and she is diagnosed with appendicitis. Answer the following questions based on knowledge of caring for clients with appendicitis.

1. What is a positive McBurney's sign?

2. What are the possible complications of untreated appendicitis?

3. What diagnostic studies will Ms. Bowman undergo?

4. Ms. Bowman undergoes an appendectomy. What should the nurse's postoperative teaching include?

NCLEX REVIEW QUESTIONS

1. Identify the medication classification that is not commonly used as an antidiarrheal.
   1. Opium derivatives
   2. Absorbants
   3. Demulcents
   4. Stimulants
2. What dietary instruction should the nurse give to the client about managing diarrhea?
   1. Eat foods high in fiber.
   2. Eat small, frequent meals.
   3. Avoid drinking electrolyte solutions such as Gatorade.
   4. Increase the intake of milk products.
3. Which statement demonstrates that the client understands teaching about managing constipation?
   1. "I should limit my fluid intake."
   2. "I should avoid bran and prunes."
   3. "I should participate in a daily form of exercise."
   4. "I should drink a glass of ice water before each meal."
4. What imaging modality is the most effective in diagnosing acute appendicitis?
   1. Ultrasound
   2. CT scan
   3. MRI
   4. Fluoroscopy
5. A urine output of less than _____ mL/hr indicates hypovolemia.
   1. 30
   2. 50
   3. 60
   4. 75
6. Identify the diarrheal illness caused by ingesting raw or improperly cooked meat, eggs, and dairy products in which symptoms develop 8 to 48 hours after ingestion.
   1. Shigellosis
   2. Traveler's diarrhea
   3. Cholera
   4. Salmonellosis
7. Identify the incorrect statement about common bowel infections.
   1. Giardiasis is a protozoal infection of the proximal small intestine.
   2. Helminths are parasitic worms capable of causing bowel infections.
   3. Amebiasis is an infection that attacks only the small bowel.
   4. Coccidiosis secretes an enterotoxin that causes watery diarrhea.

8. Which of the following indicates that the client is not correctly managing their inflammatory bowel disease (IBD)?
    1. The client has added Ensure to their diet.
    2. The client reports drinking less than one quart of fluid per day.
    3. The client takes their medication as ordered by their physician.
    4. The client has contacted the community ostomy support group.
9. How must a client with celiac sprue adjust their diet?
    1. Increase lactose in their diet.
    2. Add fats to their diet.
    3. Decrease calories in their diet.
    4. Eliminate gluten from their diet.
10. Identify the incorrect manifestation of intestinal polyps.
    1. Diarrhea
    2. Abdominal cramping
    3. Painful rectal bleeding
    4. Mucous discharge
11. Identify the incorrect statement about colorectal cancer.
    1. Ingestion of calcium and folic acid supplements can prevent colorectal cancer.
    2. Bowel cancer often produces no symptoms until it is advanced.
    3. Most recurrences of cancer occur within the first two years.
    4. Colorectal cancer is always treated by surgery.
12. Identify the correct statement about a transverse loop colostomy.
    1. It is the most common permanent colostomy performed.
    2. Two separate stomas are created.
    3. A portion of the colon is brought out onto the abdomen and is secured by a bridge or plastic rod.
    4. It is the most common temporary colostomy procedure performed.
13. Which hernia is congenital?
    1. Ventral hernia
    2. Umbilical hernia
    3. Inguinal hernia
    4. Incisional hernia
14. Which manifestation is not present in clients with a large bowel obstruction?
    1. Vomiting
    2. Constipation
    3. Colicky pain
    4. Abdominal distention
15. What portion of the gastrointestinal tract does not develop diverticuli?
    1. Stomach
    2. Jejunum
    3. Transverse colon
    4. Rectum

CHAPTER 27

ASSESSING CLIENTS WITH URINARY ELIMINATION DISORDERS

LEARNING OUTCOMES

After completing Chapter 27, you will be able to demonstrate the following objectives:

- Describe the anatomy, physiology, and functions of the urinary system.
- Explain the role of the urinary system in maintaining homeostasis.
- Identify specific topics for consideration during a health history assessment interview of the client with problems involving the urinary system.
- Describe techniques used to assess the integrity and function of the urinary system.
- Describe normal variations in assessment findings for the older adult.
- Identify manifestations of impairment of the urinary system.

CLINICAL COMPETENCIES

- Conduct and document a health history for clients who have or are at risk for alterations in urinary elimination.
- Conduct and document a physical assessment of the urinary system.
- Monitor the results of diagnostic tests and report abnormal findings.

EQUIPMENT NEEDED

- Urine specimen cup
- Disposable gloves
- Stethoscope

KEY TERMS

calculi

dysuria

glomerular filtration rate
   (GFR)

hematuria

micturition

nocturia

oliguria

polyuria

pyuria

urea

CHAPTER OUTLINE

I. Anatomy, Physiology, and Functions of the Urinary System
   A. The Kidneys
      1. Formation of Urine
      2. Maintaining Normal Composition and Volume of Urine
      3. Clearing Waste Products
      4. Renal Hormones
   B. The Ureters
   C. The Urinary Bladder
   D. The Urethra
II. Assessing Urinary Function
   A. Diagnostic Tests
   B. Genetic Considerations
   C. The Health Assessment Interview
   D. Physical Assessment
   E. Urinary Assessments

FOCUSED STUDY TIPS

1. Discuss the organs of the urinary system.

   _____

   _____

   _____

2. Summarize diagnostic tests for the urinary system.

   _____

   _____

   _____

3. Summarize the physical assessment.

   _____

   _____

   _____

4. Explain the formation of urine.

   _____

   _____

   _____

CASE STUDY

Anne Sutter is a 64-year-old female client admitted to the nursing unit. Her skin and mucous membranes are pale. She also has tenderness and pain on percussion of the costovertebral angle.

1. Explain the functions of the kidney.

2. What could tenderness and pain on percussion of the costovertebral angle suggest?

3. What could pallor of the skin and mucous membranes indicate?

NCLEX REVIEW QUESTIONS

1. The kidney is supported by which of the following?
   1. The inner renal fascia.
   2. The outer adipose capsule.
   3. The middle renal capsule.
   4. The outer renal fascia.
2. Which of the following is a function of the kidney?
   1. Form urine
   2. Conserve metabolic waste products
   3. Destroy nutrients
   4. Secrete solutes
3. Which of the following statements is true about glomerular filtration?
   1. Hydrostatic pressure forces fluid and solutes through a membrane.
   2. It is a passive, selective process.
   3. Glomerular filtration rate (GFR) is not influenced by the total surface area available for filtration.
   4. The glomerulus is less efficient than most capillary beds.
4. Urine is composed, by volume, of about _____ % water and _____% solutes.
   1. 95, 5
   2. 85, 15
   3. 75, 25
   4. 65, 35
5. Which of the following is correct about renal proteins?
   1. The stimulus for the production of erythropoietin by the kidneys is increased oxygen delivery to kidney cells.
   2. Erythropoietin stimulates the bone marrow to produce red blood cells in response to tissue hypoxia.
   3. Hormones either activated or synthesized by the kidneys include the active form of vitamin E, erythropoietin, and natriuretic hormone.
   4. Vitamin D is necessary for the absorption of calcium and phosphate by the large intestine.
6. The layers of the bladder wall (from internal to external) are the:
   1. Epithelial mucosa lining the inside, the connective tissue submucosa, the smooth muscle layer, and the fibrous outer layer.
   2. Fibrous outer layer, the connective tissue submucosa, the epithelial mucosa lining the inside, and the smooth muscle layer.
   3. Fibrous outer layer, epithelial mucosa lining the inside, the connective tissue submucosa, and the smooth muscle layer.
   4. The connective tissue submucosa, epithelial mucosa lining the inside, the smooth muscle layer, and the fibrous outer layer.
7. Which of the following statements about the bladder is correct?
   1. It holds about 600 to 800 mL of urine before internal pressure rises and signals the need to empty the bladder through micturition.
   2. It is posterior to the symphysis pubis and serves as a storage site for urine.
   3. In females, the bladder lies immediately in front of the rectum.
   4. Openings for the ureters and the urethra are outside the bladder.

8. Oliguria means:
   1. Blood in the urine.
   2. Excessive urination at night.
   3. Voiding excessive amounts of urine.
   4. Voiding scant amounts of urine.
9. Which of the following findings in the urinalysis report would the nurse consider abnormal?
   1. Light straw color
   2. A pH of 5.5
   3. WBCs 3
   4. Ketones +1
10. Which of the following statements is incorrect about age-related urinary system changes?
    1. Urinary retention is less common.
    2. Urinary frequency, urgency, and nocturia are more common with aging.
    3. Smaller amounts of residual urine are present after voiding.
    4. Urinary incontinence is a normal outcome of aging.

CHAPTER 28

NURSING CARE OF CLIENTS WITH URINARY TRACT DISORDERS

LEARNING OUTCOMES

After completing Chapter 28, you will be able to demonstrate the following objectives:

- Explain the pathophysiology of common urinary tract disorders.
- Describe the manifestations of urinary tract disorders, relating manifestations to the pathophysiology of the disorder.
- Discuss tests used to diagnose disorders affecting the urinary tract with their nursing implications.
- Discuss the nursing implications of medications and treatments prescribed for clients with urinary tract disorders.
- Describe surgical procedures used in treating urinary tract disorders.

CLINICAL COMPETENCIES

- Assess the functional health status of clients with urinary tract disorders, using data to determine priority nursing diagnoses and select individualized nursing interventions.
- Identify, report, and document abnormal or unexpected assessments, monitoring client status.
- Use evidence-based research to plan and implement nursing care for clients with urinary tract disorders.
- Integrate the interdisciplinary plan of care into care for clients with urinary tract disorders.
- Knowledgeably and safely administer prescribed medications and treatments for clients with urinary tract disorders.
- Provide effective nursing care for clients undergoing surgery of the urinary tract.
- Plan and provide appropriate teaching for prevention of and self-care of urinary tract disorders.
- Evaluate client responses, revising plan of care as needed to promote, maintain, or restore functional health of clients with urinary tract disorders.

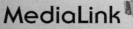

KEY TERMS

cystectomy
cystitis
dysuria
extracorporeal shock wave
   lithotripsy (EWSL)
hematuria
hydronephrosis
lithiasis
lithotripsy
neurogenic bladder
nocturia
nosocomial

pyelonephritis
reflux
renal colic
ureteral stent
ureteroplasty
urgency
urinary calculi
urinary diversion
urinary drainage system
urinary incontinence (UI)
urinary retention

CHAPTER OUTLINE

I. The Client with a Urinary Tract Infection (UTI)
   A. Risk Factors for UTI
   B. Physiology Review
   C. Pathophysiology and Manifestations
      1. Cystitis
      2. Catheter-Associated UTI
      3. Pyelonephritis
   D. Interdisciplinary Care
      1. Diagnosis
      2. Medications
      3. Surgery
   E. Nursing Care
      1. Health Promotion
      2. Assessment
      3. Nursing Diagnoses and Interventions
         a. Pain
         b. Impaired Urinary Elimination
         c. Ineffective Health Maintenance
      4. Community-Based Care
II. The Client with Urinary Calculi
   A. Incidence and Risk Factors
   B. Physiology Review
   C. Pathophysiology
   D. Manifestations
   E. Complications
      1. Obstruction
   F. Interdisciplinary Care
      1. Diagnosis
      2. Medications
      3. Nutrition and Fluid Management
      4. Surgery
   G. Nursing Care
      1. Health Promotion
      2. Assessment
      3. Nursing Diagnoses and Interventions
         a. Acute Pain
         b. Impaired Urinary Elimination
         c. Deficient Knowledge
      4. Community-Based Care

III. The Client with Urinary Tract Tumor
   A. Incidence and Risk Factors
   B. Pathophysiology
   C. Manifestations
   D. Interdisciplinary Care
      1. Diagnosis
      2. Medications
      3. Radiation Therapy
      4. Surgery
   E. Nursing Care
      1. Health Promotion
      2. Assessment
      3. Nursing Diagnoses and Interventions
         a. Impaired Urinary Elimination
         b. Risk for Impaired Skin Integrity
         c. Disturbed Body Image
         d. Risk for Infection
      4. Community-Based Care
IV. The Client with Urinary Retention
   A. Physiology Review
   B. Pathophysiology
   C. Manifestations
   D. Interdisciplinary Care
   E. Nursing Care
      1. Impaired Urinary Elimination
 V. The Client with Neurogenic Bladder
   A. Pathophysiology
      1. Spastic Bladder Dysfunction
      2. Flaccid Bladder Dysfunction
   B. Interdisciplinary Care
      1. Diagnosis
      2. Medications
      3. Nutrition
      4. Bladder Retraining
      5. Surgery
   C. Nursing Care
      1. Assessment
      2. Nursing Diagnoses and Interventions
      3. Community-Based Care
VI. The Client with Urinary Incontinence
   A. Incidence and Prevalence
   B. Pathophysiology
   C. Interdisciplinary Care
      1. Diagnosis
      2. Medications
      3. Surgery
      4. Complementary Therapies
   D. Nursing Care
      1. Health Promotion
      2. Assessment
      3. Nursing Diagnoses and Interventions
         a. Urinary Incontinence: Stress and/or Urge
         b. Self-Care Deficit: Toileting
         c. Social Isolation
      4. Linking NANDA, NIC, and NOC
      5. Community-Based Care

FOCUSED STUDY TIPS

1. Summarize the surgical procedures used in treating urinary tract disorders.

   _____

   _____

   _____

   _____

2. Discuss three diagnostic tests used to diagnose disorders that affect the urinary tract.

   _____

   _____

3. Summarize the pathophysiology of common urinary tract disorders.

   _____

   _____

4. List the risk factors of a urinary tract infection (UTI).

   _____

   _____

   _____

CASE STUDY

Christine Scott is a 37-year-old female client who came in to the clinic today. She is complaining of dysuria, urgency, hematuria, and urgency. She is diagnosed with cystitis.

1. Explain cystitis.

2. What can occur if cystitis is left untreated?

3. Why does cystitis occur more frequently in adult females?

CARE PLAN CRITICAL THINKING ACTIVITY

Define Kegel exercises and how the client should perform them.

Why is it important for Ms. Giovanni to drink decaffeinated tea and noncitrus fruit juices (grape, apple, and cranberry)?

Why should Ms. Giovanni cleanse the perineal area, wiping front to back, after each voiding or incident of urine leakage?

NCLEX REVIEW QUESTIONS

1. Which of the following statements about urinary tract infections (UTIs) is correct?
   1. More than ten million people are treated annually for UTI.
   2. Community-acquired UTIs are not common in young women, and unusual in men over the age of 50.
   3. Most community-acquired UTIs are caused by _Escherichia coli,_ a common gram-positive enteral bacteria.
   4. Catheter-associated UTIs often involve other gram-negative bacteria such as _Proteus, Klebsiella, Seratia,_ and _Pseudomonas._

2. Which of the following statements by a student nurse reflects incorrect understanding about the urinary tract?
   1. "The urinary tract is normally sterile below the urethra."
   2. "Adequate urine volume, a free flow from the kidneys through the urinary meatus, and complete bladder emptying are the most important mechanisms for maintaining sterility."
   3. "Pathogens that enter and contaminate the distal urethra are washed out during voiding."
   4. "Other defenses for maintaining sterile urine include its normal acidity and bacteriostatic properties of the bladder and urethral cells."

3. Risk factors for UTIs in females include all of the following except:
   1. Catheterization.
   2. The use of a diaphragm and spermicidal compounds for birth control.
   3. A long, straight urethra.
   4. The proximity of the urinary meatus to the vagina and anus.

4. Which of the following types of incontinence is the loss of urine associated with increased intraabdominal pressure during sneezing, coughing, and lifting, in which the quantity of urine lost is usually small?
   1. Urge
   2. Stress
   3. Overflow
   4. Functional

5. The nurse is evaluating a student nurse who is providing education to a client who is receiving a urinary antiinfective. Which of the following statements would be correct?
   1. "These drugs are used along with hygiene practices to prevent recurrent urinary tract infection (UTI). Take as directed, even when no symptoms are present."
   2. "Drink ten to twelve glasses of water or fluid per day while taking these drugs."
   3. "Take the drug before meals or food to reduce gastric effects and drink one glass of milk after taking the drug."
   4. "Nitrofurantoin (Furadantin, Nitrofan) turns the urine blue. This is not harmful and subsides when the drug is discontinued."

6. When discussing the management of urolithiasis, the nurse should recommend which of the following?
   1. Collect and strain all urine, saving any stones.
   2. It is not necessary to report stone passage to the physician and bring the stone in for analysis.
   3. Report only the changes in the amount of urine output to physician.
   4. Increase fluid intake to 3550 to 4550 mL per day.

7. The nurse is evaluating a student nurse's understanding of bladder cancer. Which of the following statements indicates a need for further teaching?
   1. An estimated 63,210 new cases of bladder cancer were diagnosed in the United States in 2005, and 13,180 people died as a result of the disease.
   2. The incidence of bladder cancer is about four times higher in women than it is in men, and about twice as high in whites as it is in blacks.
   3. Cigarette smoking is the primary risk factor for bladder cancer.
   4. Most people who develop bladder cancer are over age 60.

8. Diet modifications are often prescribed to change the character of the urine and prevent further lithiasis. The spouse of the client with lithiasis asks the nurse which of the following are foods high in oxalate?
   1. Beans and lentils, chocolate and cocoa, dried fruits, canned or smoked fish except tuna, flour, milk and milk products
   2. Asparagus, beer and colas, beets, cabbage, celery, fruits, green beans, nuts, tea, and tomatoes
   3. Goose, organ meats, sardines and herring, and venison; moderate in beef, chicken, crab, pork, salmon, and veal
   4. Cheese, eggs, grapes, meat and poultry, and whole grains

9. Which of the following actions is inappropriate for the nurse who is providing urinary stoma care?
   1. Remove old pouch, pulling gently away from skin. Warm water or adhesive solvent may be used to loosen the seal, if necessary.
   2. Gather all supplies: a clean, disposable pouch; liquid skin barrier or barrier ring; 4-by-4 gauze squares; stoma guide; adhesive solvent; clean gloves; and a clean washcloth.
   3. Cleanse skin around the stoma with soap and water, rinse, and pat or air dry.
   4. Apply the bag with an opening no more than 3 to 4 mm wider than outside of stoma.

10. The nurse is discussing with a client the following points to help prevent UTI and UI in an older adult. Which statement is correct?
    1. "Maintain a generous fluid intake. Increase fluid intake after the evening meal to reduce nocturia."
    2. "Perform pelvic muscle exercises (Kegel exercises) two times a day to increase perineal muscle tone."
    3. "Increase the consumption of caffeine-containing beverages (coffee, tea, colas), citrus juices, and artificially-sweetened beverages that contain NutraSweet."
    4. "Use behavioral techniques such as scheduled toileting, habit training, and bladder training to reduce the frequency of incontinence."

CHAPTER 29

NURSING CARE OF CLIENTS WITH KIDNEY DISORDERS

LEARNING OUTCOMES

After completing Chapter 29, you will be able to demonstrate the following objectives:

- Describe the pathophysiology of common kidney disorders, relating pathophysiology to normal physiology and manifestations of the disorder.
- Discuss risk factors for kidney disorders and nursing care to reduce these risks.
- Explain diagnostic studies used to identify disorders of the kidneys and their effects.
- Discuss the effects and nursing implications for medications and treatments used for clients with kidney disorders.
- Compare and contrast dialysis procedures used to manage acute and chronic renal failure.

CLINICAL COMPETENCIES

- Assess the functional health status of clients with kidney disorders.
- Monitor, document, and report unexpected or abnormal manifestations in clients with kidney disorders.
- Provide appropriate and effective nursing care for clients undergoing dialysis, surgery involving the kidneys, or renal transplant.
- Based on assessment data, determine priority nursing diagnoses and interventions for clients with renal disorders.
- Plan and implement evidence-based nursing care for clients with renal disorders using research and best practices.
- Collaborate with the client and other members of the interdisciplinary team to prioritize and implement care.
- Provide teaching appropriate to the client and situation for clients with kidney disorders.
- Evaluate client responses to care, revising the plan of care as needed to promote, maintain, or restore functional health status for clients with renal disorders.

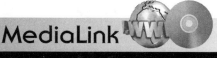

MediaLink

www.prenhall.com/lemone

Resources for this chapter can be found on the Prentice Hall Nursing MediaLink DVD accompanying this textbook, and on the Companion Website at http://www.prenhall.com/lemone. Click on Chapter 29 to select the activities for this chapter.

Prentice Hall Nursing MediaLink DVD-ROM
- Audio Glossary
- NCLEX-RN® Review

Animation/Video
- Furosemide
- The Kidney

Companion Website
www.prenhall.com/lemone
- Audio Glossary
- NCLEX-RN® Review
- Care Plan Activity: Acute Glomerulonephritis
- Case Studies
  - Acute Glomerulonephritis
  - Kidney Transplant
- MediaLink Applications
  - Kidney Disorders
  - Renal Insufficiency
- Links to Resources

KEY TERMS

acute renal failure (ARF)
acute tubular necrosis (ATN)
azotemia
chronic renal failure (CRF)
continuous renal replacement
    therapy (CRRT)
dialysate
dialysis
end-stage renal disease (ESRD)
glomerular filtration rate (GFR)
glomerulonephritis
hematuria

hemodialysis
nephrectomy
nephrotic syndrome
oliguria
peritoneal dialysis
plasmapheresis
polycystic kidney disease
proteinuria
renal artery stenosis
renal failure
ultrafiltration
uremia

CHAPTER OUTLINE

   I. Age-Related Changes in Kidney Function
  II. The Client with a Congenital Kidney Malformation
 III. The Client with Polycystic Kidney Disease
      A. Pathophysiology
      B. Manifestations
      C. Interdisciplinary Care
      D. Nursing Care
  IV. The Client with a Glomerular Disorder
      A. Physiology Review
      B. Pathophysiology
         1. Acute Proliferative Glomerulonephritis
         2. Rapidly Progressive Glomerulonephritis
         3. Nephrotic Syndrome
         4. Chronic Glomerulonephritis
         5. Diabetic Nephropathy
         6. Lupus Nephritis
      C. Interdisciplinary Care
         1. Diagnosis
         2. Medications
         3. Treatments
      D. Nursing Care
         1. Health Promotion
         2. Assessment
         3. Nursing Diagnoses and Interventions
            a. Excess Fluid Volume
            b. Fatigue
            c. Ineffective Protection
            d. Ineffective Role Performance
         4. Community-Based Care
   V. The Client with a Vascular Kidney Disorder
      A. Hypertension
      B. Renal Artery Occlusion
      C. Renal Vein Occlusion
      D. Renal Artery Stenosis
  VI. The Client with Kidney Trauma
      A. Pathophysiology and Manifestations
      B. Interdisciplinary Care
      C. Nursing Care

VII. The Client with a Renal Tumor
    A. Pathophysiology and Manifestations
    B. Interdisciplinary Care
    C. Nursing Care
        1. Nursing Diagnoses and Interventions
           a. Pain
           b. Ineffective Breathing Pattern
           c. Risk for Impaired Urinary Elimination
           d. Anticipatory Grieving
        2. Community-Based Care
VIII. Renal Failure
 IX. The Client with Acute Renal Failure
    A. Incidence and Risk Factors
    B. Physiology Review
    C. Pathophysiology
        1. Prerenal ARF
        2. Postrenal ARF
        3. Intrinsic (Intrarenal) ARF
    D. Course and Manifestations
        1. Initiation Phase
        2. Maintenance Phase
        3. Recovery Phase
    E. Interdisciplinary Care
        1. Diagnosis
        2. Medications
        3. Fluid Management
        4. Nutrition
        5. Renal Replacement Therapy: Dialysis
    F. Nursing Care
        1. Health Promotion
        2. Assessment
        3. Nursing Diagnoses and Interventions
           a. Excess Fluid Volume
           b. Imbalanced Nutrition: Less than Body Requirements
           c. Deficient Knowledge
        4. Linking NANDA, NIC and NOC
        5. Community-Based Care
  X. The Client with Chronic Renal Failure
    A. Pathophysiology
    B. Manifestations and Complications
        1. Fluid and Electrolyte Effects
        2. Cardiovascular Effects
        3. Hematologic Effects
        4. Immune System Effects
        5. Gastrointestinal Effects
        6. Neurologic Effects
        7. Musculoskeletal Effects
        8. Endocrine and Metabolic Effects
        9. Dermatologic Effects
    C. Interdisciplinary Care
        1. Diagnosis
        2. Medications
        3. Nutrition and Fluid Management
        4. Renal Replacement Therapies

D. Nursing Care
   1. Health Promotion
   2. Assessment
   3. Nursing Diagnoses and Interventions
      a. Ineffective Tissue Perfusion: Renal
      b. Imbalanced Nutrition: Less than Body Requirements
      c. Risk for Infection
      d. Disturbed Body Image
   4. Community-Based Care

FOCUSED STUDY TIPS

1. Summarize the dialysis procedures used to manage acute and chronic renal failure.

2. Define polycystic kidney disease.

3. List the diagnostic studies used to identify disorders of the kidneys.

4. List the risk factors for acute renal artery thrombosis.

CASE STUDY

Brent Brelle is a 67-year-old male client admitted to the unit this morning. The physician thinks he might have a renal tumor. His spouse Nancy has several questions about his condition for the nurse.

1. "Why didn't my husband have any signs or symptoms until the last few days?"

2. "What tests might the physician order to determine if Brent has a renal tumor?"

3. "What is the treatment of choice for a renal tumor?"

CARE PLAN CRITICAL THINKING ACTIVITY

1. Explain why Mr. Cohen is weighed daily before breakfast.

2. Explain the CAPD procedure.

3. Why should the nurse provide mouth care at least every four hours and before every meal?

NCLEX REVIEW QUESTIONS

1. Which of the following statements by a student nurse reflects correct understanding about congenital kidney malformation?
    1. Congenital kidney disorders can only affect the form of the kidney.
    2. Functional congenital kidney disorders are usually identified in infancy.
    3. Malformations include agenesis, hypoplasia, alterations in kidney position, and horseshoe kidney.
    4. Abnormal kidney position affects the ureters and urine flow, potentially leading to a decreased risk of urinary tract infection (UTI), and lithiasis, or stone formation.
2. You are evaluating a student nurse's understanding of polycystic kidney disease. Which of the following statements by the student nurse indicates a need for further teaching?
    1. It is slowly progressive.
    2. Symptoms usually develop by age 40 to 50.
    3. Common manifestations include flank pain, microscopic or gross hematuria (blood in the urine), proteinuria (proteins in the urine), and polyuria and nocturia, because the kidney's concentrating ability is impaired.
    4. The progression to end-stage renal disease tends to occur more rapidly in women than in men.
3. When discussing the nutrition and fluid management with a client who has chronic renal failure, the nurse would recommend which of the following?
    1. Water intake of 1 to 2 L per day is generally recommended to maintain water balance.
    2. Sodium is restricted to 4 g per day initially.
    3. Potassium intake is increased to more than 80 mEq/day.
    4. Daily protein intake is limited to 0.6 g/kg of body weight, or approximately 40 g/day for an average male client.
4. A nurse is planning a seminar about dialysis. Which of the following is an incorrect statement made by the nurse?
    1. For the client who is not a candidate for renal transplantation or who has had a transplant failure, dialysis is life-sustaining.
    2. Hemodialysis for end-stage renal disease (ESRD) typically is done three times a week for a total of 9 to 12 hours.
    3. Clients on long-term dialysis have a higher risk for complications and death than the general population.
    4. Serum glucose levels increase with peritoneal dialysis.
5. Risk factors for acute renal failure (ARF) include all of the following except:
    1. Major trauma or surgery.
    2. Infection.
    3. Hemorrhage.
    4. Personal hygiene practices.
6. A nurse is evaluating a client's understanding of chronic renal failure (CRF). Which of the following statements indicates a need for further teaching?
    1. The course of CRF is variable, and progresses over a period of months to many years.
    2. In end-stage renal disease (ESRD), the final stage of chronic renal failure (CRF), the glomerular filtration rate (GFR) is less than 10% of normal and renal replacement therapy is necessary to sustain life.
    3. Chronic renal failure often is not identified until its final, uremic stage is reached.
    4. Chronic renal failure affects both the pharmacokinetic and pharmacodynamic effects of drug therapy.
7. The nurse who is evaluating a kidney transplant class recognizes that further teaching is necessary when which of the following statements is made by a participant?
    1. The donor kidney is placed in the upper abdominal cavity of the recipient, and the renal artery, vein, and ureter are anastomosed.
    2. Kidney transplant improves both survival and quality of life for the client with end-stage renal disease (ESRD).

3. Most transplanted kidneys are obtained from cadavers.
4. Hypertension is a possible complication of kidney transplant.

8. Which of the following statements is false about glomerular disorders?
   1. Glomerular disorders and diseases are the leading cause of chronic renal failure in the United States.
   2. Hematuria, proteinuria, and hypertension often are late manifestations of glomerular disorders.
   3. Acute poststreptococcal glomerulonephritis (also called acute proliferative glomerulonephritis) is the least common primary glomerular disorder.
   4. Diabetes mellitus and systemic lupus erythematosus are common causes of primary glomerulonephritis.

9. Which fact about renal failure is correct?
   1. Only acute renal failure is characterized by azotemia, which is the accumulation of nitrogenous (protein) waste products in the blood.
   2. The cause of renal failure may be a primary kidney disorder, or renal failure may be secondary to a systemic disease or other urologic defects.
   3. Chronic renal failure has an abrupt onset and often is reversible with prompt treatment.
   4. Renal failure is a condition in which the kidneys are able to remove accumulated metabolites from the blood, which leads to altered fluid, electrolyte, and acid–base balance.

10. The course of acute renal failure due to acute tubular necrosis (ATN) typically includes all of the following phases except:
    1. Intrarenal.
    2. Initiation.
    3. Maintenance.
    4. Recovery.

CHAPTER 30

ASSESSING CLIENTS WITH CARDIAC DISORDERS

LEARNING OUTCOMES

After completing Chapter 30, you will be able to demonstrate the following objectives:

- Describe the anatomy, physiology, and functions of the heart.
- Trace the circulation of blood through the heart and coronary vessels.
- Identify normal heart sounds and relate them to the corresponding events in the cardiac cycle.
- Explain cardiac output and explain the influence of various factors in its regulation.
- Describe normal variations in assessment findings for the older adult.
- Identify manifestations of impaired cardiac sturcture and functions.

CLINICAL COMPETENCIES

- Assess an electrocardiogram (ECG) strip and identify normal and abnormal cardiac rhythm.
- Conduct and document a health history for clients having or at risk for having alterations in the structure and functions of the heart.
- Conduct and document a physical assessment of cardiac status.
- Monitor the results of diagnostic tests and report abnormal findings to assess cardiac function.

EQUIPMENT NEEDED

- Stethoscope with a diaphragm and a bell
- Good light source
- Watch with a second hand
- Centimeter ruler

MediaLink

www.prenhall.com/lemone

Resources for this chapter can be found on the Prentice Hall Nursing MediaLink DVD accompanying this textbook, and on the Companion Website at http://www.prenhall.com/lemone. Click on Chapter 30 to select the activities for this chapter.

Prentice Hall Nursing MediaLink DVD-ROM
- Audio Glossary
- NCLEX-RN® Review

Animation/Videos
- Cardiac A & P
- Dysrhythmias
- Heart Sounds
- Hemodynamics
- Oxygen Transport

Companion Website
www.prenhall.com/lemone
- Audio Glossary
- NCLEX-RN® Review
- Care Plan Activity: Cardiac Catheterization
- Case Study: Chest Pain
- MediaLink Application: Heart Sounds
- Links to Resources

KEY TERMS

afterload
apical impulse
cardiac index (CI)
cardiac output (CO)
cardiac reserve
contractility
dysrrhythmia
ejection fraction
heave

ischemic
lift
murmur
preload
pulsations
retraction
stroke volume (SV)
thrill
thrust

CHAPTER OUTLINE

I. Anatomy, Physiology, and Functions of the Heart
   A. The Pericardium
   B. Layers of the Heart Wall
   C. Chambers and Valves of the Heart
   D. Systemic, Pulmonary, and Coronary Circulation
     1. Systemic Circulation
     2. Pulmonary Circulation
     3. Coronary Circulation
   E. The Cardiac Cycle and Cardiac Output
     1. Heart Rate
     2. Contractility
     3. Preload
     4. Afterload
     5. Clinical Indicators of Cardiac Output
   F. The Conduction System of the Heart
   G. The Action Potential
     1. Depolarization
     2. Repolarization
II. Assessing Cardiac Function
   A. Diagnostic Tests
   B. Genetic Considerations
   C. The Health Assessment Interview
   D. Physical Assessment
III. Cardiac Assessments

FOCUSED STUDY TIPS

1. Explain the cardiac cycle.

   _____

   _____

   _____

2. List and identify manifestations of impaired cardiac structure and functions.

   _____

   _____

   _____

   _____

   _____

3. Discuss the anatomy, physiology, and functions of the heart.

_____

_____

_____

_____

4. Explain cardiac output.

_____

_____

_____

_____

CASE STUDY

Jonathan Drake is a 63-year-old male client who was brought in to the clinic by his wife Christine. Christine tells the nurse that Jonathan is here today because he needs a physical and is requesting an electrocardiogram (ECG).

1. What is an ECG?

2. How are ECG waveforms recorded?

3. What is a standard 12-lead ECG?

4. The cardiac cycle is depicted as a series of waveforms: the P, Q, R, S, and T waves. Explain each wave.

NCLEX REVIEW QUESTIONS

1. Which of the following facts about the heart is correct?
    1. Half of the heart mass lies to the left of the sternum; the upper base lies beneath the second rib, and the pointed apex is approximate with the fifth intercostal space, midpoint to the clavicle.
    2. The adult heart, a muscular pump, beats an average of 90 times per minute, or once every 0.68 seconds, every minute of a person's life.
    3. The heart is a solid, cone-shaped organ approximately the size of an adult's fist, and weighs more than 1 lb.
    4. The heart is located in the mediastinum of the thoracic cavity, between the vertebral column and the sternum, and is flanked laterally by the lungs.
2. The _____ covers the entire heart and great vessels, and then folds over to form the parietal layer that lines the pericardium and adheres to the heart surface.
    1. Endocardium
    2. Myocardium
    3. Epicardium
    4. Parietal pericardium
3. You are evaluating a student nurse's understanding of the heart. Which of the following statements indicates a need for further teaching?
    1. The right atrium receives deoxygenated blood from the veins of the body.
    2. The left ventricle receives deoxygenated blood from the left atrium and pumps it through the pulmonary artery to the pulmonary capillary bed for oxygenation.
    3. The left atrium receives freshly oxygenated blood from the lungs through the pulmonary veins.
    4. The superior vena cava returns blood from the body area above the diaphragm, the inferior vena cava returns blood from the body below the diaphragm, and the coronary sinus drains blood from the heart.

4. The greater the volume, the greater the stretch of the cardiac muscle fibers, and the greater the force with which the fibers contract to accomplish emptying. This principle is called _____ law of the heart.
   1. Stuart's
   2. Starling's
   3. Sarton's
   4. Schell's

5. Which of the following statements by a student nurse reflects correct understanding about the conduction system of the heart?
   1. The AV node acts as the normal "pacemaker" of the heart, usually generating an impulse 60 to 100 times per minute.
   2. The AV node is located at the junction of the superior vena cava and right atrium.
   3. The cellular action potential serves as the basis for electrocardiography (ECG), a diagnostic test of cardiac function.
   4. The electrical stimulus decreases the permeability of the cell membrane, which creates an action potential (electrical potential).

6. The nurse is evaluating a student nurse's understanding of electrocardiogram (ECG). Which of the following statements is correct?
   1. The electrocardiograph converts the electrical impulses it receives into a series of waveforms that represent cardiac depolarization and repolarization.
   2. ECG waveforms and patterns are examined only to detect dysrhythmias.
   3. The recording speed of the standard ECG is 5 mm/second.
   4. Placement of electrodes on different parts of the body does not allow different views of this electrical activity.

7. The _____ signifies the beginning of ventricular repolarization.
   1. T wave
   2. ST segment
   3. PR interval
   4. P wave

8. A(an) _____ is conducted in conjunction with Dopplers and color flow imaging to produce audio and graphic data about the motion, wall thickness, and chamber size of the heart; and of blood flow and velocity.
   1. Pericardiocentesis
   2. Echocardiogram
   3. Cardiac catheterization
   4. Transesophageal echocardiogram

9. Stroke volume ranges from 60 to 100 mL/beat and averages about 70 mL/beat in an adult. Which of the following is the correct formula to calculate stroke volume?
   1. CO/HR = SV
   2. CO + HR = SV
   3. CO × HR = SV
   4. BSA + CO = SV

10. Which of the following is an abnormal assessment finding?
    1. S_1 is loudest at the apex of the heart.
    2. S_2 immediately follows S1 and is loudest at the base of the heart.
    3. A splitting of S_2 is heard.
    4. No extra heart sounds are present.

CHAPTER 31

NURSING CARE OF CLIENTS WITH CORONARY HEART DISEASE

LEARNING OUTCOMES

After completing Chapter 31, you will be able to demonstrate the following objectives:

- Discuss the coronary circulation and electrical properties of the heart.
- Compare and contrast the pathophysiology and manifestations of coronary heart disease and common cardiac dysrhythmias.
- Describe interdisciplinary and nursing care for clients with coronary heart disease and/or cardiac dysrhythmias.
- Relate the outcomes of diagnostic tests and procedures to the pathophysiology of cardiac disorders and implications for client responses to the disorder.
- Discuss nursing implications for medications and treatments used to prevent and treat coronary heart disease and dysrhythmias.
- Describe nursing care for the client undergoing diagnostic testing, an interventional procedure, or surgery for coronary heart disease or a dysrhythmia.

CLINICAL COMPETENCIES

- Assess functional health status of clients with coronary heart disease and/or a dysrhythmia, including the impact of the disorder on the client's ability to perform activities of daily living and usual tasks.
- Use knowledge of the normal anatomy and physiology of the heart in caring for clients with coronary heart disease.
- Monitor clients with coronary heart disease or dysrhythmias for expected and unexpected manifestations, reporting and recording findings as indicated.

- Use assessed data to select nursing diagnoses, determine priorities of care, develop and implement individualized nursing interventions for clients with coronary heart disease and dysrhythmias.
- Administer medications and treatments for clients with coronary heart disease and dysrhythmias safely and knowledgeably.
- Integrate interdisciplinary care into nursing care planning and implementation for clients with coronary heart disease and dysrhythmias.
- Provide appropriate teaching for prevention, health promotion, and self-care related to coronary heart disease and dysrhythmias.
- Evaluate the effectiveness of nursing interventions, revising or modifying the plan of care as needed to promote, maintain, or restore functional health for clients with coronary heart disease or dysrhythmias.

KEY TERMS

acute coronary
   syndrome (ACS)
acute myocardial
   infarction (AMI)
angina pectoris
atherosclerosis
atrial kick
cardiac arrest
cardiac rehabilitation
cardiovascular disease (CVD)

collateral channels
coronary heart disease (CHD)
dysrhythmias
ectopic beats
heart block
ischemia
normal sinus rhythm (NSR)
pacemaker
paroxysmal
sudden cardiac death

CHAPTER OUTLINE

I. Disorders of Myocardial Perfusion
II. The Client with Coronary Heart Disease
   A. Incidence and Prevalence
   B. Physiology Review
   C. Pathophysiology
      1. Atherosclerosis
      2. Myocardial Ischemia
   D. Risk Factors
      1. Nonmodifiable Risk Factors
      2. Modifiable Risk Factors
   E. Interdisciplinary Care
      1. Diagnosis
      2. Risk Factor Management
      3. Medications
      4. Complementary Therapies
   F. Nursing Care
      1. Health Promotion
      2. Assessment
      3. Nursing Diagnoses and Interventions
         a. Imbalanced Nutrition: More than Body Requirements
         b. Ineffective Health Maintenance
      4. Community-Based Care
III. The Client with Angina Pectoris
   A. Pathophysiology
   B. Course and Manifestations

C. Interdisciplinary Care
   1. Diagnosis
   2. Medications
D. Nursing Care
   1. Health Promotion
   2. Assessment
   3. Nursing Diagnoses and Interventions
     a. Ineffective Tissue Perfusion: Cardiac
     b. Risk for Ineffective Therapeutic Regimen Management
   4. Community-Based Care
IV. The Client with Acute Coronary Syndrome
  A. Pathophysiology
  B. Manifestations
  C. Interdisciplinary Care
   1. Diagnosis
   2. Medications
   3. Revascularization Procedures
  D. Nursing Care
V. The Client with Acute Myocardial Infarction
  A. Pathophysiology
   1. Cocaine-Induced MI
  B. Manifestations
  C. Complications
   1. Dysrhythmias
   2. Pump Failure
   3. Infarct Extension
   4. Structural Defects
   5. Pericarditis
  D. Interdisciplinary Care
   1. Diagnosis
   2. Medications
   3. Treatments
   4. Revascularization Procedures
   5. Other Invasive Procedures
   6. Cardiac Rehabilitation
  E. Nursing Care
   1. Health Promotion
   2. Assessment
   3. Nursing Diagnoses and Interventions
     a. Acute Pain
     b. Ineffective Tissue Perfusion
     c. Ineffective Coping
     d. Fear
   4. NANDA, NIC, and NOC Linkages
   5. Community-Based Care
VI. Cardiac Rhythm Disorders
VII. The Client with a Cardiac Dysrhythmia
  A. Physiology Review
  B. Pathophysiology
   1. Supraventricular Rhythms
   2. Junctional Dysrhythmias
   3. Ventricular Dysrhythmias
   4. Atrioventricular Conduction Blocks
   5. Intraventricular Conduction Blocks

    C. Interdisciplinary Care
       1. Diagnosis
       2. Medications
       3. Countershock
       4. Pacemaker Therapy
       5. Implantable Cardioverter-Defibrillator
       6. Cardiac Mapping and Catheter Ablation
       7. Other Therapies
    D. Nursing Care
       1. Health Promotion
       2. Assessment
       3. Nursing Diagnoses and Interventions
         a. Decreased Cardiac Output
       4. Community-Based Care
VIII. The Client with Sudden Cardiac Death
    A. Pathophysiology
    B. Manifestations
    C. Interdisciplinary Care
       1. Basic Life Support
       2. Advanced Life Support
       3. Postresuscitation Care
    D. Nursing Care

FOCUSED STUDY TIPS

1. List the diagnostic testing for coronary heart disease.

_____

_____

_____

_____

2. Review the nursing implications for medications used to treat dysrhythmias.
3. Summarize the interdisciplinary and nursing care for clients with coronary heart disease.

_____

_____

_____

_____

_____

_____

_____

4. Explain coronary circulation.

_____

_____

CASE STUDY

Bradley Baldwin is scheduled to attend a seminar about the nursing care of clients with coronary heart disease. Prior to the seminar, he wrote down some questions to ask during the seminar.

1. What are modifiable and nonmodifiable risk factors for coronary heart disease (CHD)?

2. What are abnormal blood lipids?

3. What are characteristics of metabolic syndrome?

4. How is CPR performed?

CARE PLAN CRITICAL THINKING ACTIVITY

1. What were the assessment findings for Ms. Vasquez?

   _____

   _____

   _____

2. Explain synchronized cardioversion.

   _____

   _____

   _____

3. Why is it important to know that Ms. Vasquez had rheumatic fever as a child?

   _____

   _____

NCLEX REVIEW QUESTIONS

1. The nurse who is evaluating a coronary heart disease (CHD) class recognizes that further teaching is necessary when which of the following statements is made by a participant?
   1. CHD is caused by impaired blood flow to the myocardium.
   2. CHD is not asymptomatic.
   3. CHD affects 13.2 million people in the United States and causes more than 500,000 deaths annually.
   4. Accumulation of atherosclerotic plaque in the coronary arteries is the usual cause of CHD.
2. During discharge planning, the nurse is teaching the client about dietary recommendations to reduce total cholesterol, LDL levels, and CHD risk. Which of the following nursing statements is correct? "It is recommended that you:
   1. Consume 2–3 grams of dietary fiber per day."
   2. Make protein about 20% of your total daily calorie intake."
   3. Make saturated fats less than 7% of your total daily calories."
   4. Consume up to 30% of total calories as monounsaturated fat."
3. Which of the following is not a characteristic of metabolic syndrome?
   1. Hypertension
   2. Elevated fasting blood glucose
   3. High HDL
   4. Abdominal obesity

4. A nurse is providing a client education about antianginal medications. Which of the following client statements would demonstrate to the nurse that he needs further education?
   1. "If the first nitrate dose does not relieve angina within 5 minutes, take a second dose. After 5 more minutes, I may take a third dose if needed. If the pain is unrelieved or lasts for 20 minutes or longer, I'll seek medical assistance immediately."
   2. "I'll carry a supply of nitroglycerin tablets with me. I should dissolve sublingual nitroglycerin tablets under my tongue or between the upper lip and gum. Do not eat, drink, or smoke until the tablet is completely dissolved."
   3. "I'll keep the sublingual tablets in their plastic bottle to protect them from heat, light, and moisture. I'll replace the supply every 12 months."
   4. "I'll rotate the ointment or transdermal patch application sites. I'll apply to a hairless area; I'll spread ointment evenly without rubbing or massaging. I'll remove the patch or residual ointment at bedtime daily, and apply a fresh dose in the morning."

5. Which of the following is a cardiac cause of sudden cardiac death?
   1. Primary electrical disorders
   2. Choking
   3. Cerebral hemorrhage
   4. Pulmonary embolism

6. When performing CPR on an adult client, which of the following actions by the nurse would be correct?
   1. Open the airway using the-head-thrust, chin-thrust maneuvers.
   2. Check the brachial artery for a pulse.
   3. Provide 2 breaths after every 15 compressions.
   4. Assess for responsiveness by flicking the client's foot.

7. _____ is a deficient blood flow to tissue, and may be caused by partial obstruction of a coronary artery, coronary artery spasm, or a thrombus.
   1. Atrial kick
   2. Angina pectoris
   3. Ectopic beats
   4. Ischemia

8. Which of the following statements by a student nurse is correct?
   1. The normal sinus rate is 100 to 120 beats per minute. Each complex includes a P wave, QRS, and T wave.
   2. Supraventricular dysrhythmias arise in the sinus node or the atria. A P wave is always present; the QRS appears normal, and a T wave is not seen.
   3. Junctional dysrhythmias arise in tissue just above or just below the AV node. The P wave may be inverted, and may precede, follow, or be buried in the QRS complex. The QRS usually appears normal and is followed by a T wave.
   4. Ventricular dysrhythmias arise in ventricular myocardium. They do not reset the sinus node or activate the atria. QRS complexes are narrow and ordinary.

9. A nurse is presenting a seminar about myocardial infarction (MI). Which of the following statements by a client demonstrates a need for further teaching?
   1. MI occurs when blood flow to a portion of cardiac muscle is completely blocked, which results in prolonged tissue ischemia and irreversible cell damage.
   2. MI usually affects the right ventricle because it is the major "workhorse" of the heart; its muscle mass and oxygen demands are greater.
   3. MIs are described by the damaged area of the heart.
   4. Risk factors for MI are the same as those for coronary heart disease: age, gender, heredity, race, smoking, obesity, hyperlipidemia, hypertension, diabetes, sedentary lifestyle, diet, and others.

10. Which of the following is a modifiable risk factor for coronary heart disease (CHD)?
    1. Age
    2. Gender
    3. Genetic factor
    4. Lifestyle

CHAPTER 32

NURSING CARE OF CLIENTS WITH CARDIAC DISORDERS

LEARNING OUTCOMES

After completing Chapter 32, you will be able to demonstrate the following objectives:

- Compare and contrast the etiology, pathophysiology, and manifestations of common cardiac disorders, including heart failure, structural disorders, and inflammatory disorders.

- Explain risk factors and preventive measures for cardiac disorders such as heart failure, inflammatory disorders, and valve disorders.

- Discuss indications for and management of clients with hemodynamic monitoring.

- Discuss the effects and nursing implications for medications commonly prescribed for clients with cardiac disorders.

- Describe nursing care for the client undergoing cardiac surgery or cardiac transplant.

CLINICAL COMPETENCIES

- Apply knowledge of normal cardiac anatomy and physiology and assessment techniques in caring for clients with cardiac disorders.

- Assess functional health status of clients with cardiac disorders, documenting and reporting deviations for expected findings.

- Based on client assessment and knowledge of the disorder, determine priority nursing diagnoses.

- Plan, prioritize, and provide evidence-based, individualized care for clients with cardiac disorders.

- Safely and knowledgeably administer prescribed medications and treatments to clients with cardiac disorders.

- Actively participate in planning and coordinating interdisciplinary care for clients with cardiac disorders.

MediaLink

www.prenhall.com/lemone

Resources for this chapter can be found on the Prentice Hall Nursing MediaLink DVD accompanying this textbook, and on the Companion Website at http://www.prenhall.com/lemone. Click on Chapter 32 to select the activities for this chapter.

Prentice Hall Nursing MediaLink DVD-ROM
- Audio Glossary
- NCLEX-RN® Review

Animations
- Digoxin
- Hemodynamics

**Companion Website
www.prenhall.com/lemone**
- Audio Glossary
- NCLEX-RN® Review
- Care Plan Activity: Acute Pulmonary Edema
- Case Study: Rheumatic Fever
- MediaLink Applications
  - Beta Blockers
  - Heart Failure
- Links to Resources

- Provide appropriate teaching and community-based care for clients with cardiac disorders and their families.
- Evaluate the effectiveness of nursing care, revising the plan of care as needed to promote, maintain, or restore functional health status of clients with cardiac disorders.

KEY TERMS

aortic valve
cardiac tamponade
cardiomyopathy
endocarditis
heart failure
hemodynamics
mean arterial pressure (MAP)
mitral valve
murmur
myocarditis
orthopnea

paroxysmal nocturnal
   dyspnea (PND)
pericarditis
pulmonary edema
pulmonic valve
regurgitation
rheumatic fever
rheumatic heart disease (RHD)
stenosis
tricuspid valve
valvular heart disease

CHAPTER OUTLINE

  I. Heart Failure
 II. The Client with Heart Failure
    A. Incidence, Prevalence, and Risk Factors
    B. Physiology Review
    C. Pathophysiology
    D. Classifications and Manifestations of Heart Failure
      1. Systolic versus Diastolic Failure
      2. Left-Sided versus Right-Sided Failure
      3. Low-Output versus High-Output Failure
      4. Acute versus Chronic Failure
      5. Other Manifestations
    E. Complications
    F. Interdisciplinary Care
      1. Diagnosis
      2. Hemodynamic Monitoring
      3. Medications
      4. Nutrition and Activity
      5. Other Treatments
      6. Complementary Therapies
      7. End-of-Life Care
    G. Nursing Care
      1. Health Promotion
      2. Assessment
      3. Nursing Diagnoses and Interventions
        a. Decreased Cardiac Output
        b. Excess Fluid Volume
        c. Activity Intolerance
        d. Deficient Knowledge: Low-Sodium Diet
      4. NANDA, NIC, and NOC Linkages
      5. Community-Based Care
 III. The Client with Pulmonary Edema
    A. Pathophysiology
    B. Manifestations

C. Interdisciplinary Care
D. Nursing Care
   1. Nursing Diagnoses and Interventions
      a. Impaired Gas Exchange
      b. Decreased Cardiac Output
      c. Fear
   2. Community-Based Care
IV. Inflammatory Heart Disorders
V. The Client with Rheumatic Fever and Rheumatic Heart Disease
  A. Incidence, Prevalence, and Risk Factors
  B. Pathophysiology
  C. Manifestations
  D. Interdisciplinary Care
   1. Diagnosis
   2. Medications
  E. Nursing Care
   1. Health Promotion
   2. Assessment
   3. Nursing Diagnoses and Interventions
      a. Acute Pain
      b. Activity Intolerance
   4. Community-Based Care
VI. The Client with Infective Endocarditis
  A. Incidence and Risk Factors
  B. Pathophysiology
  C. Manifestations
  D. Complications
  E. Interdisciplinary Care
   1. Diagnosis
   2. Medications
   3. Surgery
  F. Nursing Care
   1. Health Promotion
   2. Assessment
   3. Nursing Diagnoses and Interventions
      a. Risk for Imbalanced Body Temperature
      b. Risk for Ineffective Tissue Perfusion
      c. Ineffective Health Maintenance
   4. Community-Based Care
VII. The Client with Myocarditis
  A. Incidence and Risk Factors
  B. Pathophysiology
  C. Manifestations
  D. Interdisciplinary Care
  E. Nursing Care
   1. Community-Based Care
VIII. The Client with Pericarditis
  A. Pathophysiology
  B. Manifestations
  C. Complications
   1. Pericardial Effusion
   2. Cardiac Tamponade
   3. Chronic Constrictive Pericarditis

FOCUSED STUDY TIPS

1. List the preventive measures for heart failure, inflammatory disorders, and valve disorders.

_____

_____

_____

_____

_____

2. Discuss the effects and nursing implications for medications that are commonly prescribed for clients with cardiac disorders.

_____

_____

_____

_____

_____

3. Describe nursing care for the client undergoing a cardiac transplant.

_____

_____

_____

_____

_____

4. Explain the etiology, pathophysiology, and manifestations of heart failure.

_____

_____

_____

_____

_____

CASE STUDY

James Hacking is a 76-year-old client who is in heart failure. A new student nurse is observing the nurse for the day; she asks the following questions.

1. "What is heart failure?"

2. "What are the causes of heart failure?"

3. "What are the stages of heart failure?"

4. "What are the complications of heart failure?"

CARE PLAN CRITICAL THINKING ACTIVITY

1. Why is it important for Ms. Snow to keep a weekly record of symptoms and their frequency for one month?

2. List three beverages and eight types of foods that contain caffeine.

3. List the symptoms of progressive mitral regurgitation.

NCLEX REVIEW QUESTIONS

1. Which of the following statements is correct about left-sided heart failure?
    1. It can lead to left-sided failure as pressures in the pulmonary vascular system increase with congestion behind the failing right ventricle.
    2. As left ventricular function fails, cardiac output increases.
    3. Pressures in the right ventricle and atrium increase as the amount of blood remaining in the ventricle after systole increases.
    4. These increased pressures impair filling, which causes congestion and increased pressures in the pulmonary vascular system.
2. A client with structural heart disease and current or prior symptoms of heart failure (shortness of breath, fatigue, decreased exercise tolerance) is in what stage of heart failure?
    1. A
    2. B
    3. C
    4. D
3. The new nurse is providing education about prosthetic heart valve to a client. Which of the following is considered an advantage of a prosthetic heart valve?
    1. Long-term durability
    2. Lifetime anticoagulation
    3. Audible click
    4. Infections are harder to treat
4. A nurse has an order for a client to receive digitalis. Which of the following nursing actions is correct?
    1. Assess apical pulse after administering.
    2. Withhold digitalis and notify the physician if heart rate is below 80 BPM and/or manifestations of decreased cardiac output are noted.
    3. Only assess serum digoxin levels before giving digitalis.
    4. Evaluate echocardiogram for scooped (spoon-shaped) ST segment, atrioventricular (AV) block, bradycardia, and other dysrhythmias (especially premature ventricular contractions (PVCs) and atrial tachycardias).
5. During discharge planning, the nurse is teaching the client with heart failure about home activity guidelines. Which of the following instructions is correct?
    1. "Eat eight small meals a day."
    2. "Lifting heavy objects is ok."
    3. "Eat a low-fiber diet."
    4. "Begin a graded exercise program."
6. A nurse is evaluating a nursing student's understanding of client education regarding mitral valve prolapse (MVP). Which of the following nursing student statements demonstrates a need for further teaching?
    1. "Discuss symptoms of progressive mitral regurgitation, and the need to report these to the cardiologist."
    2. "Teach the client about MVP, including heart valve anatomy, physiology, and function, common manifestations of MVP, and treatment rationale."
    3. "Teach the client about infective endocarditis risk and prevention with prophylactic antibiotics. Encourage the client to notify their dentist and other healthcare providers about MVP after dental or any invasive procedure."
    4. "Instruct the client to keep a weekly record of symptoms and their frequency for one month."

7. A nurse is evaluating a client's understanding about managing valvular disease. Which of the following client statements indicates a need for further teaching?
    1. "I will notify all healthcare providers about valve disease or surgery to facilitate prescription of prophylactic antibiotics before invasive procedures or dental work."
    2. "I should have adequate rest to prevent fatigue."
    3. "I need to immediately report to my healthcare provider joint pain, easy bruising, black and tarry stools, bleeding gums, or blood in the urine or sputum."
    4. "I will follow the diet restrictions to increase fluid retention and symptoms of heart failure."

8. Health promotion activities to reduce the risk for and incidence of heart failure are directed at the risk factors. Which of the following is not a correct nursing promotional activity?
    1. Teach clients about coronary heart disease (CHD), which is the primary underlying cause of heart failure.
    2. Stress the relationship between effective asthma management and reduced risk of heart failure.
    3. Discuss CHD risk factors, and ways to reduce those risk factors.
    4. Discuss the importance of effectively managing hypertension to reduce the future risk for heart failure.

9. A nurse is providing a seminar on pulmonary edema. Which of the following participant statements demonstrates a need for further teaching?
    1. "In cardiogenic pulmonary edema, the contractility of the right ventricle is severely impaired."
    2. "Pulmonary edema is a medical emergency."
    3. "Immediate treatment for acute pulmonary edema focuses on restoring effective gas exchange and reducing fluid and pressure in the pulmonary vascular system."
    4. "The client often is restless and highly anxious, although severe hypoxia may cause confusion or lethargy."

10. Which of the following statements by a student nurse reflects incorrect understanding about rheumatic fever and rheumatic heart disease?
    1. "Rheumatic heart disease frequently damages the heart valves and is a major cause of mitral and aortic valve disorders."
    2. "Rheumatic fever is a systemic inflammatory disease caused by an abnormal immune response to pharyngeal infection by group A beta-hemolytic streptococci."
    3. "The peak incidence of rheumatic fever is in clients ages 18 to 35."
    4. "Rheumatic fever and rheumatic heart disease remain significant public health problems in many developing countries."

CHAPTER 33

ASSESSING CLIENTS WITH HEMATOLOGIC, PERIPHERAL VASCULAR, AND LYMPHATIC DISORDERS

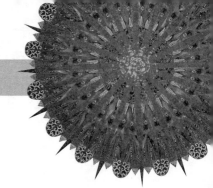

LEARNING OUTCOMES

After completing Chapter 33, you will be able to demonstrate the following objectives:
- Describe the anatomy, physiology, and functions of the hematologic, peripheral vascular, and lymphatic systems.
- Explain the physiologic dynamics of blood flow, peripheral resistance, and blood pressure.
- Compare and contrast the major factors influencing arterial blood pressure.
- Describe normal variations in assessment findings for the older adult.
- Identify manifestations of impairment in the function of the hematologic, peripheral vascular, and lymphatic systems.

CLINICAL COMPETENCIES

- Conduct and document a health history for clients having or at risk for alterations in the hematologic, peripheral vascular, and lymphatic systems.
- Conduct and document a physical assessment of hematologic, peripheral vascular, and lymphatic status.
- Monitor the results of diagnostic tests and report abnormal findings.

EQUIPMENT NEEDED

- Stethoscope
- Blood pressure cuff
- Tape measure
- Metric ruler
- Doppler ultrasound device (if unable to auscultate blood pressure or palpate pulse)
- Transducer gel for Doppler device

KEY TERMS

anemia	lymphadenopathy
auscultatory gap	lymphedema
blood flow	mean arterial pressure (MAP)
blood pressure	orthostatic hypertension
erythropoiesis	peripheral vascular resistance
hemolysis	(PVR)
hemostasis	polycythemia
Korotkoff's sounds	pulse
leukocytosis	pulse pressure
leukopenia	

CHAPTER OUTLINE

  I. Anatomy, Physiology, and Functions of the Hematologic System
    A. Red Blood Cells
    B. Red Blood Cell Production and Regulation
    C. Red Blood Cell Destruction
    D. White Blood Cells
    E. Platelets
    F. Hemostasis
      1. Vessel Spasm
      2. Formation of the Platelet Plug
      3. Development of the Fibrin Clot
      4. Clot Retraction
      5. Clot Dissolution
  II. Anatomy, Physiology, and Functions of the Peripheral Vascular System
    A. Structure of Blood Vessels
    B. Physiology of Arterial Circulation
    C. Factors Influencing Arterial Blood Pressure
 III. Anatomy, Physiology, and Functions of the Lymphatic System
 IV. Assessing Hematologic, Peripheral Vascular, and Lymphatic Function
    A. Diagnostic Tests
    B. Genetic Considerations
    C. Health Assessment Interview
      1. Peripheral Vascular System
      2. Lymphatic System
    D. Physical Assessment
  V. Hematologic, Peripheral Vascular, and Lymphatic Assessments

FOCUSED STUDY TIPS

1. Identify manifestations of impairment in the function of the hematologic system.

_____

_____

_____

_____

2. Compare and contrast the major factors that influence arterial blood pressure.

_____

_____

_____

_____

_____

3. Explain the physiologic dynamics of blood pressure.

_____

_____

_____

4. Describe the anatomy, physiology, and functions of the lymphatic system.

_____

_____

_____

_____

_____

CASE STUDY

Josh Bradley is a 32-year-old client. He tells the nurse that his physician was in early this morning and told him something about a CBC, arterial blood pressure, PVR, and MAP but he can't remember what the physician said about each of these items. Answer the following questions to help Josh understand these tests better.

1. List the normal values of a complete blood count (CBC).

2. What are the factors that influence arterial blood pressure?

3. Explain peripheral vascular resistance (PVR) and mean arterial pressure (MAP).

NCLEX REVIEW QUESTIONS

1. Which of the following statements about red blood cells (RBCs) is correct?
   1. The red blood cell is shaped like a convex disk.
   2. Abnormal numbers of RBCs, changes in their size and shape, or altered hemoglobin content or structure can adversely affect health.
   3. RBCs are the least common type of blood cell.
   4. RBCs have a lifespan of about 10 days.

2. Which of the following statements by a student nurse reflects correct understanding about platelets?
   1. "Platelets remain in the spleen for about twenty hours before entering the circulation."
   2. "Platelets live up to 120 days in circulation."
   3. "An excess of platelets is called thrombocytopenia."
   4. "There are about 250,000 to 400,000 platelets in each milliliter of blood."

3. Peripheral vascular resistance is determined by all of the following factors except:
   1. Blood viscosity.
   2. Height of the vessel.
   3. Length of the vessel.
   4. Diameter of the vessel.

4. A nurse is evaluating a nursing student's understanding of the spleen. Which of the following student nurse statements demonstrates a need for further teaching?
   1. "The spleen is the only lymphoid organ."
   2. "The spleen is in the upper left quadrant of the abdomen under the thorax."
   3. "The main function of the spleen is to filter the blood by breaking down old red blood cells."
   4. "The spleen also synthesizes lymphocytes, stores platelets for blood clotting, and serves as a reservoir of blood."

5. A nurse is planning a seminar about the structure of blood vessels. Which of the following statements needs to be corrected?
   1. All blood vessel walls have three layers: the tunica intima, the tunica media, and the tunica adventitia.
   2. The smaller arterioles are less elastic than arteries but contain more smooth muscle.
   3. Veins have a thicker tunica adventitia than do arteries.
   4. The tunica adventitia, or outermost layer, is made of connective tissue and serves to protect and anchor the vessel.

6. Which of the following is the correct formula to calculate mean arterial pressure?
   1. CO x PVR = MAP
   2. CO/PVR = MAP
   3. CO – PVR = MAP
   4. CO – PVR x 2 = MAP

7. A student nurse has just completed a client's assessment. Which of the following is a normal assessment finding?
   1. A weak and thready pulse.
   2. Capillary refill that takes more than two seconds.
   3. A bruit heard over the aorta.
   4. Non-tender lymph nodes.

8. A leg that is visibly swollen with deep pitting represents which grade of edema?
   1. 1+
   2. 2+
   3. 3+
   4. 4+

9. A pulse can be described using a scale ranging from 0 to 4+. Which of the following means a bounding pulse?
   1. 1+
   2. 2+
   3. 3+
   4. 4+

10. Which of the following statements made by a new student nurse is correct?
    1. "Veins have thicker walls."
    2. "Blood in the arteries travels at a much lower pressure than blood in the veins."
    3. "Blood pressure is the force exerted against the walls of the arteries by the blood as it is pumped from the heart."
    4. "The highest pressure exerted against the arterial walls at the peak of ventricular contraction is called the diastolic blood pressure."

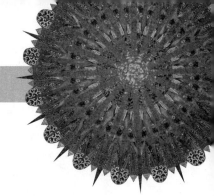

CHAPTER 34

NURSING CARE OF CLIENTS WITH HEMATOLOGIC DISORDERS

LEARNING OUTCOMES

After completing Chapter 34, you will be able to demonstrate the following objectives:

- Relate the physiology and assessment of the hematologic system and related systems (see Chapter 33) to commonly occurring hematologic disorders.
- Describe the pathophysiology of common hematologic disorders.
- Explain nursing implications for medications and other treatments prescribed for hematologic disorders.
- Discuss indications for and complications of bone marrow or stem cell transplantation, as well as related nursing care.
- Compare and contrast the pathophysiology, manifestations, and management of bleeding disorders.
- Describe the major types of leukemia and the most common treatment modalities and nursing interventions.
- Differentiate Hodgkin's disease from non-Hodgkin's lymphomas.

CLINICAL COMPETENCIES

- Assess effects of hematologic disorders and prescribed treatments on clients' functional health status.
- Monitor and document continuing assessment data, including laboratory test results, subjective and objective information, reporting data outside the normal or expected range.
- Based on knowledge of pathophysiology, prescribed treatment, and assessed data, identify and prioritize nursing diagnoses for clients with hematologic disorders.
- Use nursing research and evidence-based practice to identify and implement individualized nursing interventions for the client with a hematologic disorder.

- Safely and knowledgably administer prescribed medications and treatments for clients with hematologic disorders.
- Collaborate with the interdisciplinary care team to plan and provide coordinated, effective care for clients with hematologic disorders.
- Provide appropriate teaching for clients with hematologic disorders, evaluating learning and the need for continued reinforcement of information.
- Use continuing assessment data to revise the plan of care as needed to restore, maintain, or promote functional health in the client with a hematologic disorder.

KEY TERMS

anemia
aplastic anemia
bone marrow
   transplant (BMT)
disseminated intravascular
   coagulation (DIC)
hemolytic anemias
hemophilia
hemostasis
iron deficiency anemia

leukemia
lymphoma
multiple myeloma
pernicious anemia
polycythemia
sickle cell anemia
sickle cell crisis
stem cell transplant (SCT)
thalassemia
thrombocytopenia

CHAPTER OUTLINE

   D. Nursing Care
       1. Nursing Diagnoses and Interventions
           a. Activity Intolerance
           b. Risk for Ineffective Health Maintenance
       2. Community-Based Care
 IV. The Client with Polycythemia
   A. Pathophysiology
       1. Primary Polycythemia
       2. Secondary Polycythemia
   B. Interdisciplinary Care
       1. Diagnosis
       2. Treatments
   C. Nursing Care
  V. White Blood Cell and Lymphoid Tissue Disorders
 VI. The Client with Leukemia
   A. Incidence and Risk Factors
   B. Physiology Review
   C. Pathophysiology
   D. Manifestations
   E. Classifications
       1. Acute Myeloid Leukemia
       2. Chronic Myeloid Leukemia
       3. Acute Lymphocytic Leukemia
       4. Chronic Lymphocytic Leukemia
   F. Interdisciplinary Care
       1. Diagnosis
       2. Chemotherapy
       3. Radiation Therapy
       4. Bone Marrow Transplant
       5. Stem Cell Transplant
       6. Graft-Versus-Host Disease
       7. Biologic Therapy
       8. Complementary Therapies
   G. Nursing Care
       1. Health Promotion
       2. Assessment
       3. Nursing Diagnoses and Interventions
           a. Risk for Infection
           b. Imbalanced Nutrition: Less than Body Requirements
           c. Impaired Oral Mucous Membrane
           d. Ineffective Protection
           e. Anticipatory Grieving
       4. Linking NANDA, NIC, and NOC
       5. Community-Based Care
           a. Encouraging Self-Care
           b. Information about Leukemia and Treatment
           c. Preventing Infection and Injury
           d. Promoting Nutrition
VII. The Client with Malignant Lymphoma
   A. Incidence and Risk Factors
   B. Pathophysiology
       1. Hodgkin's Disease
       2. Non-Hodgkin's Lymphoma
   C. Course

XIII. The Client with Hemophilia
    A. Physiology Review
    B. Pathophysiology
    C. Manifestations
    D. Interdisciplinary Care
       1. Diagnosis
       2. Medications
    E. Nursing Care
       1. Health Promotion
       2. Assessment
       3. Nursing Diagnoses and Interventions
          a. Ineffective Protection
          b. Risk for Ineffective Health Maintenance
       4. Linking NANDA, NIC and NOC
       5. Community-Based Care
XIV. The Client with Disseminated Intravascular Coagulation
    A. Pathophysiology
    B. Manifestations
    C. Interdisciplinary Care
       1. Diagnosis
       2. Treatments
    D. Nursing Care
       1. Assessment
       2. Nursing Diagnoses and Interventions
          a. Ineffective Tissue Perfusion
          b. Impaired Gas Exchange
          c. Pain
          d. Fear
       3. Community-Based Care

FOCUSED STUDY TIPS

1. List the nursing implications for medications that are prescribed for hematologic disorders.

_____

_____

_____

2. Compare and contrast Hodgkin's disease from non-Hodgkin's lymphomas.

_____

_____

_____

_____

_____

3. Summarize the major types of leukemia.

_____

_____

_____

_____

_____

4. Explain the pathophysiology and manifestations of bleeding disorders.

_____

_____

_____

_____

CASE STUDY

Jonathan Obermark is a 43-year-old male client who was diagnosed today with iron-deficiency anemia. He says that his mother was just recently diagnosed with acute lymphoblastic leukemia (ALL). Answer the following questions based on knowledge of anemias and ALL:

1. List the types of anemias.

2. What are the dietary sources of heme and nonheme iron?

3. What is the classification, characteristics, manifestations, and treatments for acute lymphoblastic leukemia (ALL)?

CARE PLAN CRITICAL THINKING ACTIVITY

1. Why was an ice bag and manual pressure applied to Mr. Cruise's nose in the emergency department?

2. Why is it important for Mr. Cruise to avoid contact sports?

3. What information is available on a MedicAlert bracelet?

NCLEX REVIEW QUESTIONS

1. The amount of oxygen that reaches the tissues depends on the following factors except:
    1. The available oxygen in the alveoli.
    2. The diffusing surface and capacity of the lungs.
    3. The number of white blood cells.
    4. The ability of the cardiovascular system to transport blood and oxygen to the tissues.
2. Which of the following statements by a student nurse reflects correct understanding about iron deficiency anemia?
    1. "Iron deficiency anemia is the least common type of anemia."
    2. "The body can synthesize hemoglobin without iron."
    3. "Inadequate dietary iron intake also contributes to anemia in the older adult."
    4. "Iron deficiency anemia results in countless numbers of RBCs, microcytic and hypochromic RBCs, as well as malformed RBCs (poikilocytosis)."
3. During discharge planning, the nurse is teaching the client about the sources of heme iron. Which of the following is not a source of heme iron?
    1. Veal
    2. Clams
    3. Egg yolk
    4. Dried fruits

4. The spouse of a client (who has leukemia) is providing care. Which of the following indicates a need for further teaching? The spouse:
   1. Provides rest periods before meals.
   2. Provides medications for pain or nausea 10 minutes before meals, if prescribed.
   3. Provides liquids with different textures and tastes.
   4. Provides mouth care before and after meals.
5. The Ann Arbor Staging System is used to assess the extent and severity of lymphomas. Which stage has involvement of lymph node regions or structures on both sides of the diaphragm?
   1. Stage I
   2. Stage II
   3. Stage III
   4. Stage IV
6. During discharge planning, the nurse is teaching the client how to prevent or relieve nausea or vomiting. Which of the following instructions is incorrect?
   1. Eat soda crackers.
   2. Avoid unpleasant odors, and get fresh air.
   3. Eat soft, bland foods that are warm and above room temperature.
   4. Suck on hard candy.
7. A nurse is planning a seminar about aplastic anemia. Which of the following statements needs to be corrected before the seminar?
   1. Manifestations of aplastic anemia include fatigue, pallor, progressive weakness, exertional dyspnea, headache, and ultimately tachycardia and heart failure.
   2. In aplastic anemia, the bone marrow fails to produce both types of blood cells, which leads to pancytopenia.
   3. Aplastic anemia also may occur with viral infections such as mononucleosis, hepatitis C, and HIV disease.
   4. Aplastic anemia is rare.
8. Which of the following statements by a student nurse reflects correct understanding about polycythemia?
   1. "In primary polycythemia, RBC production is decreased."
   2. "Secondary polycythemia occurs when erythropoietin levels are elevated."
   3. "In relative polycythemia, the total RBC count is high."
   4. "In relative polycythemia, the hematocrit is abnormally low."
9. Which of the following actions is inappropriate for the nurse who is providing care for a client with acute lymphocytic leukemia?
   1. Do not restrict any visitors.
   2. Provide oral hygiene after every meal.
   3. Ensure meticulous handwashing among all people in contact with the client.
   4. Maintain protective isolation as indicated.
10. A nurse is evaluating a student's understanding of non-Hodgkin's lymphoma. Which of the following statements indicates a need for further teaching?
    1. "Non-Hodgkin's lymphomas tend to arise in peripheral lymph nodes and spread early to tissues throughout the body."
    2. "Non-Hodgkin's lymphoma is less common than Hodgkin's disease."
    3. "Non-Hodgkin's lymphoma is a diverse group of lymphoid tissue malignancies that do not contain Reed-Sternberg cells."
    4. "Older adults are more often affected, and it occurs more frequently in men than in women."

CHAPTER 35

NURSING CARE OF CLIENTS WITH PERIPHERAL VASCULAR DISORDERS

LEARNING OUTCOMES

After completing Chapter 35, you will be able to demonstrate the following objectives:

- Describe the etiology, pathophysiology, and manifestations of common peripheral vascular and lymphatic disorders.
- Compare and contrast the manifestations and effects of disorders affecting large and small vessels, arteries, and veins.
- Explain risk factors for and measures to prevent peripheral vascular disorders and their complications.
- Explain the nursing implications for medications and other interdisciplinary treatments used for clients with peripheral vascular disorders.
- Describe preoperative and postoperative nursing care of clients having vascular surgery.

CLINICAL COMPETENCIES

- Assess clients with peripheral vascular disorders, using data to select and prioritize appropriate nursing diagnoses and identify desired outcomes of care.
- Identify the effects of peripheral vascular disorders on the functional health status of assigned clients.
- Use research and an evidence-based plan to provide individualized care for clients with peripheral vascular disorders.
- Collaborate with the interdisciplinary care team in planning and providing care for clients with peripheral vascular disorders.
- Safely and knowledgably administer medications and prescribed treatments for clients with peripheral vascular disorders.
- Provide client and family teaching to promote, maintain, and restore health in clients with common peripheral vascular disorders.

MediaLink

www.prenhall.com/lemone

Resources for this chapter can be found on the Prentice Hall Nursing MediaLink DVD accompanying this textbook, and on the Companion Website at http://www.prenhall.com/lemone. Click on Chapter 35 to select the activities for this chapter.

Prentice Hall Nursing MediaLink DVD-ROM
- Audio Glossary
- NCLEX-RN® Review

Companion Website
www.prenhall.com/lemone
- Audio Glossary
- NCLEX-RN® Review
- Care Plan Activity: Lymphedema
- Case Study: Abdominal Aortic Aneurysm
- MediaLink Application
  - Calcium Channel Overdose
  - Peripheral Vascular Disease
- Links to Resources

KEY TERMS

aneurysm
atherosclerosis
blood pressure
chronic venous insufficiency
deep venous thrombosis
  (DVT)
diastolic blood pressure
dissection
embolism
hypertension
intermittent claudication
lymphedema
mean arterial pressure (MAP)
peripheral vascular disease
  (PVD)

primary hypertension
pulse pressure
Raynaud's
  disease/phenomenon
secondary hypertension
systolic blood pressure
thromboangiitis obliterans
thromboembolus
thrombus
varicose veins
vasoconstriction
vasodilation
venous thrombosis

CHAPTER OUTLINE

C. Nursing Care
  1. Assessment
  2. Nursing Diagnoses and Interventions
    a. Risk for Ineffective Tissue Perfusion
    b. Risk for Injury
    c. Anxiety
  3. Community-Based Care
VII. Disorders of the Peripheral Arteries
  A. Physiology Review
VIII. The Client with Peripheral Vascular Disease
  A. Incidence and Risk Factors
  B. Pathophysiology
  C. Manifestations and Complications
  D. Interdisciplinary Care
    1. Diagnosis
    2. Medications
    3. Treatments
    4. Revascularization
    5. Complementary Therapies
  E. Nursing Care
    1. Health Promotion
    2. Assessment
    3. Nursing Diagnoses and Interventions
      a. Ineffective Tissue Perfusion: Peripheral
      b. Pain
      c. Impaired Skin Integrity
      d. Activity Intolerance
    4. Using NANDA, NIC, and NOC
    5. Community-Based Care
IX. The Client with Thromboangiitis Obliterans
  A. Incidence and Risk Factors
  B. Pathophysiology and Course
  C. Manifestations and Complications
  D. Interdisciplinary Care
  E. Nursing Care
    1. Community-Based Care
X. The Client with Raynaud's Disease
  A. Pathophysiology and Manifestations
  B. Interdisciplinary Care
  C. Nursing Care
    1. Community-Based Care
XI. The Client with Acute Arterial Occlusion
  A. Pathophysiology
    1. Arterial Thrombosis
    2. Arterial Embolism
  B. Manifestations
  C. Interdisciplinary Care
    1. Diagnosis
    2. Medications
    3. Surgery

D. Nursing Care
 1. Assessment
 2. Nursing Diagnoses and Interventions
  a. Ineffective Tissue Perfusion: Peripheral
  b. Anxiety
  c. Altered Protection
 3. Community-Based Care
XII. Disorders of Venous Circulation
 A. Physiology Review
XIII. The Client with Venous Thrombosis
 A. Pathophysiology
  1. Deep Venous Thrombosis
  2. Superficial Venous Thrombosis
 B. Interdisciplinary Care
  1. Diagnosis
  2. Prophylaxis
  3. Medications
  4. Treatments
  5. Surgery
 C. Nursing Care
  1. Health Promotion
  2. Assessment
  3. Nursing Diagnoses and Interventions
   a. Pain
   b. Ineffective Tissue Perfusion: Peripheral
   c. Ineffective Protection
   d. Impaired Physical Mobility
   e. Risk for Ineffective Tissue Perfusion: Cardiopulmonary
  4. Using NANDA, NIC, and NOC
  5. Community-Based Care
XIV. The Client with Chronic Venous Insufficiency
 A. Pathophysiology
 B. Manifestations
 C. Interdisciplinary Care
 D. Nursing Care
XV. The Client with Varicose Veins
 A. Incidence and Risk Factors
 B. Pathophysiology
  1. Manifestations
  2. Complications
 E. Interdisciplinary Care
  1. Diagnosis
  2. Treatments
  3. Compression Sclerotherapy
  4. Surgery
 F. Nursing Care
  1. Health Promotion
  2. Assessment
  3. Nursing Diagnoses and Interventions
   a. Chronic Pain
   b. Ineffective Tissue Perfusion: Peripheral
   c. Risk for Impaired Skin Integrity
   d. Risk for Peripheral Neurovascular Dysfunction
  4. Community-Based Care

FOCUSED STUDY TIPS

1. Discuss the pathophysiology and manifestations of common peripheral vascular and lymphatic disorders.

_____

_____

_____

_____

_____

2. Summarize the manifestations of disorders that affect large and small vessels, arteries, and veins.

_____

_____

_____

_____

_____

3. List the risk factors for and measures to prevent peripheral vascular disorders and their complications.

_____

_____

_____

_____

4. Identify the nursing implications and other interdisciplinary treatments used for clients with peripheral vascular disorders.

_____

_____

_____

_____

CASE STUDY

Elizabeth Drake is a 44-year-old female client who is in the physician's office to have her blood pressure checked. Elizabeth has been diagnosed with primary hypertension.

1. Discuss the manifestations of primary hypertension.

2. Explain the complications of primary hypertension.

3. Summarize the lifestyle modifications that Elizabeth should be following.

CARE PLAN CRITICAL THINKING ACTIVITY

1. What type of hypertension does Mrs. Spezia have?

2. List the assessment findings that the nurse noted.

3. Discuss the information that the nurse should provide to Mrs. Spezia.

NCLEX REVIEW QUESTIONS

1. Which of the following is felt as the peripheral pulse and heard as the Korotkoff's sounds during blood pressure measurement?
   1. Diastolic blood pressure
   2. Systolic blood pressure
   3. Pulse pressure
   4. Mean arterial pressure
2. Your nursing instructor asks the student nurse to give the formula for MAP. Which of the following formulas should the student nurse give her?
   1. [Diastolic BP + 2 (systolic BP)] / 2
   2. [Systolic BP + 2 (diastolic BP)] / 2
   3. [Systolic BP + 2 (diastolic BP)] / 3
   4. [Diastolic BP + 2 (systolic BP)] / 3
3. Primary hypertension is thought to develop from complex interactions among factors that regulate cardiac output and systemic vascular resistance. These interactions may include all of the following except:
   1. Excess sympathetic nervous system with overstimulation of α- and β-adrenergic receptors, which results in vasodilatation and decreased cardiac output.
   2. Altered function of the renin-angiotensin-aldosterone system and its responsiveness to factors such as sodium intake and overall fluid volume.
   3. The interaction between insulin resistance, hyperinsulinemia, and endothelial function may be a primary cause of hypertension.
   4. Other chemical mediators of vasomotor tone and blood volume such as atrial natriuretic peptide (factor) also play a role by affecting vasomotor tone and sodium and water excretion.
4. Which of the following can cause primary hypertension?
   1. Kidney disease
   2. Cushing's syndrome
   3. Pregnancy
   4. Gender
5. To reduce the risk of aneurysm rupture, the nurse should implement all of the following except:
   1. Maintain bed rest with legs elevated.
   2. Maintain a calm environment and implement measures to reduce psychologic stress.
   3. Instruct client to prevent straining during defecation and avoid holding the breath while moving.
   4. Administer beta blockers and antihypertensives as prescribed.

6. Which of the following statements by a student nurse reflects correct understanding about Raynaud's disease? "Raynaud's disease:
    1. Primarily affects older women between the ages of 60 and 80."
    2. Is characterized by episodes of intense vasospasm in the small veins of the fingers and sometimes the toes."
    3. Has no identifiable cause."
    4. Has been called 'the red-yellow-white disease.'"

7. A nurse is evaluating a nursing student's understanding of preventing venous thrombosis. Which of the following statements by the student nurse indicates a need for further teaching?
    1. "Position clients to promote venous blood flow from the lower extremities, with the feet elevated and the knees slightly bent."
    2. "Place pillows under the knees and positions in which the hips and knees are sharply flexed."
    3. "The client should use a recliner chair or foot stool when sitting."
    4. "Teach ankle flexion and extension exercises, and frequently remind clients to perform them."

8. A nurse is planning a seminar about varicose veins. Which of the following statements is correct?
    1. Elastic stockings should be removed eight times a day for 15 minutes.
    2. Complications of varicose veins include venous insufficiency and stasis ulcers.
    3. Prolonged sitting, the force of gravity, lack of leg exercise, and incompetent venous valves all weaken the muscle-pumping mechanism, which reduces arteriole blood return to the heart.
    4. Varicose veins may be asymptomatic, but most cause manifestations such as severe aching leg pain, leg spasms, leg lightness, itching, or feelings of coldness in the legs.

9. During discharge planning, the nurse is teaching the client about factors that contribute to hypertension. Which of the following is considered a modifiable risk factor?
    1. Obesity
    2. Age
    3. Race
    4. Family history

10. A nurse is evaluating a client's understanding of the DASH diet. Which of the following client statements indicates a need for further teaching? "I should have:
    1. Four to five servings of fruit per day."
    2. Three to four servings of grains per day."
    3. Four to five servings of vegetables per day."
    4. Two to three servings of low-fat dairy products per day."

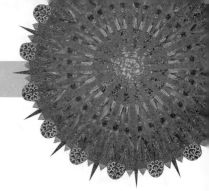

CHAPTER 36

ASSESSING CLIENTS WITH RESPIRATORY DISORDERS

LEARNING OUTCOMES

After completing Chapter 36, you will be able to demonstrate the following objectives:
- Describe the anatomy, physiology, and functions of the respiratory system.
- Explain the mechanics of ventilation.
- Compare and contrast factors affecting respiration.
- Identify specific topics for consideration during a health history interview of the client with health problems involving the respiratory system.
- Describe normal variations in assessment findings for the older adult.
- Identify manifestations of impairment of the respiratory system.

CLINICAL COMPETENCIES

- Conduct and document a health history for clients having or at risk for alterations in the respiratory system.
- Conduct and document a physical assessment of respiratory structures and functions.
- Monitor the results of diagnostic tests and report abnormal findings.

EQUIPMENT NEEDED

- Tongue blade
- Penlight
- Nasal speculum
- Metric ruler
- Marking pen
- Stethoscope with diaphragm

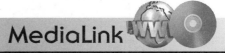

MediaLink

www.prenhall.com/lemone

Resources for this chapter can be found on the Prentice Hall Nursing MediaLink DVD accompanying this textbook, and on the Companion Website at http://www.prenhall.com/lemone. Click on Chapter 36 to select the activities for this chapter.

Prentice Hall Nursing MediaLink DVD-ROM
- Audio Glossary
- NCLEX-RN® Review

Animation/Video
- Carbon Dioxide Transport
- Oxygen Transport

Companion Website
www.prenhall.com/lemone
- Audio Glossary
- NCLEX-RN® Review
- Case Study: Respiratory Assessment
- MediaLink Applications
  - Pulmonary Function Testing
  - Wheezes and Crackles
- Links to Resources

KEY TERMS

apnea
atelectasis
bradypnea
crackles
friction rub
lung compliance
oxyhemoglobin

surfactant
tachypnea
tidal volume (TV)
vital capacity (VC)
wheezes

CHAPTER OUTLINE

I. Anatomy, Physiology, and Functions of the Respiratory System
   A. The Upper Respiratory System
      1. The Nose
      2. The Sinuses
      3. The Pharynx
      4. The Larynx
      5. The Trachea
   B. The Lower Respiratory System
      1. The Lungs
      2. The Pleura
      3. The Bronchi and Alveoli
      4. The Rib Cage and Intercostal Muscles
II. Factors Affecting Ventilation and Respiration
   A. Respiratory Volume and Capacity
   B. Air Pressures
   C. Oxygen, Carbon Dioxide, and Hydrogen Ion Concentrations
   D. Airway Resistance, Lung Compliance, and Elasticity
   E. Alveolar Surface Tension
III. Blood Gases
   A. Oxygen Transport and Unloading
   B. Carbon Dioxide Transport
IV. Assessing Respiratory Function
   A. Diagnostic Tests
   B. Genetic Considerations
   C. Health Assessment Interview
   D. Physical Assessment
V. Respiratory Assessments

FOCUSED STUDY TIPS

1. Identify manifestations of impairment of the respiratory system.

_____

_____

_____

_____

2. List the factors that affect respiration.

_____

_____

_____

3. Discuss the mechanics of ventilation.

_____

_____

_____

4. Summarize the anatomy, physiology, and functions of the respiratory system.

_____

_____

_____

_____

_____

CASE STUDY

Drake Strattman has been working as an RN for eleven years. He is the charge nurse of a respiratory floor at a local hospital. He has been asked by the nursing school to teach a class today about the respiratory system and respiratory disorders. After the class students ask the following questions:

1. "What are the factors that affect ventilation and respiration?"

2. "Where are the sinuses and what is the purpose of having sinuses?"

3. "What is the difference between inspiratory reserve volume (IRV) and expiratory reserve volume (ERV)?"

4. "What is bradypnea, tachypnea, and apnea?"

NCLEX REVIEW QUESTIONS

1. Which of the following statements by a student nurse reflects correct understanding about the respiratory system?
   1. "The internal nose is given structure by the nasal, frontal, and maxillary bones as well as plates of hyaline cartilage."
   2. "The nasal hairs filter the air as it enters the nares."
   3. "Sinuses makes the skull heavier, assist in speech, and produce mucus that drains into the nasal cavities to help trap debris."
   4. "The nasopharynx serves as a passageway for both air and food."
2. A nurse is planning a seminar about the respiratory system. Which of the following statements needs to be corrected?
   1. The laryngopharynx extends from the hyoid bone to the larynx.
   2. The right lung is smaller and has two lobes; whereas the left lung has three lobes.
   3. The parietal pleura lines the thoracic wall and mediastinum.
   4. During expiration, carbon dioxide is expelled.
3. Which of the following statements made by a student nurse is correct?
   1. There are 12 pairs of ribs that all articulate with the thoracic vertebrae.
   2. Posteriorly, the first seven ribs articulate with the body of the sternum.
   3. The seventh, eighth, and ninth ribs articulate with the cartilage immediately above the ribs.
   4. The tenth, eleventh, and twelfth ribs are called floating ribs, because they are unattached.

4. Tidal volume (TV) is the:
   1. Amount of air (approximately 500 mL) moved in and out of the lungs with each normal, quiet breath.
   2. Amount of air (approximately 2100 to 3100 mL) that can be inhaled forcibly over the tidal volume.
   3. Approximately 1000 mL of air that can be forced out over the tidal volume.
   4. Volume of air (approximately 1100 mL) that remains in the lungs after a forced expiration.
5. A nurse is evaluating a nursing student's understanding of inspiration and expiration. Which of the following statements indicates a need for further teaching?
   1. "During inspiration, the diaphragm contracts and flattens out to increase the vertical diameter of the thoracic cavity."
   2. "Expiration is primarily a passive process that occurs as a result of the elasticity of the lungs."
   3. "During expiration, the inspiratory muscles contract, the diaphragm descends, the ribs expand, and the lungs recoil."
   4. "A single inspiration lasts for about 1 to 1.5 seconds; whereas an expiration lasts for about 2 to 3 seconds."
6. A nurse is evaluating a client's understanding of some diagnostic tests that he had while in the hospital. Which of the following client statements indicates a need for further clarification?
   1. "Arterial blood gases are conducted to evaluate alterations in acid–base balances."
   2. "Pulse oximetry is used to evaluate or monitor the oxygen saturation of the blood."
   3. "A bronchoscopy is a direct visualization of the pharynx, larynx, trachea, and bronchi."
   4. "A thoracentesis, when done for diagnostic purposes, is conducted to obtain a specimen of pleural fluid."
7. Two nurses are discussing a client's respiratory condition. Which of the following statements by a nurse is correct?
   1. "Dullness is heard in clients with atelectasis, lobar pneumonia, and pleural effusion."
   2. "Retraction of intercostal spaces may be seen in pneumothorax."
   3. "Bulging of intercostal spaces may be seen in asthma."
   4. "Bilateral chest expansion is increased in emphysema."
8. Carbon dioxide is transported in all of the following forms except:
   1. Dissolved in plasma.
   2. Bound to hemoglobin.
   3. As bicarbonate ions in the plasma.
   4. Dissociated from hemoglobin.
9. The lower respiratory tract includes which of the following?
   1. Nose
   2. Trachea
   3. Pleura
   4. Sinuses
10. Which of the following is part of the upper respiratory tract?
    1. Larynx
    2. Lungs
    3. Bronchi
    4. Rib cage

CHAPTER 37

NURSING CARE OF CLIENTS WITH UPPER RESPIRATORY DISORDERS

LEARNING OUTCOMES

After completing Chapter 37, you will be able to demonstrate the following objectives:

- Relate anatomy and physiology of the upper respiratory tract to commonly occurring disorders and risk factors for these disorders.
- Describe the pathophysiology of common upper respiratory tract disorders, relating their manifestations to the pathophysiologic process.
- Discuss nursing implications for medications and other interdisciplinary care measures to treat upper respiratory disorders.
- Describe surgical procedures used to treat upper respiratory disorders and their implications for client care and recovery.
- Identify health promotion activities related to reducing the incidence of upper respiratory disorders, describing the appropriate population and setting for implementing identified measures.
- Discuss treatment options for oral and laryngeal cancers with their implications for the client's body image and functional health.

CLINICAL COMPETENCIES

- Assess functional health status of clients with upper respiratory disorders, using data to identify and prioritize holistic nursing care needs.
- Use nursing research and evidence-based practice to plan and implement nursing care for clients with upper respiratory disorders.
- Provide safe and effective nursing care for clients having surgery involving the upper respiratory system and/or with a tracheostomy.
- Safely and knowledgably administer medications and prescribed treatments for clients with disorders of the upper respiratory tract.
- Provide appropriate teaching for the client and family affected by upper respiratory tract disorders.
- Evaluate the effectiveness of care, reassessing and modifying the plan of care as needed to achieve desired client outcomes.

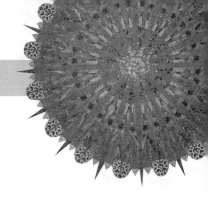

MediaLink

www.prenhall.com/lemone

Resources for this chapter can be found on the Prentice Hall Nursing MediaLink DVD accompanying this textbook, and on the Companion Website at http://www.prenhall.com/lemone. Click on Chapter 37 to select the activities for this chapter.

Prentice Hall Nursing MediaLink DVD-ROM
- Audio Glossary
- NCLEX-RN® Review

Companion Website
www.prenhall.com/lemone
- Audio Glossary
- NCLEX-RN® Review
- Care Plan Activity: Epistaxis
- Case Study: Sleep Apnea
- MediaLink Applications
  - Laryngectomy
  - Pulse Oximetry
- Links to Resources

KEY TERMS

coryza
epistaxis
influenza
laryngectomy
laryngitis
pertussis
pharyngitis

rhinitis
rhinoplasty
sinusitis
sleep apnea
tonsillitis

CHAPTER OUTLINE

I. Infectious or Inflammatory Disorders
II. The Client with Viral Upper Respiratory Infection
   A. Pathophysiology
   B. Manifestations and Complications
   C. Interdisciplinary Care
      1. Medications
      2. Complementary Therapies
   D. Nursing Care
      1. Health Promotion
      2. Community-Based Care
III. The Client with Respiratory Syncytial Virus
IV. The Client with Influenza
   A. Pathophysiology
   B. Manifestations
   C. Complications
   D. Interdisciplinary Care
      1. Prevention
      2. Diagnosis
      3. Medications
   E. Nursing Care
      1. Health Promotion
      2. Assessment
      3. Nursing Diagnoses and Interventions
         a. Ineffective Breathing Pattern
         b. Ineffective Airway Clearance
         c. Disturbed Sleep Pattern
         d. Risk for Infection
      4. Using NANDA, NIC, and NOC
      5. Community-Based Care
V. The Client with Sinusitis
   A. Physiology Review
   B. Pathophysiology
   C. Manifestations and Complications
   D. Interdisciplinary Care
      1. Diagnosis
      2. Medications
      3. Surgery
      4. Complementary Therapies
   E. Nursing Care
      1. Health Promotion
      2. Assessment

C. Nursing Care
　　1. Community-Based Care
XIV. The Client with Obstructive Sleep Apnea
　　A. Risk Factors
　　B. Pathophysiology
　　C. Manifestations
　　D. Complications
　　E. Interdisciplinary Care
　　　　1. Diagnosis
　　　　2. Treatments
　　　　3. Surgery
　　F. Nursing Care
　　　　1. Community-Based Care
XV. Upper Respiratory Tumors
XVI. The Client with Nasal Polyps
　　A. Pathophysiology and Manifestations
　　B. Interdisciplinary Care
　　C. Nursing Care
XVII. The Client with a Laryngeal Tumor
　　A. Risk Factors
　　B. Pathophysiology and Manifestations
　　　　1. Benign Tumors
　　　　2. Laryngeal Cancer
　　C. Interdisciplinary Care
　　　　1. Diagnosis
　　　　2. Treatments
　　　　3. Surgery
　　　　4. Speech Rehabilitation
　　D. Nursing Care
　　　　1. Health Promotion
　　　　2. Assessment
　　　　3. Nursing Diagnoses and Interventions
　　　　　　a. Risk for Impaired Airway Clearance
　　　　　　b. Impaired Verbal Communication
　　　　　　c. Impaired Swallowing
　　　　　　d. Imbalanced Nutrition: Less than Body Requirements
　　　　　　e. Anticipatory Grieving
　　　　4. Using NANDA, NIC, and NOC
　　　　5. Community-Based Care

FOCUSED STUDY TIPS

1. Explain the treatment options for oral and laryngeal cancers.

　　_____

　　_____

　　_____

2. List the health promotion activities related to reducing the incidence of upper respiratory disorders.

　　_____

　　_____

　　_____

3. Explain the surgical procedures used to treat upper respiratory disorders.

_____

_____

_____

_____

4. Discuss nursing implications for medications used to treat upper respiratory disorders.

_____

_____

_____

_____

CASE STUDY

Nathaniel Smith is a 37-year-old male client who has been diagnosed with obstructive sleep apnea. Part of the nursing responsibilities is to provide Nathaniel with education about sleep apnea before he leaves the clinic. Answer the following questions based on your knowledge of sleep apnea.

1. Explain the pathophysiology of sleep apnea.

2. List the manifestations of obstructive sleep apnea.

3. Review the complications of obstructive sleep apnea.

4. Review the treatments for obstructive sleep apnea.

CARE PLAN CRITICAL THINKING ACTIVITY

1. Why is it important for Ms. Wunderman to drink ice-cold fluids?

2. List the types of beverages and foods that Ms. Wunderman should avoid.

3. Discuss various pain management strategies that Ms. Wunderman could use.

NCLEX REVIEW QUESTIONS

1. A nurse is evaluating a client's understanding of preventing the spread of acute viral URI. Which of the following client statements indicates a need for further teaching?
   1. "I'll use disposable tissues to cover my mouth and nose while coughing or sneezing to reduce airborne spread of the virus."
   2. "I'll blow my nose with one nostril open to prevent infected matter from being forced into the eustachian tubes."
   3. "I'll wash my hands frequently, especially after coughing or sneezing, to limit viral transmission."
   4. "I'll limit use of nasal decongestants to every four hours for only a few days at a time to prevent rebound effect."

2. Which type of influenza is found in humans?
   1. A only
   2. A and C
   3. B and C
   4. A, B, and C

3. Which of the following statements by a student nurse reflects correct understanding about tonsillitis?
   1. "The tonsils appear yellow and edematous."
   2. "Pressing on a tonsil may produce purulent drainage."
   3. "Yellow exudate is present on the tonsils."
   4. "The uvula is white and swollen."

4. Infectious mononucleosis is caused by which virus?
   1. Epstein-Barr
   2. Influenza
   3. Rotavirus
   4. Norwalk virus

5. A nurse is teaching a client about home care following a polypectomy. Which of the following statements by the nurse is correct?
   1. "Apply heat or hot compresses to the nose to decrease swelling, promote comfort, and prevent bleeding."
   2. "Avoid blowing the nose for 1 hour after nasal packing is removed."
   3. "Avoid straining during bowel movements, vigorous coughing, and strenuous exercise."
   4. "Rest for one day after surgery to reduce the risk of bleeding."

6. A nurse is conducting discharge teaching for a client about tracheostomy stoma care and preventing respiratory infection. Which of the following nursing instructions demonstrates that the nurse requires further education?
   1. Water sports are not contraindicated with a permanent tracheostomy.
   2. Increase fluid intake to maintain mucosal moisture and loosen secretions.
   3. Shield the stoma with a stoma guard, such as a gauze square on a tie around the neck, to prevent particulate matter from entering the lower respiratory tract.
   4. Use a humidifier or vaporizer to add humidity to inspired air.

7. Which of the following actions is inappropriate for the nurse caring for a client who has an epistaxis (nosebleed)?
   1. Pinch the client's nares or bridge of the nose.
   2. Apply ice to the client's nose.
   3. Have the client sit upright and lean forward.
   4. Have the client tilt the head backwards.

8. A nurse is discussing risk factors of laryngeal cancer with a client. Which of the following is a major risk factor of laryngeal cancer?
   1. Tobacco use
   2. Alcohol consumption
   3. Poor nutrition
   4. Exposure to asbestos

9. A nurse is planning a seminar about nasal polyps. Which of the following statements needs to be corrected?
   1. Polyps form in areas of dependent mucous membrane, and present as pale, edematous masses that are covered with mucous membrane.
   2. Nasal polyps are benign grape-like growths of the mucous membrane that lines the nose.
   3. Polyps are unilateral and have a firm base, which makes them rigid.
   4. Polyps may be asymptomatic, although large polyps may cause nasal obstruction, rhinorrhea, and loss of sense of smell.

10. When discussing the management of sleep apnea with the nurse, the client asks, "How can I manage sleep apnea?" The nurse should discuss or recommend which of the following?
    1. Discuss the relationship of alcohol and sedatives to sleep apnea, and refer to an alcohol treatment program or Alcoholics Anonymous as indicated.
    2. Recommend the use of the CPAP intermittently throughout the night.
    3. Discuss the relationship between obesity and sleep apnea.
    4. Recommend an adequate fluid intake to maintain moist mucous membranes.

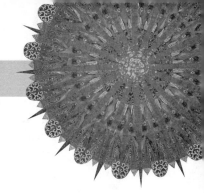

CHAPTER 38

Nursing Care of Clients with Ventilation Disorders

LEARNING OUTCOMES

After completing Chapter 38, you will be able to demonstrate the following objectives:

- Relate the pathophysiology and manifestations of lower respiratory infections and inflammation, lung cancer, chest wall disorders, and trauma to the ability to maintain effective ventilation and respiration (gas exchange).
- Compare and contrast the etiology, risk factors, and vulnerable populations for lower respiratory infections, lung cancer, chest wall disorders, and trauma.
- Describe interdisciplinary care and the nursing role in health promotion and caring for clients with lower respiratory infections, lung cancer, chest wall disorders, and trauma.
- Discuss surgery and other invasive procedures used to treat lung cancer, chest wall disorders, and trauma, and nursing responsibilities in caring for clients undergoing these procedures.
- Describe the nursing implications for oxygen therapy and medications used to treat respiratory disorders.

CLINICAL COMPETENCIES

- Assess functional health status and the effects of lower respiratory and chest wall disorders on ventilation and gas exchange.
- Use assessed data and knowledge of the effects of the disorder and prescribed treatment to identify priority nursing diagnoses and plan care for clients with lower respiratory disorders.
- Use the nursing process and evidence-based nursing research to plan and implement individualized nursing care, including measures to promote ventilation and gas exchange, for clients with lower respiratory disorders.
- Plan and provide appropriate teaching for health promotion among vulnerable populations and to prepare clients and families for community-based care.

MediaLink

www.prenhall.com/lemone

Resources for this chapter can be found on the Prentice Hall Nursing MediaLink DVD accompanying this textbook, and on the Companion Website at http://www.prenhall.com/lemone. Click on Chapter 38 to select the activities for this chapter.

Prentice Hall Nursing MediaLink DVD-ROM
- Audio Glossary
- NCLEX-RN® Review

Animation
- Tuberculosis

Companion Website
www.prenhall.com/lemone
- Audio Glossary
- NCLEX-RN® Review
- Care Plan Activity: Pneumonia
- Case Study: TB Medication and Compliance
- MediaLink Applications
  - Health Promotion Among Vulnerable Populations
  - SARS
- Links to Resources

- Evaluate the effectiveness of nursing interventions and teaching, revising strategies and teaching plans as needed.
- Safely and knowledgeably coordinate interdisciplinary care and administer prescribed medications and treatments for clients with lower respiratory disorders.

KEY TERMS

asphyxiation
bronchitis
cyanosis
dyspnea
empyema
flail chest
hemoptysis
hemothorax
hypoxemia

lung abscess
pleural effusion
pleuritis
pneumonia
pneumothorax
severe acute respiratory
   syndrome (SARS)
thoracentesis
tuberculosis (TB)

CHAPTER OUTLINE

    F. Nursing Care
       1. Health Promotion
       2. Assessment
       3. Nursing Diagnoses and Interventions
          a. Ineffective Breathing Pattern
          b. Activity Intolerance
          c. Pain
          d. Anticipatory Grieving
       4. Using NANDA, NIC, and NOC
       5. Community-Based Care

FOCUSED STUDY TIPS

1. List the nursing implications for medications used to treat respiratory disorders.

   _____

   _____

   _____

   _____

2. Summarize invasive procedures used to treat lung cancer, chest wall disorders, and trauma.

   _____

   _____

   _____

   _____

   _____

3. Compare and contrast the etiology, risk factors, and vulnerable populations for lower respiratory infections, lung cancer, chest wall disorders, and trauma.

   _____

   _____

   _____

   _____

   _____

4. Discuss the nursing role in health promotion for clients with lower respiratory infections.

CASE STUDY

Mimi Sutter is a 37-year-old female client who complains of moderate fever, general malaise, nonproductive cough, and substernal chest pain. The physician has diagnosed her with acute bronchitis. Answer the following questions based on knowledge of acute bronchitis.

1. What are the manifestations of acute bronchitis?

2. How is acute bronchitis diagnosed?

3. How is acute bronchitis treated?

CARE PLAN CRITICAL THINKING ACTIVITY

1. Discuss Mr. Mueller's assessment findings.

2. What are the possible effects of lung cancer that should be discussed with Mr. and Mrs. Mueller?

3. What methods are available to assist Mr. Mueller to stop smoking?

NCLEX REVIEW QUESTIONS

1. Which of the following statements by a student nurse reflects correct understanding about pneumonia?
   1. "Inflammation of the bronchi is known as pneumonia."
   2. "Bacteria, viruses, fungi, protozoa, and other microbes can lead to infectious pneumonia."
   3. "Infectious causes of pneumonia include aspiration of gastric contents and inhalation of toxic or irritating gases."
   4. "The most common causative organism for community-acquired pneumonia is *Staphylococcus aureus* (also called pneumococcus), a gram-negative bacterium."

2. Which of the following statements by a student nurse is correct?
   1. "The incubation period for SARS is generally one day."
   2. "A lower grade fever lower than 98.2°F (38°C) is typically the initial manifestation of the disease."
   3. "The primary population affected by SARS is previously healthy children from age 5 to 10 years."
   4. "The infective agent responsible for SARS is a coronavirus not previously identified in humans."

3. A nurse is planning a seminar about tuberculosis (TB). Which of the following statements needs to be corrected?
   1. Primary or secondary tuberculosis lesions may affect other body systems such as the kidneys, genitalia, bone, and brain.
   2. Worldwide, TB continues to be a significant health problem.
   3. A previously-healed tuberculosis lesion may not be reactivated.
   4. *Mycobacterium tuberculosis* is a relatively slow-growing, slender, rod-shaped, acid-fast organism with a waxy outer capsule that increases its resistance to destruction.

4. During discharge planning, the nurse is teaching the client who has tuberculosis how to limit transmitting the disease to others. Which of the following actions or statements is incorrect?
   1. Always cough and expectorate into tissues.
   2. Dispose of tissues properly and place them in a closed bag.
   3. Wear a mask if you are sneezing or unable to control respiratory secretions.
   4. Because the disease is spread by touching inanimate objects, follow special precautions for eating utensils, clothing, books, or other objects used.

5. A nurse is evaluating a client's understanding of histoplasmosis. Which of the following statements by the client indicates a need for further teaching?
   1. "The *Histoplasma capsulatum* organism is found in the soil and is linked to exposure to bird droppings and bats."
   2. "Initial chest X-rays are nonspecific; later ones show areas of calcification."
   3. "Histoplasmosis is the most common bacterial lung infection in the United States."
   4. "Infection occurs when the spores are inhaled and reach the alveoli."

6. A client is scheduled for a thoracentesis. Which of the following is not a correct action by the nurse?
   1. Verify the presence of a signed informed consent for the procedure.
   2. Ensure that the client has been fasting.
   3. Position the client upright and leaning forward with arms and head supported on an anchored overbed table.
   4. Administer a cough suppressant if indicated.

7. The nursing care of a client with chest tubes includes all of the following except:
   1. Keep the collection apparatus above the level of the chest.
   2. Check tubes frequently for kinks or loops.
   3. Tape all connections and secure the chest tube to the chest wall.
   4. Assess respiratory status at least every four hours.

8. The nurse is interpreting a client's tuberculin test results. Which of the following could be considered a negative response?
    1. Less than 5 mm
    2. 5 to 9 mm
    3. 10 to 15 mm
    4. Greater than 15 mm
9. Which of the following is the correct definition of hemothorax?
    1. Blood in the pleural space, usually occurs as a result of chest trauma, surgery, or diagnostic procedures.
    2. Develops when an air-filled bleb, or blister, on the lung surface ruptures.
    3. Accumulation of air in the pleural space.
    4. A collection of excess fluid in the pleural space.
10. The pleural space normally contains only about _____ of serous fluid.
    1. 1 to 5 mL
    2. 10 to 20 mL
    3. 25 to 30 mL
    4. 35 to 45 mL

CHAPTER 39

NURSING CARE OF CLIENTS WITH GAS EXCHANGE DISORDERS

LEARNING OUTCOMES

After completing Chapter 39, you will be able to demonstrate the following objectives:

- Relate the pathophysiology and manifestations of obstructive, pulmonary vascular, and critical respiratory disorders to their effects on ventilation and respiration (gas exchange).

- Compare and contrast the etiology, risk factors, and vulnerable populations for disorders affecting ventilation and gas exchange within the lungs.

- Describe interdisciplinary care and the nursing role in health promotion and caring for clients with disorders that affect the ability to ventilate the lungs and exchange gases with the environment.

- Discuss interdisciplinary interventions to provide airway and ventilatory support for the client with respiratory failure, and nursing responsibilities in caring for clients requiring airway and ventilatory support.

- Describe the nursing implications for medications used to promote ventilation and gas exchange.

CLINICAL COMPETENCIES

- Assess functional health status of clients with disorders affecting ventilation and gas exchange.

- Use assessed data and knowledge of the effects of the disorder and prescribed treatment to identify priority nursing diagnoses and plan care for clients with disorders affecting ventilation and gas exchange.

- Use the nursing process and evidence-based nursing research to plan and implement individualized nursing care for clients, including measures to promote ventilation and gas exchange.

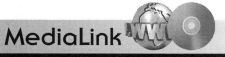

MediaLink

www.prenhall.com/lemone

Resources for this chapter can be found on the Prentice Hall Nursing MediaLink DVD accompanying this textbook, and on the Companion Website at http://www.prenhall.com/lemone. Click on Chapter 39 to select the activities for this chapter.

Prentice Hall Nursing MediaLink DVD-ROM
- Audio Glossary
- NCLEX-RN® Review

Animation/Video
- ARDS
- Asthma
- Metered-Dose Inhalers
- Using a Nebulizer

Companion Website
www.prenhall.com/lemone
- Audio Glossary
- NCLEX-RN® Review
- Care Plan Activity: Acute Asthma Attack
- Case Study: Acute Asthma Attack
- Exercise: Compare and Contrast
- MediaLink Application: Respiratory Disorders
- Links to Resources

- Plan and provide appropriate teaching for health promotion among vulnerable populations and to prepare clients and families for community-based care.
- Evaluate the effectiveness of nursing interventions and teaching, revising strategies and teaching plans as needed.
- Safely and knowledgeably coordinate interdisciplinary care and administer prescribed medications and treatments for clients with disorders affecting ventilation and gas exchange.

KEY TERMS

acute respiratory distress
   syndrome (ARDS)
asthma
atelectasis
bronchiectasis
chronic bronchitis
chronic obstructive
   pulmonary disease
   (COPD)

cor pulmonale
cystic fibrosis (CF)
emphysema
pulmonary embolism
pulmonary hypertension
respiratory failure
sarcoidosis
status asthmaticus
weaning

CHAPTER OUTLINE

FOCUSED STUDY TIPS

1. List the nursing implications for medications used to promote ventilation and gas exchange.

   _____

   _____

   _____

2. Discuss the etiology, risk factors, and vulnerable populations for disorders affecting gas exchange within the lungs.

   _____

   _____

   _____

   _____

   _____

3. Summarize interdisciplinary interventions to provide airway support for the client with respiratory failure.

   _____

   _____

   _____

   _____

4. Explain the nursing responsibilities in caring for clients with ventilatory support.

   _____

   _____

   _____

CASE STUDY

Isabella Hitt is a 12-year-old client who is brought to the clinic by her mother Anne. Isabella is coughing, wheezing, and stating that her chest hurts. Anne is very agitated and tells the nurse, "My daughter is having an asthma attack and needs an inhaler right away." Answer the following questions based on knowledge of asthma.

1. Summarize the triggers of asthma.

2. List the manifestations of acute asthma.

3. Explain how to use a metered-dose inhaler and a dry powder inhaler.

4. Discuss preventive measures for asthma.

CARE PLAN CRITICAL THINKING ACTIVITY

1. Explain ARDS.

2. Why is it important to monitor Ms. Adamson's urine output hourly and to report output of less than 30 mL per hour?

3. Define synchronized intermittent mandatory ventilation (SIMV) and continuous positive airway pressure (CPAP).

NCLEX REVIEW QUESTIONS

1. A nurse is conducting a seminar about asthma. Which of the following statements by a participant indicates a need for further instruction?
   1. "Airways within the lungs contain vertical strips of rough muscle that control their diameter."
   2. "Asthma is a chronic inflammatory disorder of the airways characterized by recurrent episodes of wheezing, breathlessness, chest tightness, and coughing."
   3. "Common triggers for an acute asthma attack include exposure to allergens, respiratory tract infection, exercise, inhaled irritants, and emotional upsets."
   4. "The frequency of attacks and severity of symptoms vary greatly from person to person."

2. Which of the following statements about chronic bronchitis is false?
   1. Chronic bronchitis is a disorder of excessive bronchial mucus secretion. It is characterized by a productive cough that lasts three or more months in two consecutive years.
   2. Cigarette smoke is the major factor implicated in the development of chronic bronchitis.
   3. Chronic bronchitis is insidious in onset.
   4. Chronic bronchitis affected an estimated 8.6 million Americans in 2003.

3. The hallmark pathophysiologic effects of cystic fibrosis (CF) include all of the following except:
   1. Secretions in affected organs become very thin and runny.
   2. Excess mucus production in the respiratory tract with impaired ability to clear secretions and progressive chronic obstructive pulmonary disease (COPD).
   3. Pancreatic enzyme deficiency and impaired digestion.
   4. Abnormal elevation of sodium and chloride concentrations in sweat.

4. Which of the following statements by a student nurse reflects correct understanding about atelectasis?
   1. "The least common cause of atelectasis is obstruction of the bronchus that ventilates a segment of lung tissue."
   2. "It is a state of partial or total lung collapse and airlessness."
   3. "It is only a chronic condition."
   4. "The secondary therapy for atelectasis is prevention."

5. Which of the following actions is appropriate for the nurse when teaching a client how to use a metered-dose inhaler?
   1. Firmly insert a charged metered-dose inhaler (MDI) canister into the mouthpiece unit or spacer (if used).
   2. Hold the canister upright, place the mouthpiece in the mouth, and close lips around it if a spacer is being used.
   3. Press and hold the canister down while inhaling deeply and slowly for 5 to 7 seconds.
   4. Remove mouthpiece cap. Do not shake canister vigorously.

6. A nurse is evaluating a client's performance when using a dry powder inhaler. Which of the following client actions indicates a need for further teaching?
   1. The client removed the cap and held the inhaler upright.
   2. The client held the inhaler level with the mouthpiece end facing up.
   3. The client removed the inhaler from his mouth and held his breath for 10 seconds.
   4. The client exhaled slowly through pursed lips.

7. Which of the following statements about cigarette smoking and tobacco use is false?
   1. Widespread use of tobacco among the male population of the industrialized world began during World War II.
   2. At one time, tobacco was thought to have medicinal qualities effective against all common diseases.
   3. Tobacco is now recognized as the leading cause of preventable illness in the world.
   4. The link between tobacco use and lung cancer was reported as early as 1912.

8. A nurse is teaching a client about effective coughing and breathing techniques. Which of the following statements by the nurse is correct?
   1. "Pursed-lip and diaphragmatic breathing techniques increase air trapping and fatigue."
   2. "Pursed-lip breathing helps maintain open airways by maintaining positive pressures longer during exhalation."
   3. "Diaphragmatic or abdominal breathing helps conserve energy by using the smaller and less efficient muscles of respiration."
   4. "Pursed-lip breathing maintains negative pressure during exhalation."

9. Which nursing intervention for a client with chronic obstructive pulmonary disease (COPD) is correct?
   1. Increase fluid intake to 3500 mL per day and provide a bedside humidifier.
   2. Elevate head of bed to at least 90 degrees at all times.
   3. Teach the "huff" coughing technique.
   4. Assess respiratory status and level of consciousness every 4 to 6 hours until stable, then at least every 12 hours.
10. The common manifestations of pulmonary embolism include all of the following except:
    1. Chest pain.
    2. Anxiety.
    3. Cough.
    4. Bradypnea.

CHAPTER 40

ASSESSING CLIENTS WITH MUSCULOSKELETAL DISORDERS

LEARNING OUTCOMES

After completing Chapter 40, you will be able to demonstrate the following objectives:

- Describe the anatomy, physiology, and functions of the musculoskeletal system.
- Explain the normal movements allowed by synovial joints.
- Identify specific topics for consideration during a health history interview of the client with health problems involving the musculoskeletal system.
- Describe normal variations in assessment findings for the older adult.
- Identify manifestations of impairment of the musculoskeletal system.

CLINICAL COMPETENCIES

- Conduct and document a health history for clients having or at risk for alterations in the mulsculoskeletal system.
- Conduct and document a physical assessment of musculoskeletal structures and functions.
- Monitor the results of diagnostic tests and report abnormal findings.

EQUIPMENT NEEDED

- Tape measure
- Goniometer

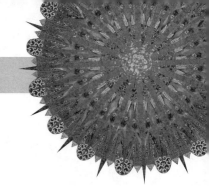

MediaLink

www.prenhall.com/lemone

Resources for this chapter can be found on the Prentice Hall Nursing MediaLink DVD accompanying this textbook, and on the Companion Website at http://www.prenhall.com/lemone. Click on Chapter 40 to select the activities for this chapter.

Prentice Hall Nursing MediaLink DVD-ROM
- Audio Glossary
- NCLEX–RN® Review

Animation
- Joint Movement

Companion Website
www.prenhall.com/lemone
- Audio Glossary
- NCLEX-RN® Review
- Care Plan Activity: Musculoskeletal Disorders
- Case Study: Knee Pain
- MediaLink Application: Musculoskeletal Injuries of Health Care Providers
- Links to Resources

KEY TERMS

bursitis	ossification
crepitation	scoliosis
hematopoiesis	synovitis
kyphosis	tendonitis
lordosis	

CHAPTER OUTLINE

I. Anatomy, Physiology, and Functions of the Musculoskeletal System
   A. The Skeleton
      1. Bone Structure
      2. Bone Shapes
      3. Bone Remodeling in Adults
   B. Muscles
   C. Joints, Ligaments, and Tendons
      1. Fibrous Joints
      2. Cartilaginous Joints
      3. Synovial Joints
II. Assessing Musculoskeletal Function
   A. Diagnostic Tests
   B. Genetic Considerations
   C. Health Assessment Interview
   D. Physical Assessment
III. Musculoskeletal Assessments

FOCUSED STUDY TIPS

1. List manifestations of impairment of the musculoskeletal system.

   _____

   _____

   _____

2. List specific topics for consideration during a health history interview of the client with health problems that involve the musculoskeletal system.

   _____

   _____

   _____

3. Summarize the anatomy, physiology, and functions of the musculoskeletal system.

   _____

   _____

   _____

   _____

4. Describe the normal movements allowed by synovial joints.

   _____

   _____

   _____

CASE STUDY

Michael Baldwin, RN, is preparing for a seminar about the musculoskeletal system. To assess the participants' understanding of the material he is presenting, Michael decided to develop the following questions. Answer the questions based on knowledge of the musculoskeletal system.

1. Bones are classified by which shapes?

2. Summarize bone remodeling in adults.

3. What are the different types of joints?

NCLEX REVIEW QUESTIONS

1. A nurse is evaluating a client's understanding of the musculoskeletal system. Which of the following statements by the client indicates a need for further teaching?
   1. The musculoskeletal system is composed of bones of the skeletal system and ligaments, tendons and muscles of the muscular system, and joints.
   2. The bones serve as the framework for the body and for the attachment of muscles, tendons, and ligaments.
   3. The musculoskeletal system has two subsystems: the bones and joints of the skeleton, and the skeletal muscles.
   4. The tissues and structures of the musculoskeletal system perform one function, which is movement.
2. Which of the following statements about bones is false?
   1. Bones store minerals.
   2. The human skeleton is made up of 226 bones.
   3. Bones of the skeletal system are divided into the axial and the appendicular skeleton.
   4. Bones protect vital organs from injury and serve to move body parts by providing points of attachment for muscles.
3. Which type of bone is longer than it is wide?
   1. Short
   2. Long
   3. Irregular
   4. Flat
4. The bones of the wrist and ankle are considered which type of bone?
   1. Irregular
   2. Long
   3. Flat
   4. Short
5. Which of the following is not a type of muscle tissue in the body?
   1. Rough muscle
   2. Skeletal muscle
   3. Smooth muscle
   4. Cardiac muscle
6. The body has approximately _____ muscles.
   1. 200
   2. 400
   3. 600
   4. 800
7. Which type of joint is freely moveable, allows many kinds of movements, and is found at all articulations of the limbs?
   1. Amphiarthroses
   2. Cartilaginous
   3. Fibrous
   4. Synovial

8. During a client assessment, which of the following instructions by the nurse assesses abduction?
    1. "Make a fist."
    2. "Open your hand."
    3. "Spread your fingers."
    4. "Close your fingers."
9. A lateral, S-shaped curvature of the spine is called:
    1. Lordosis
    2. Scoliosis
    3. Kyphosis
    4. Synovitis
10. Numbness and burning in the fingers during the _____ test may indicate carpal tunnel syndrome.
    1. Bulge
    2. Thomas
    3. Phalen's
    4. McMurray's

CHAPTER 41

NURSING CARE OF CLIENTS WITH MUSCULOSKELETAL TRAUMA

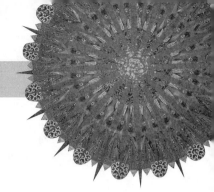

LEARNING OUTCOMES

After completing Chapter 41, you will be able to demonstrate the following objectives:

- Compare and contrast the causes, risk factors, pathophysiology, manifestations, interdisciplinary care, and nursing care of contusions, strains, sprains, joint dislocations, and fractures.
- Describe the stages of bone healing.
- Explain the pathophysiology, manifestations, and related treatment for complications of bone fractures: compartment syndrome, fat embolism syndrome, deep venous thrombosis, infection, delayed union and nonunion, and reflex sympathetic dystrophy.
- Discuss the purposes and related nursing interventions for casts, traction, and stump care.
- Explain the causes, levels, types, and potential complications (infection, delayed healing, chronic stump pain, phantom pain, and contractures) of an amputation.
- Describe the pathophysiology, interdisciplinary care, and nursing care for repetitive use injuries: carpal tunnel syndrome, bursitis, and epicondylitis.

CLINICAL COMPETENCIES

- Assess functional health status of clients with musculoskeletal injuries, and monitor, document, and report abnormal manifestations.
- Use evidence-based research to plan and implement nursing care for clients with skeletal pin sites.
- Determine priority nursing diagnoses, based on assessed data, to select and implement individualized nursing interventions for clients with musculoskeletal injuries.
- Provide skilled cast care, traction care, and stump care.

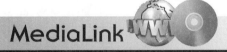

MediaLink

www.prenhall.com/lemone

Resources for this chapter can be found on the Prentice Hall Nursing MediaLink DVD accompanying this textbook, and on the Companion Website at http://www.prenhall.com/lemone. Click on Chapter 41 to select the activities for this chapter.

Prentice Hall Nursing MediaLink DVD-ROM
- Audio Glossary
- NCLEX-RN® Review

Animation/Video
- Bone Healing
- Crutch Instruction

Companion Website
www.prenhall.com/lemone
- Audio Glossary
- NCLEX-RN® Review
- Care Plan Activity: Below-the-Knee Amputation
- Case Study: A Client with Fractures
- MediaLink Applications
  - Compartment Syndrome
  - Preventing Musculoskeletal Injuries
- Links to Resources

- Integrate interdisciplinary care into care of clients with musculoskeletal trauma.
- Provide teaching appropriate for prevention and self-care of traumatic injuries of the musculoskeletal system.
- Revise plan of care as needed to provide effective interventions to promote, maintain, or restore functional health status to clients with traumatic injuries of the musculoskeletal system.

KEY TERMS

amputation	flail chest
bursitis	fracture
compartment syndrome	nonunion
contracture	phantom limb pain
contusion	sprain
dislocation	strain
fat embolism	subluxation
syndrome (FES)	Volkmann's contracture

CHAPTER OUTLINE

F. Fractures of Specific Bones or Bony Areas
1. Fracture of the Skull
2. Fracture of the Face
3. Fracture of the Spine
4. Fracture of the Clavicle
5. Fracture of the Humerus
6. Fracture of the Elbow
7. Fracture of the Radius and/or Ulna
8. Fractures in the Wrist and Hand
9. Fracture of the Ribs
10. Fracture of the Pelvis
11. Fracture of the Shaft of the Femur
12. Fracture of the Hip
13. Fracture of the Tibia and/or Fibula
14. Fracture in the Ankle and Foot
G. Nursing Care
1. Health Promotion
2. Assessment
3. Nursing Diagnoses and Interventions
a. Acute Pain
b. Risk for Peripheral Neurovascular Dysfunction
c. Risk for Infection
d. Impaired Physical Mobility
e. Risk for Disturbed Sensory Perception: Tactile
4. Using NANDA, NIC, and NOC
5. Community-Based Care
VI. The Client with an Amputation
A. Causes of Amputation
B. Levels of Amputation
C. Types of Amputation
D. Amputation Site Healing
E. Complications
1. Infection
2. Delayed Healing
3. Chronic Stump Pain and Phantom Pain
4. Contractures
F. Interdisciplinary Care
1. Diagnosis
2. Medications
3. Prosthesis
G. Nursing Care
1. Health Promotion
2. Assessment
3. Nursing Diagnoses and Interventions
a. Acute Pain
b. Risk for Infection
c. Risk for Impaired Skin Integrity
d. Risk for Dysfunctional Grieving
e. Disturbed Body Image
f. Impaired Physical Mobility
4. Using NANDA, NIC, and NOC
5. Community-Based Care

VII. The Client with a Repetitive Use Injury
    A. Pathophysiology
        1. Carpal Tunnel Syndrome
        2. Bursitis
        3. Epicondylitis
    B. Interdisciplinary Care
        1. Diagnosis
        2. Medications
        3. Treatments
    C. Nursing Care
        1. Nursing Diagnoses and Interventions
            a. Acute Pain
            b. Impaired Physical Mobility
        2. Community-Based Care

FOCUSED STUDY TIPS

1. Explain the interdisciplinary care and nursing care for repetitive use injuries: carpal tunnel syndrome, bursitis, and epicondylitis.

2. Describe the nursing interventions for casts, traction, and stump care.

3. Summarize the stages of bone healing.

4. List the potential complications (infection, delayed healing, chronic stump pain, phantom pain, and contractures) of an amputation.

CASE STUDY

Georgene Smith, a 12-year-old female client, presented at the clinic after experiencing an injury while ice skating. Georgene states that she heard her right knee "pop" after she landed from an axle jump. Her knee is swollen with slight discoloration. Her pain assessment score is 9 out of 10. Answer the following questions based on knowledge of sprains and strains.

1. Define strain and sprain.

2. Give examples of how a strain or sprain could occur.

3. What are the manifestations of a strain or a sprain?

4. Explain RICE therapy.

NCLEX REVIEW QUESTIONS

1. Which of the following statements about a strain is correct?
   1. The most common sites for a muscle strain are the wrist and ankle.
   2. The manifestations of a strain include pain, limited motion, muscle spasms, swelling, and possible muscle weakness.
   3. Severe strains that partially or completely tear the ligament are very painful and disabling.
   4. A strain is a stretch and/or tear of one or more ligaments that surround a joint.
2. What does the R in RICE therapy for musculoskeletal injuries mean?
   1. Rest
   2. Relax
   3. Raise
   4. Rub
3. A _____ is an injury of a joint in which the ends of bones are forced from their normal position.
   1. Dislocation
   2. Strain
   3. Sprain
   4. Fracture
4. Which of the following statements about fractures is correct?
   1. Fractures do not vary in severity.
   2. A fracture occurs when the bone is subjected to less kinetic energy than it can absorb.
   3. Not all of the 206 bones in the body can be fractured.
   4. Two basic mechanisms produce fractures: direct force and indirect force.
5. A nurse is evaluating a student's understanding of compartment syndrome. Which of the following statements by the student indicates a need for further teaching?
   1. "Compartment syndrome usually develops within the first 24 hours of injury, when edema is at its peak."
   2. "Compartment syndrome occurs when excess pressure in a limited space constricts the structures within a compartment, which reduces circulation to muscles and nerves."
   3. "Acute compartment syndrome may result from hemorrhage and edema within the compartment following a fracture or from a crush injury, or from external compression of the limb by a cast that is too tight."
   4. "Increased pressure within the confined space of the compartment results in entrapment of nerves, blood vessels, and muscles."
6. _____ traction is the application of a pulling force through placement of pins into the bone.
   1. Skin
   2. Skeletal
   3. Balanced suspension
   4. Manual

7. Which of the following statements by a student nurse reflects correct understanding about casts?
   1. "The cast is applied to immobilize the joint above and the joint below the fractured bone so that the bone will not move during healing."
   2. "A plaster cast may require up to 24 hours to dry; whereas a fiberglass cast dries in 2 hours."
   3. "Casts are applied on clients who have unstable fractures."
   4. "The cast must be allowed to partially dry before any pressure is applied to it."
8. During discharge planning, the nurse is teaching the client about cast care. Which of the following statements is incorrect?
   1. "Scratch under a cast with a dull object."
   2. "Do not get a plaster cast wet."
   3. "Elevate the injured extremity below the level of the heart."
   4. "Break off any rough edges on the cast."
9. All of the following guidelines may help preserve the amputated part until it can be surgically reattached except:
   1. Put the amputated part into direct contact with the ice or water.
   2. Apply firm pressure to the bleeding area with a towel or article of clothing.
   3. Send the amputated part to the emergency department with the injured person, and be sure the emergency personnel know what it is.
   4. Wrap the amputated part in a clean cloth.
10. Which of the following is a correct statement about fractures?
    1. An uncomplicated fracture of the arm or foot can heal in 3 to 4 weeks.
    2. A fractured vertebra will take at least 6 weeks to heal.
    3. Healing of a fractured hip may take from 8 to 10 weeks.
    4. The age, physical condition of the client, and the type of fracture sustained influence the healing of fractures.

CHAPTER 42

NURSING CARE OF CLIENTS WITH MUSCULOSKELETAL DISORDERS

LEARNING OUTCOMES

After completing Chapter 42, you will be able to demonstrate the following objectives:

- Explain the pathophysiology, manifestations, complications, interdisciplinary care, and nursing care of metabolic, degenerative, autoimmune, inflammatory, infectious, neoplastic, connective tissue, and structural musculoskeletal disorders.

- Compare and contrast the pathophysiology, manifestations, diagnosis, and treatments for osteoporosis, osteoarthritis, Paget's disease, and rheumatoid arthritis.

- Discuss the purposes, nursing implications, and health education for the client and family for medications used to treat osteoporosis, Paget's disease, gout, osteomalacia, osteoarthritis, rheumatoid arthritis, systemic lupus erythematosus, osteomyelitis, bone tumors, scleroderma, and low back pain.

- Describe the surgical procedures used to treat clients with arthritis.

CLINICAL COMPETENCIES

- Assess functional status of clients with musculoskeletal disorders, and monitor, document, and report abnormal manifestations.

- Use evidence-based research to assess clients at risk for osteoporosis and to evaluate the effectiveness of Internet use to teach older adults with rheumatoid arthritis.

- Determine priority nursing diagnoses, based on assessed data, to select and implement individualized nursing interventions for clients with musculoskeletal disorders.

- Administer topical, oral, and injectable medications used to treat musculoskeletal disorders knowledgeably and safely.

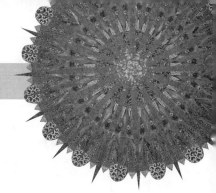

MediaLink

- Provide skilled care of clients having a surgical debridement for osteomyelitis and a total joint replacement.
- Integrate interdisciplinary care into care of clients with musculoskeletal disorders.
- Provide teaching appropriate for community-based self-care of musculoskeletal disorders.
- Revise plan of care as needed to provide effective interventions to promote, maintain, or restore functional health status to clients with musculoskeletal disorders.

KEY TERMS

ankylosing spondylitis
arthritis
fibromyalgia
gout
Lyme disease
muscular dystrophy (MD)
osteoarthritis (OA)
osteomalacia
osteomyelitis
osteoporosis
Paget's disease

polymyositis
reactive arthritis (ReA)
rheumatic disorders
rheumatoid arthritis (RA)
scleroderma
septic arthritis
Sjögren's syndrome
systemic lupus
    erythematosus (SLE)
tophi

CHAPTER OUTLINE

E. Nursing Care
  1. Nursing Diagnoses and Interventions
     a. Chronic Pain
     b. Impaired Physical Mobility
  2. Community-Based Care
IV. The Client with Gout
  A. Pathophysiology
  B. Manifestations
     1. Asymptomatic Hyperuricemia
     2. Acute Gouty Arthritis
     3. Tophaceous (Chronic) Gout
  C. Complications
  D. Interdisciplinary Care
     1. Diagnosis
     2. Medications
  E. Complementary and Alternative Therapy
  F. Treatments
  G. Nursing Care
     1. Nursing Diagnoses and Interventions
        a. Acute Pain
     2. Community-Based Care
V. The Client with Osteomalacia
  A. Pathophysiology
  B. Manifestations
  C. Interdisciplinary Care
     1. Diagnosis
     2. Medications
  D. Nursing Care
VI. Degenerative Disorders
VII. The Client with Osteoarthritis
  A. Risk Factors
  B. Pathophysiology
  C. Manifestations
  D. Complications
  E. Interdisciplinary Care
     1. Diagnosis
     2. Medications
     3. Treatments
  F. Nursing Care
     1. Health Promotion
     2. Assessment
     3. Nursing Diagnoses and Interventions
        a. Chronic Pain
        b. Impaired Physical Mobility
        c. Self-Care Deficit
     4. Using NANDA, NIC, and NOC
     5. Community-Based Care
VIII. The Client with Muscular Dystrophy
  A. Pathophysiology
  B. Manifestations
  C. Interdisciplinary Care
  D. Nursing Care
     1. Nursing Diagnoses and Interventions
        a. Self-Care Deficit
     2. Community-Based Care

XVII. The Client with Osteomyelitis
    A. Pathophysiology
        1. Hematogenous Osteomyelitis
        2. Osteomyelitis from a Contiguous Infection
        3. Osteomyelitis Associated with Vascular Insufficiency
    B. Manifestations
    C. Interdisciplinary Care
        1. Diagnosis
        2. Medications
        3. Surgery
    D. Nursing Care
        1. Nursing Diagnoses and Interventions
            a. Risk for Infection
            b. Hyperthermia
            c. Impaired Physical Mobility
            d. Acute Pain
        2. Community-Based Care
XVIII. The Client with Septic Arthritis
    A. Pathophysiology
    B. Manifestations
    C. Interdisciplinary Care
    D. Nursing Care
  XIX. Neoplastic Disorders
  XX. The Client with Bone Tumors
    A. Pathophysiology
    B. Manifestations
    C. Interdisciplinary Care
        1. Diagnosis
        2. Treatments
    D. Nursing Care
        1. Nursing Diagnosis and Interventions
            a. Risk for Injury
            b. Acute Pain, Chronic Pain
            c. Impaired Physical Mobility
            d. Decisional Conflict
        2. Community-Based Care
  XXI. Connective Tissue Disorders
XXII. The Client with Systemic Sclerosis (Scleroderma)
    A. Pathophysiology
    B. Manifestations
    C. Interdisciplinary Care
        1. Diagnosis
        2. Medications
        3. Physical Therapy
    D. Nursing Care
        1. Nursing Interventions
        2. Community-Based Care
XXIII. The Client with Sjögren's Syndrome
    A. Pathophysiology
    B. Interdisciplinary Care
    C. Nursing Care
XXIV. The Client with Fibromyalgia
    A. Pathophysiology
    B. Manifestations
    C. Interdisciplinary Care
    D. Nursing Care

XXV. Structural Disorders
XXVI. The Client with Spinal Deformities
    A. Pathophysiology
        1. Scoliosis
        2. Kyphosis
    B. Interdisciplinary Care
        1. Diagnosis
        2. Treatments
    C. Nursing Care
        1. Nursing Diagnoses and Interventions
            a. Risk for Injury
            b. Risk for Peripheral Neurovascular Dysfunction
        2. Community-Based Care
XXVII. The Client with Low Back Pain
    A. Pathophysiology
    B. Manifestations
    C. Interdisciplinary Care
        1. Diagnosis
        2. Medications
        3. Conservative Treatment
    D. Nursing Care
        1. Health Promotion
        2. Nursing Diagnoses and Interventions
            a. Acute Pain
            b. Deficient Knowledge
            c. Risk for Impaired Adjustment
        3. Community-Based Care
XXVIII. The Client with Common Foot Disorders
    A. Pathophysiology
        1. Hallux Valgus
        2. Hammertoe
        3. Morton's Neuroma
    B. Interdisciplinary Care
    C. Nursing Care
        1. Nursing Diagnoses and Interventions
            a. Chronic Pain
            b. Risk for Infection
        2. Community-Based Care

FOCUSED STUDY TIPS

1. Discuss the surgical procedures used to treat clients with arthritis.

_____

_____

_____

2. Summarize the treatments for osteoporosis, osteoarthritis, Paget's disease, and rheumatoid arthritis.

_____

_____

_____

_____

_____

3. Describe the health education for the client and family for medications used to treat osteoporosis, Paget's disease, gout, osteomalacia, osteoarthritis, rheumatoid arthritis, systemic lupus erythematosus, osteomyelitis, bone tumors, scleroderma, and low back pain.

_____

_____

_____

_____

_____

_____

_____

_____

_____

_____

4. List the manifestations and complications of metabolic, degenerative, autoimmune, inflammatory, infectious, neoplastic, connective tissue, and structural musculoskeletal disorders.

_____

_____

_____

_____

_____

_____

_____

_____

_____

CASE STUDY

Christine Scott is a 37-year-old client in today for her yearly physical. She tells the nurse that her mother was diagnosed with osteoporosis two weeks ago. Christine then asks the following questions:

1. "What are the unmodifiable risk factors for osteoporosis?"

2. "What are the modifiable risk factors for osteoporosis?"

3. "What are the most common signs and symptoms of osteoporosis?"

4. "Are there complications of osteoporosis?"

CARE PLAN CRITICAL THINKING ACTIVITY

1. Ms. James is diagnosed with rheumatoid arthritis at age 42. At what age does rheumatoid arthritis typically occur?

2. List the causes of rheumatoid arthritis.

3. Where can Ms. James obtain information about rheumatoid arthritis?

NCLEX REVIEW QUESTIONS

1. During discharge planning, the nurse is teaching the client about osteoporosis. Which of the following statements is correct?
    1. Vitamin D deficiency is an important modifiable risk factor that contributes to osteoporosis.
    2. The most common manifestations of osteoporosis are loss of height, progressive curvature of the spine, low back pain, and fractures of the forearm, spine, or hip.
    3. Fractures are not the most common complication of osteoporosis.
    4. Osteoporosis is not preventable or treatable.
2. Which of the following is not a food source of calcium?
    1. Sardines
    2. Collard greens
    3. Clams
    4. Carrots
3. Which of the following statements by a student nurse reflects correct understanding about Paget's disease?
    1. "The most common manifestation in Paget's disease is localized pain of the short bones."
    2. "Paget's disease is a progressive metabolic skeletal disorder of the osteoclast that results from excessive metabolic activity in bone, with excessive bone resorption followed by excessive bone formation."
    3. "The bones decrease in size and thickness in Paget's disease."
    4. "Paget's disease is also called osteoporosis."
4. A nurse is evaluating a nursing student's understanding of gout. Which of the following statements by the nursing student indicates a need for further teaching?
    1. "Over time, urate deposits in subcutaneous tissues cause the formation of small white nodules called tophi."
    2. "Gout has an acute onset, usually at night, and often involves the fifth metatarsophalangeal joint."
    3. "Kidney disease may occur in clients with untreated gout, particularly when hypertension is also present."
    4. "Serum uric acid is nearly always elevated (usually above 7.5 mg/dL)."
5. A nurse is planning a seminar about osteomalacia. Which of the following statements on a handout needs to be corrected?
    1. Osteomalacia may be difficult to differentiate from osteoporosis because the manifestations are very similar.
    2. The manifestations of osteomalacia include bone pain and tenderness.
    3. The primary causes of osteomalacia are calcium deficiency and hyperphosphatemia.
    4. Osteomalacia is a metabolic bone disorder characterized by inadequate or delayed mineralization of bone matrix in mature compact and spongy bone, which results in softening of bones.
6. A nurse is evaluating a nursing student's understanding of osteoarthritis. Which of the following statements by the nursing student demonstrates a need for further teaching?
    1. "The onset of osteoarthritis is usually gradual and insidious, and the course is slowly progressive."
    2. "Osteoarthritis is the most common of all forms of arthritis, and is a leading cause of pain and disability in older adults."
    3. "The onset of osteoarthritis is usually gradual and insidious."
    4. "Women are affected more than men and at an earlier age, but the rate of osteoarthritis in men exceeds women by the middle adult years."
7. Which of the following is not a manifestation of systemic lupus erythematosus (SLE)?
    1. Unexplained fever
    2. White skin discoloration, especially on the face
    3. Extreme fatigue
    4. Painful or swollen joints
8. Hallux valgus, commonly called a_____, is the enlargement and lateral displacement of the first metatarsal (the great toe).
    1. Bunion
    2. Hammertoe
    3. Claw toe
    4. Morton's neuroma

9. Which of the following is a lateral curvature of the spine?
   1. Scoliosis
   2. Kyphosis
   3. Hunchback
   4. Lordosis
10. _____ is a common rheumatic syndrome characterized by musculoskeletal pain, stiffness, and tenderness.
    1. Osteomyelitis
    2. Fibromyalgia
    3. Polymyositis
    4. Sjögren's syndrome

CHAPTER 43

ASSESSING CLIENTS WITH NEUROLOGIC DISORDERS

LEARNING OUTCOMES

After completing Chapter 43, you will be able to demonstrate the following objectives:

- Describe the anatomy, physiology, and functions of the nervous system.
- Identify specific topics for consideration during a health history assessment interview of the client with neurologic disorders.
- Explain techniques for assessment of neurologic function, including examinations of mental status, cranial nerves, sensory nerves, motor nerves, cerebellar function, and reflexes.
- Identify manifestations of impairment of neurologic function.
- Describe normal variations in assessment findings for the older adult.

CLINICAL COMPETENCIES

- Conduct and document a health history for clients having or at risk for alterations in the neurologic system.
- Conduct and document a physical assessment of neurologic structures and functions.
- Perform specific neurologic assessments for clients with suspected meningeal irritation and for disoriented or comatose clients.
- Monitor the results of diagnostic tests and report abnormal findings.

EQUIPMENT NEEDED

- Cotton balls
- Safety pin
- Tongue depressor
- Tuning fork
- Reflex hammer

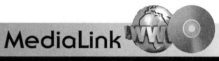

- Pencil and paper
- Penlight
- Printed materials
- Substances to test the senses of smell and taste

KEY TERMS

anosmia
aphasia
ataxia
decerebrate posturing
decorticate posturing
diaphoresis
dysarthria
dysphagia

dysphonia
fasciculations
flaccidity
kinesthesia
nystagmus
ptosis
spasticity
tremors

CHAPTER OUTLINE

I. Anatomy, Physiology, and Functions of the Nervous System
  A. Nerve Cells, Action Potentials, and Neurotransmitters
    1. Neurons
    2. Action Potentials
    3. Neurotransmitters
  B. The Central Nervous System
    1. The Brain
    2. The Spinal Cord
  C. The Peripheral Nervous System
    1. Spinal Nerves
    2. Cranial Nerves
    3. Reflexes
  D. The Autonomic Nervous System
    1. Sympathetic Division
    2. Parasympathetic Division
II. Assessing Neurologic Function
  A. Diagnostic Tests
  B. Genetic Considerations
  C. Health Assessment Interview
  D. Physical Assessment
  E. Neurologic Assessments
  F. Reflex Assessments
  G. Special Neurologic Assessments

FOCUSED STUDY TIPS

1. List manifestations of impairment of neurologic function.

_____

_____

_____

_____

_____

2. Summarize the assessment of neurologic function.

_____

_____

_____

_____

3. List specific topics to consider during a health history assessment interview of the client with neurologic disorders.

_____

_____

_____

_____

_____

4. Discuss the anatomy, physiology, and functions of the nervous system.

_____

_____

_____

_____

_____

_____

CASE STUDY

James Smith is a new nursing student who is attending a seminar about the central nervous system today. At the end of the seminar he asks the following questions:

1. "What are the four major regions of the brain?"

2. "What does the brainstem consist of?"

3. "What protects and surrounds the spinal cord?"

4. "How many pairs of spinal nerves are there and where are they located?"

NCLEX REVIEW QUESTIONS

1. Which of the following is not a part of a neuron?
   1. Dendrite
   2. Cell body
   3. Axon
   4. Nucleus
2. Which of the following statements by a student nurse reflects correct understanding about neurons?
   1. "The dendrite is a short process from the cell body that conducts impulses away (efferent) from the cell body."
   2. "Many axons are covered with a myelin sheath, which is a gray thick substance."
   3. "Cell bodies, most of which are located within the CNS, are clustered in ganglia or nuclei."
   4. "The myelin sheath serves to decrease the speed of nerve impulse conduction in axons and is essential for the survival of larger nerve processes."

3. Which of the following statements about neurotransmitters is false?
   1. The neurotransmitter may either be inhibitory or excitatory.
   2. The inhibitory neurotransmitter is almost always acetylcholine (ACh).
   3. Norepinephrine (NE), which may be either excitatory or inhibitory, is another major neurotransmitter.
   4. Neurotransmitters are the chemical messengers of the nervous system.
4. A nurse is evaluating a client's understanding of the brain. Which of the following statements by the client indicates a need for further teaching?
   1. The brain is the control center of the nervous system and also generates thoughts, emotions, and speech.
   2. The brain weighs an average of 24 to 36 ounces.
   3. The brain has four major regions: the cerebrum, the diencephalon, the brainstem, and the cerebellum.
   4. The brain is surrounded by the skull.
5. Which of the following is not part of the brainstem?
   1. Midbrain
   2. Pons
   3. Medulla oblongata
   4. Ventricles
6. The brain contains _____ ventricles, which are chambers filled with cerebrospinal fluid (CSF).
   1. Two
   2. Three
   3. Four
   4. Five
7. Which statement about cerebrospinal fluid (CSF) is false?
   1. Cerebrospinal fluid is a clear and colorless liquid.
   2. Cerebrospinal fluid is formed by the choroid plexus, which are groups of specialized capillaries located in the brain ventricles.
   3. The usual amount of cerebrospinal fluid ranges from 20 to 80 mL, and averages about 40 mL,
   4. Cerebrospinal fluid is normally produced and absorbed in equal amounts.
8. Which metabolic factor does not affect cerebral blood flow?
   1. Carbon dioxide
   2. Hydrogen ion
   3. Oxygen concentrations
   4. Potassium
9. The spinal cord is surrounded and protected by _____ vertebrae.
   1. 13
   2. 23
   3. 33
   4. 43
10. During a client assessment, the nurse notes that the client can smile, frown, wrinkle forehead, show teeth, puff out cheek, purse lips, raise eyebrows, and close eyes against resistance. Which cranial nerve is the nurse assessing?
    1. II
    2. III
    3. V
    4. VII

CHAPTER 44

NURSING CARE OF CLIENTS WITH INTRACRANIAL DISORDERS

LEARNING OUTCOMES

After completing Chapter 44, you will be able to demonstrate the following objectives:

- Compare and contrast the pathophysiology, manifestations, interdisciplinary care, and nursing care of clients with alterations in level of consciousness and increased intracranial pressure.
- Explain the pathophysiology, manifestations, complications, interdisciplinary care, and nursing care of intracranial disorders, including headaches, epilepsy, traumatic brain injury, central nervous system infections, and brain tumors.
- Describe criteria for diagnosing persistent vegetative state and brain death.
- Discuss the purposes, nursing implications, and health education for the client and family for medications used to treat altered cerebral function, headaches, epilepsy, traumatic brain injury, central nervous system infections, and brain tumors.
- Discuss surgical options for the treatment of increased intracranial pressure, epilepsy, traumatic brain injury, and brain tumors.

CLINICAL COMPETENCIES

- Assess functional status of clients with intracranial disorders and monitor, document, and report abnormal manifestations.
- Determine priority nursing diagnoses, based on assessed data, to select and implement individualized nursing interventions for clients with intracranial disorders.
- Administer oral and injectable medications used to treat intracranial disorders knowledgeably and safely.
- Provide skilled care to clients having intracranial pressure monitoring, tonic-clonic seizures, and intracranial surgery.
- Integrate interdisciplinary care into care of clients with intracranial disorders.

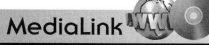

MediaLink

www.prenhall.com/lemone

Resources for this chapter can be found on the Prentice Hall Nursing MediaLink DVD accompanying this textbook, and on the Companion Website at http://www.prenhall.com/lemone. Click on Chapter 44 to select the activities for this chapter.

Prentice Hall Nursing MediaLink DVD-ROM
- Audio Glossary
- NCLEX-RN® Review

Animations
- Complex Seizure
- Coup-Contrecoup Injury
- Epilepsy
- Grand Mal Seizure

Companion Website
www.prenhall.com/lemone
- Audio Glossary
- NCLEX-RN® Review
- Care Plan Activity: Subdural Hematoma
- Case Study: Bacterial Meningitis
- MediaLink Applications
  - Meningitis Prevention
  - Paralysis
- Links to Resources

- Provide appropriate teaching and evidence-based practice to facilitate community-based care to promote safety and prevent injury, and to provide information and support necessary for long-term care of clients with intracranial disorders.
- Revise plan of care as needed to provide effective interventions to promote, maintain, or restore functional health status to clients with intracranial disorders.

KEY TERMS

brain death
cerebral edema
concussion
consciousness
encephalitis
epidural hematoma
epilepsy
hydrocephalus

increased intracranial
    pressure (IICP)
locked-in syndrome
meningitis
persistent vegetative state
seizures
subdural hematoma
traumatic brain injury (TBI)

CHAPTER OUTLINE

I. Altered Cerebral Function
II. The Client with Altered Level of Consciousness
   A. Pathophysiology
      1. Arousal and Cognition
      2. Patterns of Respirations
      3. Pupillary and Oculomotor Responses
      4. Motor Responses
      5. Coma States and Brain Death
   B. Prognosis
   C. Interdisciplinary Care
      1. Diagnosis
      2. Medications
      3. Surgery
      4. Other Treatments
      5. Nutrition
   D. Nursing Care
      1. Support of the Family
      2. Nursing Diagnoses and Interventions
         a. Ineffective Airway Clearance
         b. Risk for Aspiration
         c. Risk for Impaired Skin Integrity
         d. Impaired Physical Mobility
         e. Risk for Imbalanced Nutrition: Less than Body Requirements
III. The Client with Increased Intracranial Pressure
   A. Pathophysiology
   B. Manifestations
      1. Level of Consciousness
      2. Motor Responses
      3. Vision and Pupils
      4. Vital Signs
      5. Other Manifestations
   C. Cerebral Edema
   D. Hydrocephalus
   E. Brain Herniation
   F. Interdisciplinary Care
      1. Diagnosis
      2. Medications

1. Focal Brain Injuries
2. Diffuse Brain Injury
   B. Interdisciplinary Care
   1. Diagnosis
   2. Managing IICP
   3. Surgery
   C. Nursing Care
   1. Health Promotion
   2. Assessment
   3. Nursing Diagnoses and Interventions
      a. Decreased Intracranial Adaptive Capacity
      b. Ineffective Airway Clearance
      c. Ineffective Breathing Pattern
   4. Using NANDA, NIC, and NOC
   5. Community-Based Care
      a. Concussion
      b. Acute Brain Injury
IX. Central Nervous System Infections
X. The Client with a Central Nervous System Infection
   A. Pathophysiology
   1. Meningitis
   2. Encephalitis
   3. Brain Abscess
   B. Interdisciplinary Care
   1. Diagnosis
   2. Medications
   3. Surgery
   C. Nursing Care
   1. Health Promotion
   2. Assessment
   3. Nursing Diagnoses and Interventions
      a. Ineffective Protection
      b. Risk for Deficient Fluid Volume
   4. Using NANDA, NIC, and NOC
   5. Community-Based Care
XI. Tumors of the Brain
XII. The Client with a Brain Tumor
   A. Incidence and Prevalence
   B. Pathophysiology
   C. Manifestations
   D. Interdisciplinary Care
   1. Diagnosis
   2. Medications
   3. Surgery
   4. Radiation Therapy
   5. Specialty Procedures
   E. Nursing Care
   1. Nursing Diagnoses and Interventions
      a. Anxiety
      b. Risk for Infection
      c. Ineffective Protection
      d. Acute Pain
      e. Situational Low Self-Esteem
   2. Using NANDA, NIC, and NOC
   3. Community-Based Care

FOCUSED STUDY TIPS

1. Summarize the surgical options for the treatment of increased intracranial pressure, epilepsy, and brain tumors.

   _____

   _____

   _____

   _____

   _____

2. Discuss the interdisciplinary care and nursing care of clients with alterations in level of consciousness and increased intracranial pressure.

   _____

   _____

   _____

   _____

3. Discuss the nursing implications for the client with altered cerebral function, headaches, epilepsy, traumatic brain injury, central nervous system infections, and brain tumors.

   _____

   _____

   _____

   _____

   _____

4. Describe criteria for diagnosing persistent vegetative state and brain death.

   _____

   _____

   _____

CASE STUDY

Joshua Hacking is a 9-year-old male client in the clinic. His mother Michelle tells the nurse that he has been complaining of a headache, nasal congestion, and nausea. Joshua states, "I'm seeing those bright spots again." Answer the following questions based on knowledge of migraines.

1. Explain the stages of a classic migraine.

2. What factors are believed to trigger an onset of a migraine?

3. Discuss the therapeutic management of migraines.

CARE PLAN CRITICAL THINKING ACTIVITY

1. What are the manifestations of seizures?

2. List and define the types of seizures.

3. Explain the nursing care to be given to a client who is experiencing a seizure.

NCLEX REVIEW QUESTIONS

1. With compression of cranial nerve _____ at the midbrain, the pupils may become oval or eccentric (off center).
   1. I
   2. II
   3. III
   4. IV
2. Doll's eye movements are reflexive movements of the eyes in the _____ direction of head rotation.
   1. Opposite
   2. Parallel
   3. Same
   4. Identical
3. Which of the following statements by a student nurse reflects correct understanding about brain death?
   1. "Brain death is the cessation and irreversibility of all brain functions, including the brainstem."
   2. "The exact criteria for establishing brain death does not vary from state to state."
   3. "The electrocardiogram (ECG) may be used to establish the absence of cardiac activity when brain death is suspected."
   4. "It is generally agreed that brain death has occurred when there is no evidence of cerebral or brainstem function for an extended period (usually 48 to 72 hours) in a client who has an abnormal body temperature and is not affected by a depressant drug or alcohol poisoning."
4. Cerebral edema _____ ICP, which in turn _____ cerebral blood flow.
   1. Increases, decreases
   2. Decreases, increases
   3. Increases, increases
   4. Decreases, decreases
5. A nurse is planning a seminar about headaches. Which of the following statements on a handout for the seminar needs to be corrected?
   1. Tension headache is characterized by bilateral pain, with a sensation of a band of tightness or pressure around the head.
   2. There are two types of migraine headaches: common migraine (with an aura) and classic migraine (without an aura).
   3. Migraine headache is a recurring vascular headache that lasts from 4 to 72 hours, often initiated by a triggering event and usually accompanied by a neurologic dysfunction.
   4. A cluster headache is an extremely severe, unilateral, burning pain located behind or around the eyes.
6. The nurse is providing first aid to a client who is having a seizure. Which of the following actions by the nurse is incorrect?
   1. Turn the client on his side.
   2. Cushion the client's head.
   3. Place a tongue blade in the client's mouth.
   4. Loosen items around the client's neck.
7. During discharge planning, the nurse is teaching the client's spouse about when she needs to call for medical assistance when her husband is having a seizure. Which of the following actions is incorrect?
   1. If the seizure lasts for less than 4 minutes.
   2. There is slow recovery from the seizure.
   3. There is a second seizure.
   4. There are signs of injury.

8. Which of the following information about hematomas is false?
    1. An epidural hematoma (also called an extradural hematoma) develops in the potential space between the dura and the skull, which normally adhere to one another.
    2. Acute subdural hematomas develop over weeks or months.
    3. Subdural hematoma is a localized mass of blood that collects between the dura mater and the arachnoid mater.
    4. Intracerebral hematomas may be single or multiple, and are associated with contusions.
9. Meningitis is an inflammation of all the following except:
    1. Dura mater.
    2. Pia mater.
    3. Arachnoid.
    4. Subarachnoid space.
10. During discharge planning, the nurse is teaching the client how to decrease incidents of migraine headaches. Which of the following suggestions is incorrect?
    1. Wake up at the same time each morning.
    2. No artificial sweeteners.
    3. No MSG (monosodium glutamate).
    4. Consume a food source or beverage with caffeine before 6 p.m.

CHAPTER 45

NURSING CARE OF CLIENTS WITH CEREBROVASCULAR AND SPINAL CORD DISORDERS

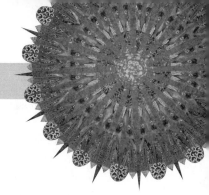

MediaLink

www.prenhall.com/lemone

Resources for this chapter can be found on the Prentice Hall Nursing MediaLink DVD accompanying this textbook, and on the Companion Website at http://www.prenhall.com/lemone. Click on Chapter 45 to select the activities for this chapter.

Prentice Hall Nursing MediaLink DVD-ROM
- Audio Glossary
- NCLEX-RN® Review

Companion Website
www.prenhall.com/lemone
- Audio Glossary
- NCLEX-RN® Review
- Care Plan Activity: Hemorrhagic Stroke
- Case Study: Spinal Cord Injury
- MediaLink Applications
  - Intracranial Pressure
  - Spinal Cord Injury
  - Stroke
  - Stroke Lifestyle Changes
- Links to Resources

LEARNING OUTCOMES

After completing Chapter 45, you will be able to demonstrate the following objectives:
- Identify prevalence, incidence, and risk factors responsible for disorders of cerebral blood flow and spinal cord structure and function.
- Explain the pathophysiology, manifestations, complications, interdisciplinary care, and nursing care of clients with stroke, ruptured intracranial aneurysm, arteriovenous malformation, spinal cord injury, herniated intervertebral disk, and spinal cord tumor.
- Compare and contrast the acute treatment and care of the client with a stroke or ruptured intracranial aneurysm and spinal cord injury.
- Discuss the pathophysiologic effects of injuries and tumors of the spinal cord by level of injury.
- Discuss the purposes, nursing implications, and health education for the client and family for medications used to treat stroke, ruptured intracranial aneurysm, and spinal cord injury.
- Describe the methods used to stabilize and immobilize spinal cord injuries.
- Describe the surgical procedures used to treat cerebrovascular and spinal cord disorders.

CLINICAL COMPETENCIES

- Assess functional status of clients with cerebrovascular and spinal cord disorders, and monitor, document, and report abnormal manifestations.
- Use evidence-based research to promote early recognition and treatment of the warning signs of a stroke.
- Determine priority nursing diagnoses, based on assessed data, to select and implement individualized nursing interventions for clients with cerebrovascular and spinal cord disorders.

- Administer oral and injectable medications used to treat cerebrovascular and spinal cord disorders knowledgeably and safely.
- Provide skilled care to clients having a carotid endarterectomy, halo fixation, or a posterior laminectomy.
- Integrate interdisciplinary care into care of clients with cerebrovascular and spinal cord disorders.
- Provide appropriate teaching to facilitate self-catheterization, self-care of a ruptured intervertebral disk, and community-based self-care of disabilities resulting from cerebrovascular and spinal cord disorders.
- Revise plan of care as needed to provide effective interventions to promote, maintain, or restore functional health status to clients with cerebrovascular and spinal cord disorders.

KEY TERMS

agnosia	neglect syndrome
aphasia	paraplegia
apraxia	quadriplegia
autonomic dysreflexia	sciatica
contralateral deficit	spasticity
flaccidity	spinal cord injury (SCI)
hemianopia	spinal shock
hemiparesis	stroke
hemiplegia	transient ischemic
hydrocephalus	attack (TIA)

CHAPTER OUTLINE

I. Cerebrovascular Disorders
II. The Client with a Stroke
  A. Incidence and Prevalence
  B. Risk Factors
  C. Pathophysiology
    1. Ischemic Stroke
    2. Hemorrhagic Stroke
  D. Manifestations
  E. Complications
    1. Sensoriperceptual Deficits
    2. Cognitive and Behavioral Changes
    3. Communication Disorders
    4. Motor Deficits
    5. Elimination Disorders
  F. Interdisciplinary Care
    1. Diagnosis
    2. Medications
    3. Treatments
  G. Nursing Care
    1. Health Promotion
    2. Assessment
    3. Nursing Diagnoses and Interventions
      a. Ineffective Tissue Perfusion: Cerebral
      b. Impaired Physical Mobility
      c. Self-Care Deficit
      d. Impaired Verbal Communication
      e. Impaired Urinary Elimination and Risk for Constipation
      f. Impaired Swallowing
    4. Using NANDA, NIC, and NOC
    5. Community-Based Care

III. The Client with an Intracranial Aneurysm
    A. Incidence and Prevalence
    B. Pathophysiology
    C. Manifestations
    D. Complications
       1. Rebleeding
       2. Vasospasm
       3. Hydrocephalus
    E. Interdisciplinary Care
       1. Diagnosis
       2. Medications
       3. Procedures Used to Treat Aneurysm
    F. Nursing Care
       1. Nursing Diagnoses and Interventions
          a. Ineffective Tissue Perfusion: Cerebral

IV. The Client with an Arteriovenous Malformation
    A. Pathophysiology
    B. Interdisciplinary Care
    C. Nursing Care

V. Spinal Cord Disorders

VI. The Client with a Spinal Cord Injury
    A. Incidence and Prevalence
    B. Risk Factors
    C. Pathophysiology
       1. Forces Resulting in SCI
       2. Sites of Pathology
       3. Classification of SCI
    D. Manifestations
    E. Complications
       1. Upper and Lower Motor Neuron Deficits
       2. Paraplegia and Quadriplegia
       3. Autonomic Dysreflexia
    F. Interdisciplinary Care
       1. Emergency Care
       2. Diagnosis
       3. Medications
       4. Treatments
    G. Nursing Care
       1. Health Promotion
       2. Assessment
       3. Nursing Diagnoses and Interventions
          a. Impaired Physical Mobility
          b. Impaired Gas Exchange
          c. Ineffective Breathing Patterns
          d. Dysreflexia
          e. Impaired Urinary Elimination and Constipation
          f. Sexual Dysfunction
          g. Low Self-Esteem
       4. Using NANDA, NIC, and NOC
       5. Community-Based Care

VII. The Client with a Herniated Intervertebral Disk
    A. Incidence and Prevalence
    B. Pathophysiology
    C. Lumbar Disk Manifestations
    D. Cervical Disk Manifestations

    E. Interdisciplinary Care
       1. Diagnosis
       2. Medications
       3. Treatments
    F. Nursing Care
       1. Health Promotion
       2. Assessment
       3. Nursing Diagnoses and Interventions
         a. Acute Pain
         b. Chronic Pain
         c. Constipation
       4. Community-Based Care
VIII. The Client with a Spinal Cord Tumor
    A. Classification
    B. Pathophysiology
    C. Manifestations
    D. Interdisciplinary Care
       1. Diagnosis
       2. Medications
       3. Surgery
       4. Radiation Therapy
    E. Nursing Care

FOCUSED STUDY TIPS

1. Summarize the surgical procedures used to treat cerebrovascular and spinal cord disorders.

2. Discuss the acute treatment and care of the client with a stroke, ruptured intracranial aneurysm, and spinal cord injury.

3. Explain the methods used to stabilize and immobilize spinal cord injuries.

4. Identify the risk factors responsible for disorders of cerebral blood flow and spinal cord structure and function.

CASE STUDY

Jonathan Baldwin is a 63-year-old client who experienced a stroke last night. His daughter Anne asks the nurse the following questions:

1. "What is a stroke?"

2. "What type of complications can occur from a stroke?"

3. "What are the manifestations of a stroke?"

NCLEX REVIEW QUESTIONS

1. Which of the following is not another name or abbreviation used to mean stroke?
   1. Cerebral vascular accident
   2. CVA
   3. Brain attack
   4. Heart attack
2. A (an) _____ stroke results from blockage of a cerebral artery, which decreases or stops blood flow and ultimately causes a brain infarction.
   1. Embolic
   2. Thrombotic
   3. Ischemic
   4. Hemorrhagic
3. _____ is a sensory speech problem in which one cannot understand the spoken (and often written) word.
   1. Receptive aphasia
   2. Dysarthria
   3. Expressive aphasia
   4. Broca's aphasia
4. The Hunt-Hess classification of subarachnoid manifestations is frequently used to classify nontraumatic subarachnoid hemorrhages. Which of the following grades includes a moderate to severe headache, neck rigidity, and cranial nerve deficits?
   1. Grade 1
   2. Grade 2
   3. Grade 3
   4. Grade 4
5. A nurse is instituting aneurysm precautions to prevent rebleeding on the client. Which action by the nurse is correct?
   1. Keep the client in an active, well-lit room.
   2. Allow visitors to visit at any time.
   3. Prevent the client from having constipation and straining to have a bowel movement.
   4. Does not elevate the head of the bed.
6. A nurse is planning a seminar about spinal cord injuries (SCI). Which of the following statements on a handout for the seminar needs to be corrected?
   1. The three major risk factors for SCIs are age, gender, and alcohol or drug abuse.
   2. The major causes of SCI are contusion, laceration, transection, hemorrhage, and damage to blood vessels that supply the spinal cord.
   3. Although SCIs occur in people of all ages, they are most often seen in adults age 35 to 45.
   4. The most common cause of abnormal spinal column movements are acceleration and deceleration.

7. _____ is paralysis of the lower portion of the body, which sometimes involves the lower trunk.
   1. Autonomic dysreflexia
   2. Paraplegia
   3. Quadriplegia
   4. Tetraplegia
8. Guidelines for emergency care for a client who sustained trauma to the head or spine includes all of the following except:
   1. Avoid flexing, extending, or rotating the neck.
   2. Immobilize the neck, using rolled towels or blankets, or apply a cervical collar before moving the client onto a backboard.
   3. Secure the head by placing a belt or tape across the forehead and securing it to the stretcher.
   4. Maintain the client in the prone position.
9. A bowel retraining program includes the following actions except:
   1. Maintain a low-fluid, low-fiber diet.
   2. Maintain upright position if at all possible and ensure privacy.
   3. Use stool softeners as prescribed.
   4. Rectal suppositories and enemas may be used 30 minutes after meals to stimulate stronger peristalsis and facilitate evacuation.
10. Which of the following statements by a client reflects correct understanding about a herniated intervertebral disk?
    1. "A herniated intervertebral disk is also called a ruptured disk, herniated nucleus pulposus, or a slipped disk."
    2. "A herniated intervertebral disk only occurs in adults."
    3. "The intervertebral disks, located between the vertebral bodies, are made of an outer nucleus pulposus and an inner collar."
    4. "The herniation only occurs gradually."

CHAPTER 46

Nursing Care of Clients with Neurologic Disorders

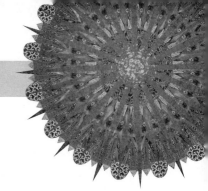
LEARNING OUTCOMES

After completing Chapter 46, you will be able to demonstrate the following objectives:
- Identify prevalence, incidence, and risk factors for degenerative neurologic, peripheral nervous system, cranial nerve, infection- and neurotoxin-caused neurologic disorders.
- Explain the pathophysiology, manifestations, complications, interdisciplinary care, and nursing care of clients with neurologic disorders.
- Compare and contrast the manifestations of the progressive stages of Alzheimer's disease.
- Discuss the purposes, nursing implications, and health education for the client and family for medications used to treat Alzheimer's disease, multiple sclerosis, Parkinson's disease, and myasthenia gravis.
- Describe the procedures (thymectomy, percutaneous rhizotomy, plasmapheresis) used to treat selected neurologic disorders.

CLINICAL COMPETENCIES

- Assess functional status of clients with neurologic disorders, and monitor, document, and report abnormal manifestations.
- Use evidence-based research to design nursing interventions specific to the needs of aging clients with multiple sclerosis.
- Determine priority nursing diagnoses, based on assessed data, to select and implement individualized nursing interventions for clients with neurologic disorders.
- Administer oral and injectable medications used to treat neurologic disorders knowledgeably and safely.
- Provide skilled care to clients having a thymectomy, percutaneous rhizotomy, or plasmapheresis.

- Integrate interdisciplinary care into care of clients with neurologic disorders.
- Provide appropriate teaching to facilitate safety and communication, prevent neurologic infections and toxins (rabies, tetanus, and botulism), and facilitate community-based acute and chronic self-care for healthcare needs resulting from neurologic disorders.
- Revise plan of care as needed to provide effective interventions to promote, maintain, or restore functional health status to clients with neurologic disorders.

KEY TERMS

Alzheimer's disease (AD)
amyotrophic lateral
   sclerosis (ALS)
Bell's palsy
botulism
Creutzfeldt-Jakob
   disease (CJD)
dementia
Guillain-Barré
   syndrome (GBS)

Huntington's disease
multiple sclerosis (MS)
myasthenia gravis
Parkinson's disease (PD)
postpoliomyelitis syndrome
rabies
sundowning
tetanus
trigeminal neuralgia

CHAPTER OUTLINE

   I. Degenerative Neurologic Disorders
  II. Dementia
 III. The Client with Alzheimer's Disease
    A. Incidence and Prevalence
    B. Risk Factors and Warning Signs
    C. Pathophysiology
    D. Manifestations
       1. Stage 1 AD
       2. Stage 2 AD
       3. Stage 3 AD
    E. Interdisciplinary Care
       1. Diagnosis
       2. Medications
       3. Alternative and Complementary Therapy
    F. Nursing Care
       1. Health Promotion
       2. Assessment
       3. Nursing Diagnoses and Interventions
          a. Impaired Memory
          b. Chronic Confusion
          c. Anxiety
          d. Hopelessness
          e. Caregiver Role Strain
       4. Using NANDA, NIC, and NOC
       5. Community-Based Care
  IV. The Client with Multiple Sclerosis
    A. Incidence and Prevalence
    B. Pathophysiology
    C. Manifestations
    D. Interdisciplinary Care
       1. Diagnosis
       2. Medications

       3. Surgery
       4. Nutrition and Fluids
       5. Rehabilitation
    E. Nursing Care
       1. Health Promotion
       2. Assessment
       3. Nursing Diagnoses and Interventions
          a. Fatigue
          b. Self-Care Deficit
       4. Using NANDA, NIC, and NOC
       5. Community-Based Care
  V. The Client with Parkinson's Disease
    A. Incidence and Prevalence
    B. Pathophysiology
    C. Manifestations
       1. Tremor
       2. Rigidity and Bradykinesia
       3. Abnormal Posture
       4. Autonomic and Neuroendocrine Effects
       5. Mood and Cognition
       6. Sleep Disturbances
       7. Interrelated Effects
    D. Complications
    E. Interdisciplinary Care
       1. Diagnosis
       2. Medications
       3. Deep Brain Stimulation
       4. Surgery
       5. Rehabilitation
    F. Nursing Care
       1. Health Promotion
       2. Assessment
       3. Nursing Diagnoses and Interventions
          a. Impaired Physical Mobility
          b. Impaired Verbal Communication
          c. Imbalanced Nutrition: Less than Body Requirements
          d. Disturbed Sleep Pattern
       4. Using NANDA, NIC, and NOC
       5. Community-Based Care
 VI. The Client with Huntington's Disease
    A. Pathophysiology
    B. Manifestations
    C. Interdisciplinary Care
       1. Diagnosis
       2. Medications
    D. Nursing Care
       1. Nursing Diagnoses and Interventions
          a. Risk for Aspiration
          b. Imbalanced Nutrition: Less than Body Requirements
          c. Impaired Skin Integrity
          d. Impaired Verbal Communication
       2. Community-Based Care
VII. The Client with Amyotrophic Lateral Sclerosis
    A. Pathophysiology
    B. Manifestations

FOCUSED STUDY TIPS

1. Discuss the procedures used to treat plasmapheresis.

_____

_____

_____

2. List manifestations and complications of clients with neurologic disorders.

_____

_____

_____

_____

3. Summarize the manifestations of the progressive stages of Alzheimer's disease.

_____

_____

_____

_____

4. Explain the nursing implications for Alzheimer's disease, multiple sclerosis, Parkinson's disease, and myasthenia gravis.

_____

_____

_____

_____

_____

CASE STUDY

MiMi Bradley is a 73-year-old female client in today for a physical examination. Her daughter Christine tells the nurse that her mother has been experiencing memory loss, difficulty performing familiar tasks, appears disoriented at times, is misplacing things, and a change in personality. Christine then asks the nurse the following questions:

1. "What are the risk factors of Alzheimer's disease?"

2. "What the warning signs of Alzheimer's disease?"

3. "What are the stages of Alzheimer's disease?"

NCLEX REVIEW QUESTIONS

1. All of the following are warning signs of Alzheimer's disease except:
   1. Misplacing things.
   2. Loss of initiative.
   3. Performing familiar tasks.
   4. Change in personality.
2. Which of the following statements by a student nurse reflects incorrect understanding about multiple sclerosis (MS)?
   1. "It is a chronic demyelinating neurologic disease of the central nervous system (brain, optic nerves, and spinal cord) associated with an abnormal immune response to an environmental factor."
   2. "The initial onset cannot be followed by a total remission."
   3. "The manifestations of MS does not vary according to the area of the nervous system affected."
   4. "The onset of MS is usually between 40 and 60 years of age, with a peak at age 50."
3. During discharge planning, the nurse is teaching the client about Parkinson's disease. Which of the following statements is correct?
   1. "Parkinson's disease is one of the least common neurologic disorders that affects older adults."
   2. "The disorder usually develops after the age of 75 years, but 25% of those diagnosed are under 50 years of age."
   3. "Women and men are affected equally."
   4. "Parkinson's disease begins with subtle manifestations."
4. All of the following statements about Parkinson's disease are true except:
   1. In Parkinson's disease, neurons in the cerebral cortex atrophy and are lost, the dopaminergic nigrostriatal (pigmented) pathway degenerates, and the number of specific dopamine receptors in the basal ganglia decreases.
   2. Parkinson's disease has three stages.
   3. Both depression and dementia are pathologies associated with Parkinson's disease.
   4. Clients with Parkinson's disease commonly have sleep disturbances, although they may experience decreased manifestations during sleep in the early stages.

5. Which of the following is not a complication associated with Parkinson's disease?
   1. Falls from balance, posture, and motor changes.
   2. Depression and social isolation.
   3. Skin breakdown and pressure ulcers associated with urinary incontinence, malnutrition, and sweat reflex changes.
   4. Obesity related to dysphagia.
6. A nurse is evaluating a client's understanding of Huntington's disease (HD). Which of the following statements indicates a need for further teaching?
   1. HD is a progressive, degenerative, inherited neurologic disease characterized by increasing dementia and chorea (jerky, rapid, involuntary movements).
   2. HD is a single-gene autosomal-dominant inherited disease that causes localized death of neurons of the basal ganglia.
   3. HD is a familial disease, and each child of an HD parent has a 25% chance of inheriting the HD gene.
   4. HD causes destruction of cells in the caudate nucleus and putamen areas of the basal ganglia.
7. A nurse is planning a seminar about amyotrophic lateral sclerosis (ALS). Which of the following statements is correct?
   1. ALS is a slow and fatal degenerative neurologic disease characterized by weakness and wasting of tissue, with accompanying sensory or cognitive changes.
   2. ALS is also known as Babe Ruth's disease.
   3. ALS is the least common motor neuron disease in the United States.
   4. ALS results from the degeneration and demyelination of both upper and lower motor neurons in the anterior horn of the spinal cord, brainstem, and cerebral cortex.
8. The nurse is evaluating a myasthenia gravis class. During the class she recognizes that further teaching is necessary when which of the following statements is made by a participant?
   1. "Myasthenia gravis is an acute inflammatory demyelinating disorder of the peripheral nervous system characterized by an acute onset of motor paralysis that is usually ascending."
   2. "The manifestations of myasthenia gravis correspond to the muscles involved. Initially, the eye muscles are affected and the client experiences either diplopia (unilateral or bilateral double vision) or ptosis (drooping of the eyelid)."
   3. "In myasthenia gravis, antibodies destroy or block neuromuscular junction receptor sites, which results in a decreased number of acetylcholine receptors."
   4. "Myasthenia gravis is sometimes associated with a tumor of the thymus, thyrotoxicosis (hyperthyroidism), rheumatoid arthritis, and lupus erythematosus."
9. Which of the following statements by a student nurse reflects incorrect understanding about trigeminal neuralgia?
   1. "Trigeminal neuralgia occurs more commonly in younger adults and affects men more often than women."
   2. "Trigeminal neuralgia, also called facial paralysis, is a chronic disease of the trigeminal cranial nerve (V) that causes severe facial pain."
   3. "There are three specific diagnostic tests for trigeminal neuralgia."
   4. "Trigeminal neuralgia is characterized by brief (lasting a few seconds to a few minutes), repetitive episodes of sudden severe (usually unilateral) facial pain."
10. All of the following are names or abbreviations used to describe a rapidly progressive, degenerative neurologic disease that causes brain degeneration without inflammation except:
    1. CJD.
    2. Spongiform encephalopathy.
    3. Creutzfeldt-Jakob disease.
    4. SE.

CHAPTER 47

ASSESSING CLIENTS WITH EYE AND EAR DISORDERS

LEARNING OUTCOMES

After completing Chapter 47, you will be able to demonstrate the following objectives:

- Describe the anatomy, physiology, and functions of the eye and the ear.
- Explain the physiologic processes involved in vision, hearing, and equilibrium.
- Identify specific topics for consideration during a health history interview of the client with health problems of the eye or ear.
- Describe normal variations in assessment findings for the older adult.
- Identify abnormal findings that may indicate impairment in the function of the eye and the ear.

CLINICAL COMPETENCIES

- Conduct and document a health history for clients having or at risk for alterations in the structure or functions of the eye and ear.
- Monitor the results of diagnostic tests and report abnormal findings.
- Conduct and document a physical assessment of the structure or functions of the eye and ear.

EQUIPMENT NEEDED

- Visual acuity charts
- Opaque eye cover
- Pen
- Penlight

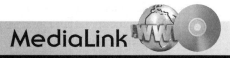

MediaLink
www.prenhall.com/lemone

Resources for this chapter can be found on the Prentice Hall Nursing MediaLink DVD accompanying this textbook, and on the Companion Website at http://www.prenhall.com/lemone. Click on Chapter 47 to select the activities for this chapter.

Prentice Hall Nursing MediaLink DVD-ROM
- Audio Glossary
- NCLEX-RN® Review

Companion Website www.prenhall.com/lemone
- Audio Glossary
- NCLEX-RN® Review
- Care Plan Activity: Ear Pain
- Case Studies
  - Identifying Common Pathologies
  - Otitis Media
- MediaLink Applications: Nystagmus
- Links to Resources

- Cotton-tipped applicator
- Ophthalmoscope
- Otoscope
- Tuning fork

KEY TERMS

accommodation
cerumen
convergence
corneal reflex
hyperopia
myopia

nystagmus
presbyopia
ptosis
pupillary light reflex
refraction

CHAPTER OUTLINE

I. Anatomy, Physiology, and Functions of the Eyes
  A. Extraocular Structures
  B. Intraocular Structures
    1. Sclera and Cornea
    2. Iris
    3. Aqueous Fluid
    4. Internal Chamber
  C. The Visual Pathway
  D. Refraction
II. Assessing the Eyes
  A. Diagnostic Tests
  B. Genetic Considerations
  C. Health Assessment Interview
  D. Physical Assessment of the Eyes and Vision
    1. Assessing Visual Fields
  E. Eye and Vision Assessments
    1. Vision Assessment
    2. Eye Movement Assessment
    3. Pupillary Assessment
    4. External Eye Assessment
    5. Internal Eye Assessment
III. Anatomy, Physiology, and Functions of the Ears
  A. The External Ear
  B. The Middle Ear
  C. The Inner Ear
  D. Sound Conduction
  E. Equilibrium
IV. Assessing the Ears
  A. Diagnostic Tests
  B. Genetic Considerations
  C. Health Assessment Interview
  D. Physical Assessment of the Ears and Hearing
  E. Ear and Hearing Assessments
    1. Hearing Assessment
    2. External Ear Assessment

FOCUSED STUDY TIPS

1. List abnormal findings that may indicate impairment in the function of the eye and the ear.

_____

_____

_____

_____

_____

2. Discuss specific topics for consideration during a health history interview of the client with health problems of the eye or ear.

_____

_____

_____

_____

_____

3. Summarize the physiologic processes involved in vision, hearing, and equilibrium.

_____

_____

_____

4. Explain the functions of the eye and the ear.

_____

_____

_____

_____

CASE STUDY

Michael Scott RN, BSN is preparing his notes for a class about eye and ear disorders. He has developed the following questions to ask the nursing students after his lecture.

1. What is the colored part of the eye? What is its function?

2. What does the external ear consist of?

3. Explain equilibrium.

NCLEX REVIEW QUESTIONS

1. The_____ gives the eye its color and regulates light entry by controlling the size of the_____.
   1. Iris, cornea
   2. Pupil, iris
   3. Iris, sclera
   4. Sclera, cornea

2. Which of the following statements about aqueous humor is correct?
   1. Aqueous humor is a cloudy fluid.
   2. Aqueous humor provides nutrients and oxygen to the pupil and the iris.
   3. Aqueous humor is constantly formed and drained to maintain a relatively constant pressure of 25 to 30 mmHg in the eye.
   4. Aqueous humor fills the anterior cavity.
3. When the eye focuses on an image, it is called:
   1. Accommodation.
   2. Refraction.
   3. Convergence.
   4. Pupillary light reflex.
4. Which of the following actions is correct for the nurse who is measuring a client's visual fields?
   1. Move the penlight from the periphery toward the center from right to left, above and below, and from the middle of each of these directions.
   2. Ask the client to look directly at a point behind and to the side of you.
   3. Ask the client to cover one eye with the opaque cover while you cover your own eye corresponding to the client's.
   4. Sit directly opposite the client at a distance of 36 to 48 inches.
5. Which of the following is a correct statement about a Snellen chart?
   1. The Snellen chart contains rows of letters in various sizes, with inconsistent numbers at the end of each row.
   2. The number at the end of the row indicates the visual acuity of a client who can read the row at a distance of 30 feet.
   3. The top number is the distance (in feet) at which a person with normal vision can read the line.
   4. A person with normal vision can read the row marked 20/20.
6. Which of the following is not part of the middle ear?
   1. Incus
   2. Stapes
   3. Malleus
   4. Tympanic membrane
7. All of the following statements pertain to the inner ear except:
   1. The inner ear, also called the labyrinth, is a maze of bony chambers located deep within the temporal bone, just behind the eye socket.
   2. The malleus attaches to the tympanic membrane and articulates with the stapes, which in turn articulates with the incus.
   3. Within the chambers of the membranous labyrinth is a fluid called endolymph.
   4. The bony labyrinth has three regions: the vestibule, the semicircular canals, and the cochlea.
8. Which of the following statements about sound conduction is false?
   1. Hearing is the perception and interpretation of sound.
   2. Sound is produced when the molecules of a medium are compressed, which results in a pressure disturbance evidenced as a sound wave.
   3. Sound waves enter the external auditory canal and cause the tympanic membrane to vibrate at the same frequency.
   4. The human ear is most sensitive to sound waves with frequencies between 100 and 400 cycles per second, but can detect sound waves with frequencies between 2 and 200 cycles per second.
9. Which of the following assessment findings of the tympanic membrane should be reported to the physician?
   1. It appears shiny.
   2. The color is pearly gray.
   3. It is translucent.
   4. It is bulging.
10. The_____ test places the base of a vibrating tuning fork on the midline vertex of the client's head.
    1. Rinne
    2. Weber
    3. Whisper
    4. Caloric

CHAPTER 48

NURSING CARE OF CLIENTS WITH EYE AND EAR DISORDERS

LEARNING OUTCOMES

After completing Chapter 48, you will be able to demonstrate the following objectives:

- Relate knowledge of normal anatomy, physiology, and sensory functions of the eye and ear to the effects of disorders of these organs on the cognitive/perceptual functional health pattern.
- Describe the pathophysiology of commonly occurring disorders of the eyes and ears, relating their manifestations to the pathophysiologic process.
- Explain the risk factors for selected disorders of the eyes and ears, identifying the nursing implications for these risk factors.
- Identify diagnostic tests used for specific eye and ear disorders.
- Discuss the effects of and nursing implications for medications prescribed to treat eye and ear disorders.
- Describe surgical and other invasive procedures used to treat eye and ear disorders, identifying their implications for nursing care.
- Discuss the nurse's role in caring for clients with impaired vision or hearing loss.

CLINICAL COMPETENCIES

- Assess vision, hearing, and functional health of clients with eye and ear disorders.
- Using assessed data, determine priority nursing diagnoses and interventions for clients with eye and ear disorders.
- Collaborate with other members of the healthcare team to provide effective care for clients with eye and ear disorders.
- Plan and implement appropriate and individualized evidence-based nursing interventions and teaching for the client with an eye or ear disorder.
- Safely and effectively administer eye and ear medications and prescribed treatments.

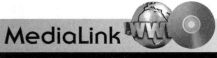

MediaLink

www.prenhall.com/lemone

Resources for this chapter can be found on the Prentice Hall Nursing MediaLink DVD accompanying this textbook, and on the Companion Website at http://www.prenhall.com/lemone. Click on Chapter 48 to select the activities for this chapter.

Prentice Hall Nursing MediaLink DVD-ROM
- Audio Glossary
- NCLEX-RN® Review

Animations/Video
- Middle Ear Dynamics
- Pilocarpine

Companion Website www.prenhall.com/lemone
- Audio Glossary
- NCLEX-RN® Review
- Care Plan Activity: The Client with a Hearing Aid
- Case Study: Retinal Detachment
- MediaLink Application: Cataracts
- Links to Resources

- Provide appropriate care and teaching for the client having eye or ear surgery.
- Evaluate the effectiveness of nursing care provided for clients with eye and ear disorders, revising plan of care as indicated.

KEY TERMS

acoustic neuroma
astigmatism
cataract
chalazion
conjunctivitis
corneal ulcer
diabetic retinopathy
enophthalmos
enucleation
glaucoma

hordeolum (sty)
hyperopia
hyphema
keratitis
labyrinthitis
macular degeneration
mastoiditis
Ménière's disease
myopia
myringotomy

nystagmus
otitis externa
otitis media
otosclerosis
presbycusis
ptosis
retinal detachment
tinnitus
tympanoplasty
vertigo

CHAPTER OUTLINE

FOCUSED STUDY TIPS

1. Summarize the nurse's role in caring for clients with impaired vision or hearing loss.

   _____

   _____

2. List the risk factors for selected disorders of the eyes and ears.

   _____

   _____

   _____

3. Explain the nursing implications for medications prescribed to treat eye and ear disorders.

   _____

   _____

   _____

4. Discuss the diagnostic tests used for specific eye and ear disorders.

_____

_____

_____

CASE STUDY

Drake Smith is a 21-year-old male client who has redness and itching of the right eye. He was diagnosed with conjunctivitis. Just as he is about to leave the clinic he asks the nurse the following questions.

1. "Is conjunctivitis the same thing as 'pink eye'?"

2. "Is pink eye contagious?"

3. "What are the signs and symptoms of conjunctivitis?"

CARE PLAN CRITICAL THINKING ACTIVITY

1. Explain how to administer eye drops.

2. How could a nurse assist Mrs. Rainey to express her fears related to the surgery and recovery?

3. Why is it important for Mrs. Rainey to avoid shutting her eyelids tightly, sneezing, coughing, laughing, bending over, lifting, or straining to have a bowel movement?

NCLEX REVIEW QUESTIONS

1. When a client tells the nurse that he or she is nearsighted, the nurse realizes that this means that he or she:
    1. Is having rapid involuntary eye movements.
    2. Has an opacification (clouding) of the lens of the eye.
    3. Sees objects in close range clearly but those at a distant are blurred.
    4. Sees objects clearer at a distance than objects that are closer.
2. Which of the following statements by a student nurse reflects correct understanding about conjunctivitis?
    1. "It is also known as 'red eye'."
    2. "It is not very contagious."
    3. "It is often caused by _Streptococcus_."
    4. "It may be bacterial, viral, or fungal in origin."
3. Laser eye surgery is commonly performed to correct refractive errors such as myopia, hyperopia, and astigmatism. Which of the following is not a type of laser eye surgery?
    1. LASIK
    2. PRK
    3. LASEK
    4. LKT
4. During an educational seminar, the nurse is teaching participants about preventing corneal disorders. Which of the following statements by a participant indicates a need for further education? "I should:
    1. Not share towels and makeup."
    2. Avoid rubbing or scratching my eyes."
    3. Prevent trauma and infection of my eyes."
    4. Never remove my extended-wear contact lenses to clean them."

5. A granulomatous cyst or nodule of the lid is a:
   1. Hordeolum.
   2. Chalazion.
   3. Hyphema.
   4. Cataract.
6. Which of the following is not a stage of diabetic retinopathy?
   1. Mild nonproliferative or background retinopathy
   2. Moderate nonproliferative retinopathy
   3. Severe nonproliferative retinopathy
   4. Critical proliferative retinopathy
7. A nurse is evaluating a client's understanding of otitis externa. Which of the following statements indicates a need for further teaching?
   1. "It is inflammation of the ear canal."
   2. "It is commonly known as diver's ear."
   3. "It is most prevalent in people who spend significant time in the water."
   4. "Wearing a hearing aid or ear plugs, which hold moisture in the ear canal, is an additional risk factor."
8. Which of the following statements by a student nurse reflects correct understanding about otosclerosis?
   1. "Otosclerosis occurs most commonly in Caucasians and in males."
   2. "Otosclerosis is not a cause of conductive hearing loss."
   3. "Otosclerosis is a hereditary disorder with an autosomal dominant pattern of inheritance."
   4. "Otosclerosis is a hearing loss that typically begins in older adulthood and seems to be reduced by pregnancy."
9. Which of the following is a chronic disorder characterized by recurrent attacks of vertigo with tinnitus and a progressive unilateral hearing loss?
   1. Acoustic neuroma
   2. Labyrinthitis
   3. Ménière's disease
   4. Otitis externa
10. A nurse is planning a seminar about presbycusis. Which of the following statements on a handout for the seminar needs to be corrected?
    1. Hearing loss of presbycusis is gradual.
    2. Lower-pitched tones and conversational speech are lost initially.
    3. It is associated with aging.
    4. Hearing aids and other amplification devices are useful for most clients with presbycusis.

CHAPTER 49

ASSESSING CLIENTS WITH REPRODUCTIVE SYSTEM AND BREAST DISORDERS

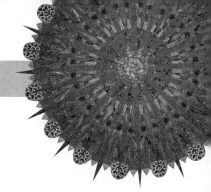

MediaLink

www.prenhall.com/lemone

Resources for this chapter can be found on the Prentice Hall Nursing MediaLink DVD accompanying this textbook, and on the Companion Website at http://www.prenhall.com/lemone. Click on Chapter 49 to select the activities for this chapter.

Prentice Hall Nursing MediaLink DVD-ROM
- Audio Glossary
- NCLEX-RN® Review

Companion Website
www.prenhall.com/lemone
- Audio Glossary
- NCLEX-RN® Review
- Care Plan Activity: STDs
- Case Studies
  - Assessing Sexual Function
  - Irregular Menstrual Cycle
- Exercise: Sexual Function Health History
- MediaLink Applications: Breast Cancer Screening
- Links to Resources

LEARNING OUTCOMES

After completing Chapter 49, you will be able to demonstrate the following objectives:
- Describe the anatomy, physiology, and functions of the male and female reproductive systems, including the breasts.
- Explain the functions of the male and female sex hormones.
- Identify specific topics for consideration during a health history interview of the client with health problems involving reproductive and breast structures and/or functions.
- Describe normal variations in assessment findings for the older adult.
- Identify manifestations of impairment in male and female reproductive system and breast structure or function.

CLINICAL COMPETENCIES

- Conduct and document a health history for men and women having or at risk for alterations of the reproductive system, including the breasts.
- Conduct and document a physical assessment of male and female reproductive system structures and functions, including the breasts.
- Monitor the results of diagnostic tests and report abnormal findings.

EQUIPMENT NEEDED

- Disposable gloves
- Water-soluble lubricant
- A good light source
- Sterile cotton swabs (for culture)

- Culture media (for culture)
- A spatula, cotton swab or endocervical brush, slides, and cytologic fixative (for Pap smear)
- Vaginal speculum of appropriate size

KEY TERMS

androgens
anorgasmia
dyspareunia
estrogen
gynecomastia
impotence
menstrual cycle

menstruation
ovarian cycle
phimosis
progesterone
semen
testosterone

CHAPTER OUTLINE

I. Anatomy, Physiology, and Functions of the Male Reproductive System
  A. The Breasts
  B. The Penis
  C. The Scrotum
  D. The Testes
  E. The Ducts and Semen
  F. The Prostate Gland
  G. Spermatogenesis
  H. Male Sex Hormones

II. Assessing the Male Reproductive System
  A. Diagnostic Tests
  B. Genetic Considerations
  C. Health Assessment Interview
  D. Physical Assessment
  E. Male Reproductive System Assessments
    1. Breast and Lymph Node Assessment
    2. External Genitalia Assessment
    3. Prostate Assessment

III. Anatomy, Physiology, and Functions of the Female Reproductive System
  A. The Breasts
  B. The External Genitalia
  C. The Internal Organs
    1. The Vagina and Cervix
    2. The Uterus
    3. The Fallopian Tubes
    4. The Ovaries
  D. Female Sex Hormones
  E. Oogenesis and the Ovarian Cycle
  F. The Menstrual Cycle

IV. Assessing the Female Reproductive System
  A. Diagnostic Tests
  B. Genetic Considerations
  C. Health Assessment Interview
  D. Physical Assessment
  E. Female Reproductive System Assessments
    1. Breast Assessment
    2. Axillary Assessment
    3. External Genitalia Assessment
    4. Vaginal and Cervical Assessment

FOCUSED STUDY TIPS

1. Identify the manifestations of impairment in male and female reproductive and breast structure or function.

   _____

   _____

   _____

   _____

   _____

2. Discuss the specific topics for consideration during a health history interview of the client with health problems involving reproductive and breast structures or functions.

   _____

   _____

   _____

   _____

   _____

3. Summarize the anatomy and physiology of the male and female reproductive systems.

   _____

   _____

   _____

   _____

4. Explain the functions of the male and female sex hormones.

   _____

   _____

   _____

   _____

CASE STUDY

Holly Anne is a 15-year-old female client. She attended a class about the female reproduction system a few days ago and asks the nurse the following questions.

1. "What is the ovarian cycle?"

2. "Why do I need estrogen?"

3. "What is the difference between the vagina and cervix?"

NCLEX REVIEW QUESTIONS

1. Which of the following statements about the testes is false? The testes:
   1. Are surrounded by two coverings: an outer tunica albuginea and an inner tunica vaginalis.
   2. Produce sperm and testosterone.
   3. Develop in the abdominal cavity of the fetus and then descend through the inguinal canal into the scrotum.
   4. Are homologous to the female's ovaries.

2. Which of the following statements by a student nurse reflects correct understanding about the prostate gland?
   1. "The prostate gland is about the size of a pea."
   2. "The prostate encircles the urethra just above the urinary bladder."
   3. "The prostate is made of 40 to 50 tubuloalveolar glands surrounded by smooth muscle."
   4. "Secretions from the prostate gland make up about one-third of the volume of semen."
3. A student nurse is preparing a presentation about the scrotum. Which of the following statements needs to be corrected?
   1. The scrotum is a sac or pouch made of two layers.
   2. When the testicular temperature is too low, the scrotum contracts to bring the testes up against the body.
   3. The optimum temperature for sperm production is about 4 to 5 degrees below body temperature.
   4. The scrotum hangs at the base of the penis, anterior to the anus, and regulates the temperature of the testes.
4. Which of the following is not a function of seminal fluid?
   1. Nourishes the sperm
   2. Decreases alkalinity
   3. Provides bulk
   4. Increases alkalinity
5. Which of the following statements by a student nurse reflects correct understanding about female external genitalia?
   1. "The female internal genitalia include the mons pubis, the labia, the clitoris, the vaginal and urethral openings, and glands."
   2. "The clitoris is an erectile organ that is analogous to the penis in the male."
   3. "The labia minora, which are folds of skin and adipose tissue covered with hair, are outermost; they begin at the base of the mons pubis and end at the anus."
   4. "After puberty, the mons is covered with hair with a square-shaped distribution."
6. Which of the following statements about the vagina is false?
   1. The vagina is a fibromuscular tube about 3 to 4 inches (8 to 10 cm) in length that is located posterior to the bladder and urethra and anterior to the rectum.
   2. The walls of the vagina are membranes that form folds, called rugae.
   3. The vagina serves as a route for the excretion of secretions, including menstrual fluid, and also is an organ of sexual response.
   4. The walls of the vagina are usually moist and maintain a pH that ranges from 4.8 to 6.2.
7. The ovarian cycle has three consecutive phases that occur cyclically each 28 days (although the cycle normally may be longer or shorter). Which of the following is not characteristic of a phase of the ovarian cycle?
   1. The luteal phase lasts from the 14th to the 28th days.
   2. The follicular phase lasts from the 1st to the 10th day of the cycle.
   3. The luteal phase lasts from the 5th to the 10th day of the cycle.
   4. The ovulatory phase lasts from the 11th to the 14th day of the cycle and ends with ovulation.
8. Which of the following is a blood test used to diagnose prostate cancer and to monitor treatment of prostate cancer?
   1. PSA
   2. VDRL
   3. RPR
   4. FTA-ABS
9. Which female organ(s) is (are) homologous to the male's testes?
   1. Fallopian tubes
   2. Ovaries
   3. Mons pubis
   4. Labia minora
10. Which of the following statements about the ovaries is false?
   1. A woman's total number of ova is present at birth.
   2. Each ovary contains many small structures called ovarian follicles.
   3. The ovaries in the young adult woman are flat, apple-shaped structures located on either side of the uterus above the fallopian tubes.
   4. The ovaries store the female germ cells and produce the female hormones estrogen and progesterone.

CHAPTER 50

Nursing Care of Men with Reproductive System and Breast Disorders

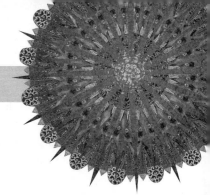

LEARNING OUTCOMES

After completing Chapter 50, you will be able to demonstrate the following objectives:

- Explain the pathophysiology, manifestations, complications, interdisciplinary care, and nursing care of disorders of the male reproductive system, including disorders of sexual function, the penis, the testes and scrotum, the prostate gland, and the breast.

- Compare and contrast the risk factors for cancer of the penis, testes, and prostate gland.

- Discuss the purposes, nursing implications, and health education for medications and treatments used to treat disorders of sexual function, the penis, the testes and scrotum, the prostate gland, and the breast.

- Describe the various surgical procedures used to treat disorders of the male reproductive system.

CLINICAL COMPETENCIES

- Assess functional health status of men with reproductive system and breast disorders and monitor, document, and report abnormal manifestations.

- Use evidence-based research to provide appropriate discharge teaching to men having a radical prostatectomy.

- Determine priority nursing diagnoses, based on assessed data, to select and implement individualized nursing interventions for men with disorders of the reproductive system and breast.

MediaLink

www.prenhall.com/lemone

Resources for this chapter can be found on the Prentice Hall Nursing MediaLink DVD accompanying this textbook, and on the Companion Website at http://www.prenhall.com/lemone. Click on Chapter 50 to select the activities for this chapter.

Prentice Hall Nursing MediaLink DVD-ROM
- Audio Glossary
- NCLEX-RN® Review

Animation/Video
- Testicular Self-Examination

Companion Website
www.prenhall.com/lemone
- Audio Glossary
- NCLEX-RN® Review
- Care Plan Activity: Radical Prostatectomy
- Case Studies
  - Benign Prostatic Hyperplasia
  - Prostatitis
- Teaching Plan: ED Medication and Safety
- MediaLink Applications
  - Prostate Cancer Prevention
  - Sleep Apnea and Erectile Dysfunction
- Links to Resources

- Administer, or teach clients how to administer, topical, oral, and injectable medications used to treat disorders of the male reproductive system knowledgeably and safely.
- Provide skilled care to men having prostate surgery.
- Revise plan of care as needed to provide effective interventions to promote, maintain, or restore functional health status to men with disorders of the reproductive system and breast.

KEY TERMS

benign prostatic hyperplasia (BPH)
epididymitis
erectile dysfunction (ED)
gynecomastia
hydrocele
impotence
libido

orchitis
phimosis
priapism
prostatitis
retrograde ejaculation
spermatocele
testicular torsion
varicocele

CHAPTER OUTLINE

3. Nursing Diagnoses and Interventions
   a. Urinary Incontinence (Reflex, Stress, Total)
   b. Sexual Dysfunction
   c. Acute/Chronic Pain
4. Using NANDA, NIC, and NOC
5. Community-Based Care
XVII. Male Breast Disorders
XVIII. The Man with Gynecomastia
XIX. The Man with Breast Cancer

FOCUSED STUDY TIPS

1. List the risk factors for cancer of the penis, testes, and prostate gland.

   _____

   _____

   _____

2. Summarize the various surgical procedures used to treat disorders of the male reproductive system.

   _____

   _____

   _____

3. Discuss manifestations and complications of the disorders of the male reproductive system.

   _____

   _____

   _____

4. Explain the nursing implications and treatments used to treat disorders of sexual function, the penis, the testes and scrotum, the prostate gland, and the breast.

   _____

   _____

   _____

CASE STUDY

Nathaniel Obermark is a 22-year-old male client who states, "I have slight enlargement of my right testicle with some discomfort and I have a feeling of heaviness in the scrotum." He then asks the nurse the following questions.

1. "What is the cause of testicular cancer?"

2. "What are the risk factors for testicular cancer?"

3. "What are the manifestations of testicular cancer?"

NCLEX REVIEW QUESTIONS

1. Which of the following statements is false?
   1. Erectile dysfunction is the male's inability to attain and maintain an erection sufficient to permit satisfactory sexual intercourse.
   2. Impotence is a term often used synonymously with erectile dysfunction.
   3. Erectile dysfunction has many possible causes.
   4. Erectile dysfunction can only be treated with oral medications.
2. The oral medications used to treat erectile dysfunction (ED) include all of the following except:
   1. Vardenafil hydrochloride (Levitra).
   2. Sildenafil citrate (Viagra).
   3. Minoxidil (Rogaine).
   4. Tadalafil (Cialis).
3. Which condition is constriction of the foreskin that it cannot be retracted over the glans penis?
   1. Paraphimosis
   2. Phimosis
   3. Priapism
   4. Hydrocele
4. What is the most common cause of scrotal swelling that is a collection of fluid within the tunica vaginalis?
   1. Testicular torsion
   2. Spermatocele
   3. Hydrocele
   4. Varicocele
5. Which of the following statements by a student nurse reflects correct understanding about orchitis?
   1. "Orchitis is a chronic infection of the testes."
   2. "Orchitis most commonly occurs as a complication of a systemic illness or as an extension of epididymitis."
   3. "The most common infectious cause of orchitis in postpubertal men is measles."
   4. "The manifestations of orchitis has a gradual onset, usually within 3 to 4 weeks after the swelling of the parotid glands."
6. A nurse is evaluating a client's understanding of testicular cancer. Which of the following statements indicates a need for further teaching?
   1. "Testicular cancer is more common on the left side, which parallels the incidence of cryptorchidism."
   2. "Testicular cancer is the most common cancer in men between the ages of 15 and 40."
   3. "The first sign of testicular cancer may be a slight enlargement of one testicle with some discomfort."
   4. "Testicular cancer is more common on the right side, which parallels the incidence of cryptorchidism."
7. A nurse is planning a seminar about benign prostatic hyperplasia (BPH). Which of the following statements on an educational handout needs to be corrected?
   1. The two necessary preconditions for BPH are age of 50 or greater and the presence of testes.
   2. BPH, which is the twisting of the spermatic cord with scrotal swelling and pain, is a potential medical emergency.
   3. The exact cause of BPH is unknown.
   4. Risk factors of BPH include age, family history, race (highest in African Americans and lowest in native Japanese), and a diet high in meat and fats.
8. Which of the following statements is false?
   1. Gynecomastia, which is the abnormal enlargement of the male breast, is thought to result from a high ratio of estradiol to testosterone.
   2. No treatment is necessary for the transient gynecomastia of puberty.
   3. Gynecomastia is usually unilateral.
   4. Drugs such as digitalis, opiates, and chemotherapeutic agents are also associated with gynecomastia.
9. A _____ is a mobile, usually painless, mass that forms when efferent ducts in the epididymis dilate and form a cyst.
   1. Spermatocele
   2. Testicular torsion
   3. Hydrocele
   4. Varicocele

10. Select the false statement:
    1. Testicular torsion, which is the twisting of the spermatic cord with scrotal swelling and pain, is a potential medical emergency.
    2. Orchitis is an acute inflammation or infection of the testes.
    3. Testicular torsion is caused only by trauma.
    4. Epididymitis is an infection or inflammation of the epididymis, which is the structure that lies along the posterior border of the testis.

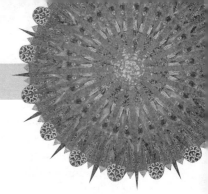

CHAPTER 51

NURSING CARE OF WOMEN WITH REPRODUCTIVE SYSTEM AND BREAST DISORDERS

LEARNING OUTCOMES

After completing Chapter 51, you will be able to demonstrate the following objectives:

- Explain the pathophysiology, manifestations, complications, interdisciplinary care, and nursing care of disorders of female sexual function, menstrual disorders, structural disorders, reproductive tissue disorders, and breast disorders.
- Describe the physiologic process of menopause.
- Compare and contrast the incidence, risk factors, pathophysiology, manifestations, diagnosis, treatment, and nursing care for cancer of the cervix, endometrium, ovary, vulva, and breast.
- Discuss the purposes, nursing implications, and health education for clients and their families for cancer screening, medications, and treatments for women with disorders of the reproductive system and breast.
- Discuss alternative and complementary therapies used by women to relieve manifestations associated with menopause and menstrual disorders.
- Describe the surgical procedures used to treat female reproductive system and breast disorders.

CLINICAL COMPETENCIES

- Assess functional status of women with reproductive system and breast disorders, and monitor, document, and report abnormal manifestations.

MediaLink

- Use evidence-based research to design interventions to promote early diagnosis and treatment of African American women with breast cancer.
- Determine priority nursing diagnoses, based on assessed data, to select and implement individualized nursing interventions for women with reproductive system and breast disorders.
- Administer medications used to treat female reproductive system and breast disorders knowledgeably and safely.
- Provide skilled care for the woman having a D&C, laparoscopy, hysterectomy, mastectomy, and breast reconstruction.
- Integrate interdisciplinary care into care of women with reproductive system and breast disorders.
- Provide teaching appropriate for community-based self-care of female reproductive and breast disorders.
- Revise plan of care as needed to provide effective interventions to promote, maintain, or restore functional health status to women with reproductive system and breast disorders.

KEY TERMS

amenorrhea
anorgasmia
dysfunctional uterine
  bleeding (DUB)
dysmenorrhea
dyspareunia
endometriosis

fibrocystic changes (FCC)
leiomyoma
lymphedema
menopause
menorrhagia
metrorrhagia
premenstrual syndrome (PMS)

CHAPTER OUTLINE

  I. Disorders of Female Sexual Function
    A. Pathophysiology
      1. Dyspareunia
      2. Inhibited Sexual Desire
      3. Orgasmic Dysfunction
    B. Nursing Care
  II. The Perimenopausal Woman
    A. The Physiology of Menopause
    B. Manifestations
    C. Interdisciplinary Care
      1. Diagnosis
      2. Medications
      3. Alternative and Complementary Therapies
    D. Nursing Care
      1. Health Promotion
      2. Assessment
      3. Nursing Diagnoses and Interventions
        a. Deficient Knowledge
        b. Ineffective Sexuality Pattern
        c. Situational Low Self-Esteem
        d. Disturbed Body Image
  III. Menstrual Disorders
  IV. The Woman with Premenstrual Syndrome
    A. Pathophysiology
    B. Manifestations
    C. Interdisciplinary Care
      1. Medications
      2. Alternative and Complementary Therapies

XIII. The Woman with Endometriosis
    A. Pathophysiology
    B. Manifestations
    C. Interdisciplinary Care
        1. Diagnosis
        2. Medications
        3. Surgery
    D. Nursing Care
        1. Nursing Diagnoses and Interventions
           a. Anxiety
        2. Using NANDA, NIC, and NOC
        3. Community-Based Care
XIV. The Woman with Cervical Cancer
    A. Risk Factors
    B. Pathophysiology
    C. Manifestations
    D. Interdisciplinary Care
        1. Diagnosis
        2. Medications
        3. Surgery
        4. Radiation Therapy
    E. Nursing Care
        1. Health Promotion
        2. Assessment
        3. Nursing Diagnoses and Interventions
           a. Fear
           b. Impaired Tissue Integrity
        4. Using NANDA, NIC, and NOC
        5. Community-Based Care
XV. The Woman with Endometrial Cancer
    A. Risk Factors
    B. Pathophysiology
    C. Manifestations
    D. Interdisciplinary Care
        1. Diagnosis
        2. Medications
        3. Surgery
        4. Radiation Therapy
    E. Nursing Care
        1. Health Promotion
        2. Assessment
        3. Nursing Diagnoses and Interventions
           a. Acute Pain
           b. Disturbed Body Image
           c. Ineffective Sexuality Pattern
        4. Community-Based Care
XVI. The Woman with Ovarian Cancer
    A. Risk Factors
    B. Pathophysiology
    C. Manifestations
    D. Complications
    E. Interdisciplinary Care
        1. Diagnosis
        2. Medications
        3. Surgery
        4. Radiation Therapy

FOCUSED STUDY TIPS

1. List alternative and complementary therapies used by women to relieve manifestations associated with menopause and menstrual disorders.

---

2. Summarize the surgical procedures used to treat female reproductive system and breast disorders.

---

3. Discuss the physiologic process of menopause.

_____

_____

_____

4. List the risk factors, manifestations, and nursing care for cancer of the cervix, endometrium, ovary, vulva, and breast.

_____

_____

_____

_____

CASE STUDY

Elizabeth Baldwin is a 21-year-old female client. She is in today to have her first Pap test and breast examination. Answer the following questions based on knowledge of Pap tests and breast examinations.

1. How often does the American Cancer Society recommend Pap tests?

2. What are risk factors for cervical cancer?

3. What are the instructions for how to perform a breast self-examination?

NCLEX REVIEW QUESTIONS

1. Select the false statement:
   1. The sexual response cycle has four phases: excitement, plateau, orgasm, and resolution.
   2. Sexual stimulation results in vasocongestion of the blood vessels that surround the vagina, which causes engorgement, increased lubrication, and genital swelling and enlargement.
   3. Multiple orgasms are physically possible in all women.
   4. The sexual response phases always occur in the same sequence and duration.
2. A nurse is planning a seminar about menopause. Which of the following statements made by a participant is correct and indicates a need for further teaching?
   1. Menopause is a disease and is not a normal physiologic process.
   2. Menopause is the permanent cessation of menses.
   3. Late menopause is associated with genetics, smoking, higher altitude, and obesity.
   4. The average woman will live one-fourth of her life after menopause.
3. Which term means bleeding between menstrual periods?
   1. Menorrhagia
   2. Metrorrhagia
   3. Oligomenorrhea
   4. Amenorrhea
4. Which of the following is an exaggerated forward tilting of the uterus?
   1. Retroversion
   2. Retroflexion
   3. Anteversion
   4. Anteflexion

5. A nurse is evaluating a client's understanding of breast self-examination (BSE). Which of the following statements indicates a need for further teaching?
   1. "Lie down on your back and place your right arm behind your head."
   2. "Use three different levels of pressure to feel all the breast tissue."
   3. "Use overlapping quarter-sized circular motions of the finger pads to feel the breast tissue."
   4. "Look at your breasts for any changes in size, shape, contour, or dimpling."
6. A nurse is planning a seminar about ovarian cancer. Which of the following statements by a participant is correct?
   1. "Ovarian cancer is the first most common gynecologic cancer in women in the United States."
   2. "An enlarged abdomen with ascites signals early-stage disease."
   3. "There are several types of ovarian cancers: epithelial tumors, germ cell tumors, and gonadal stromal tumors."
   4. "In early stages, ovarian cancer generally causes several warning signs or manifestations."
7. A nurse is evaluating a client's understanding of fibrocystic changes (FCC), or fibrocystic breast disease. Which of the following statements indicates a need for further teaching?
   1. "FCC is the physiologic nodularity and breast tenderness that increases and decreases with the menstrual cycle."
   2. "FCC is most common in women 20 to 30 years of age, and is common in postmenopausal women who are not taking hormone replacement."
   3. "FCC includes many different lesions and breast changes."
   4. "Women with fibrocystic changes experience bilateral or unilateral pain or tenderness in the upper, outer quadrants of their breasts, and report that their breasts feel particularly thick and lumpy the week prior to menses."
8. Select the correct statement about premenstrual syndrome (PMS).
   1. PMS is never a factor in absenteeism at school or work, decreased productivity, interpersonal relationship difficulties, and lifestyle disruption.
   2. Manifestations of PMS occur during the follicular phase of the menstrual cycle (3 to 6 days prior to the onset of the menstrual flow), and abate when the menstrual flow begins.
   3. The treatment of PMS integrates a self-monitored record of manifestations, regular exercise, caffeine, and a diet low in simple sugars and low in lean proteins.
   4. Alternative and complementary therapies that the woman with PMS may find helpful focus on diet, exercise, relaxation, and stress management.
9. A _____ uterine prolapse is complete prolapse of the uterus outside the body, with inversion of the vaginal canal.
   1. Mild
   2. First-degree
   3. Second-degree
   4. Third-degree
10. A _____ is a highly vascular, solid tumor attached by a pedicle or stem.
    1. Polyp
    2. Cyst
    3. Fistula
    4. Prolapse

CHAPTER 52

NURSING CARE OF CLIENTS WITH SEXUALLY TRANSMITTED INFECTIONS

LEARNING OUTCOMES

After completing Chapter 52, you will be able to demonstrate the following objectives:
- Explain the incidence, prevalence, characteristics, and prevention/control of sexually transmitted infections (STIs).
- Compare and contrast the pathophysiology, manifestations, interdisciplinary care, and nursing care of genital herpes, genital warts, vaginitis, chlamydia, gonorrhea, syphilis, and pelvic inflammatory disease.
- Explain the risk factors for and complications of STIs.
- Discuss the effects and nursing implications of medications and treatments used to treat STIs.

CLINICAL COMPETENCIES

- Assess functional health status of clients with STIs and monitor, document, and report abnormal manifestations.
- Determine priority nursing diagnoses and select and implement individualized nursing interventions for clients with STIs.
- Administer topical, oral, and injectable medications knowledgeably and safely.
- Integrate interdisciplinary care into care of clients with STIs.
- Provide teaching appropriate for prevention, control, and self-care of STIs.
- Revise plan of care as needed to provide effective interventions to promote, maintain, or restore functional health status to clients with STIs.

KEY TERMS

bacterial vaginosis
candidiasis
chancre
chlamydia
dyspareunia
genital herpes
genital warts

gonorrhea (GC)
pelvic inflammatory disease
   (PID)
sexually transmitted
   infections (STIs)
syphilis
trichomoniasis

CHAPTER OUTLINE

   I. Overview of Sexually Transmitted Infections
       A. Incidence and Prevalence
       B. Characteristics
       C. Prevention and Control
  II. The Client with Genital Herpes
       A. Pathophysiology
       B. Manifestations
       C. Interdisciplinary Care
           1. Diagnosis
           2. Medications
       D. Nursing Care
           1. Nursing Diagnoses and Interventions
               a. Acute Pain
               b. Sexual Dysfunction
           2. Community-Based Care
 III. The Client with Genital Warts
       A. Pathophysiology
       B. Manifestations
       C. Interdisciplinary Care
           1. Medications
           2. Other Treatments
       D. Nursing Care
           1. Nursing Diagnoses and Interventions
               a. Deficient Knowledge
               b. Fear
               c. Anxiety
           2. Community-Based Care
  IV. The Client with a Vaginal Infection
       A. Pathophysiology and Manifestations
           1. Bacterial Vaginosis
           2. Candidiasis
           3. Trichomoniasis
       B. Interdisciplinary Care
           1. Diagnosis
           2. Medications
       C. Nursing Care
           1. Nursing Diagnoses and Interventions
               a. Deficient Knowledge
               b. Acute Pain
           2. Community-Based Care
   V. The Client with Chlamydia
       A. Pathophysiology
       B. Manifestations

FOCUSED STUDY TIPS

1. Explain the nursing implications of medications and treatments used to treat STIs.

---

2. List the risk factors for and complications of STIs.

_____

_____

3. Discuss the interdisciplinary care and nursing care of genital warts, genital herpes, vaginitis, chlamydia, gonorrhea, syphilis, and pelvic inflammatory disease.

_____

_____

_____

_____

_____

4. Summarize the prevention/control of sexually transmitted infections (STIs).

_____

_____

CASE STUDY

John Bradley, RN is teaching a class about sexual transmitted infections (STIs). After the class one of the participants asks the following questions.

1. "What cause genital herpes?"

2. "What are the three clinical stages of syphilis?"

3. "Which STIs are reportable?"

NCLEX REVIEW QUESTIONS

1. Sexually transmitted infections (STIs) have reached epidemic proportions in the United States and continue to increase worldwide. Select the false statement about STIs.
    1. Many STIs are more easily transmitted from a woman to a man than from a man to a woman.
    2. The incidence of STIs is highest in young adults ages 15 to 24.
    3. STIs include those caused by bacteria, chlamydiae, viruses, fungi, protozoa, and parasites.
    4. Infections that are transmitted by vaginal, oral, and anal intimate contact and intercourse are referred to as sexually transmitted infections (STIs).
2. _____ is associated with cold sores, but may be transmitted to the genital area by oral intercourse or by self-inoculation through poor hand-washing practices.
    1. HSV-2
    2. HPV
    3. HSV-1
    4. GC
3. Which of the following is not a reportable disease?
    1. Genital warts
    2. Gonorrhea
    3. Syphilis
    4. AIDS

4. Which of the following statements about chlamydia is false?
    1. Because chlamydia is asymptomatic in most women until the uterus and fallopian tubes have been invaded, treatment may be delayed, which results in devastating long-term complications.
    2. Chlamydia can only be present for days to weeks without producing noticeable symptoms in women.
    3. The infections caused by chlamydia include acute urethral syndrome, nongonococcal urethritis, mucopurulent cervicitis, and pelvic inflammatory disease (PID).
    4. Complications of chlamydial infections in men include epididymitis, prostatitis, sterility, and Reiter's syndrome.
5. A nurse is evaluating a client's understanding of gonorrhea (GC). Which of the following statements by the client indicates a need for further teaching?
    1. "GC is caused by *Neisseria gonorrhoeae,* a gram-negative diplococcus."
    2. "GC is a reportable communicable disease."
    3. "Humans are not the only host for the organism."
    4. "Manifestations of gonorrhea in men include dysuria and serous, milky, or purulent discharge from the penis."
6. The_____ stage of syphilis is characterized by the appearance of a chancre and by regional enlargement of lymph nodes; little or no pain accompanies these warning signs.
    1. Secondary
    2. Latent
    3. Primary
    4. Tertiary
7. A nurse is planning a seminar about pelvic inflammatory disease (PID). Which of the following statements on an educational handout needs to be corrected?
    1. PID is a reportable disease in the United States.
    2. PID is usually polymicrobial (caused by more than one microbe) in origin; gonorrhea and chlamydia are common causative organisms.
    3. Manifestations of PID include fever, purulent vaginal discharge, severe lower abdominal pain, and a painful cervical movement.
    4. Complications include pelvic abscess, infertility, ectopic pregnancy, chronic pelvic pain, pelvic adhesions, dyspareunia, and chronic pelvic pain. Abscess formation is common.
8. _____ are slightly raised lesions that are often invisible to the naked eye, and also develop on keratinized skin.
    1. Keratotic warts
    2. Papular warts
    3. Flat warts
    4. Condyloma acuminata
9. Which of the following statements by a student nurse reflects correct understanding about trichomoniasis?
    1. "Trichomoniasis is caused by *Trichomonas vaginalis,* a protozoan parasite."
    2. "Trichomoniasis is the least common noncurable STI in young, sexually active women."
    3. "Symptoms of trichomoniasis usually appear within 1 to 4 days of exposure."
    4. "Women with trichomoniasis have a non-frothy, red-orange vaginal discharge with a strong fishy odor that is often accompanied by itching and irritation of the genitalia."
10. Which of the following diagnostic tests would you expect to see ordered for a client who may have syphilis?
    1. VDRL
    2. RPR
    3. FTA-ABS
    4. Gram stain

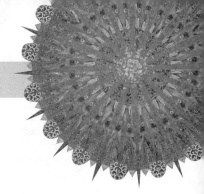

Answer Key

Chapter 1

Case Study Answers

1. *Explain the concept of heroic measures with regard to the administration of insulin. Does this constitute a dilemma for the nursing staff?* Heroic measures are defined as extraordinary, emergent life-saving measures used to prolong life when death is imminent. While diabetes is a chronic condition and the administration of insulin is life-saving this does not meet the criterion as a heroic measure because death is not imminent.

   The dilemma for the nursing staff is the discrepancy between the client's understanding of what constitutes a heroic measure and the true definition. Through education and additional support, the client will hopefully come to understand that this is a controllable process.

2. *While Jacob's reaction to a new chronic diagnosis may be common, what is he really saying?* The client is really saying that he is overwhelmed. He needs education, support, and possibly even some sleep.

3. *What role or roles might the nurse play in helping both Jacob and his wife at this time?* In caring for this client, the nurse will take on the roles of caregiver, especially during the acute care admission; and educator, both in the hospital and after discharge. The nurse may also play act as client advocate, both in and out of the acute care setting, by looking for an assisted living facility that will meet the needs of the client and his wife and facilitating any changes the client wants to make to his advanced directive after he adapts to his disease. A case manager would hopefully be assigned to help coordinate this client's long-term care needs.

NCLEX Review Question Answers

1. Answer: 2 & 5
   Rationale: Errors and misuse of services are becoming more common but they are system problems, they are not caused by healthcare professionals. Misuse or overuse of diagnostic tests and errors effect thousands of clients every year, and cause injury and/or death. The nursing shortage is both a system problem within a facility

and an international problem, but it is the system problem that allows the high nurse-to-client ratio. Lack of focus is only one component that can introduce error; typically, there are many other issues that lead to an error. Breakdowns in the system, from the time of the assessment to the administration of a treatment or diagnostic test, allow errors to occur or the misuse of services.
   Nursing Process: Planning
   Client Need: Safe, Effective Care Environment

2. Answer: 1
   Rationale: Critical thinking allows the nurse to focus his or her own thoughts on a specific situation. It is only by examining one's attitudes and prejudices that the nurse is able to identify those variables and limit their effects on client care. Critical thinking requires practice and experience—it is not innate. Critical thinking helps to identify the independent practice domain; it is not a matter of restriction.
   Nursing Process: Planning
   Client Need: Psychosocial Integrity

3. Answer: 3
   Rationale: Exploring divergent opinions allows the nurse to explore options for this situation and care in the future. While critical thinking is important in all situations, reflection cannot take place in emergency situations. After the emergency there will be time for reflection. Clarification includes validating information as well as noting similarities and differences in information and previous situations. While critical thinking is predominantly an independent process, discussion with peers and mentors can be an essential part of the process.
   Nursing Process: Planning
   Client Need: Health Promotion and Maintenance

4. Answer: 2
   Rationale: Developing nursing diagnoses is part of the second step of the nursing process, diagnosis. Diagnosis is driven by assessment findings but is not part of the assessment step. Clarification of subjective data is part of the question and answer period of every nursing assessment. Planning client care is the third step in the nursing process and is based on assessment

findings. Evaluation is the final step of the nursing process. While evaluation is based on measurable objectives which are based on assessment findings, it is not a part of the assessment process.
Nursing Process: Assessment
Client Need: Physiological Integrity

5. Answer: 4
Rationale: Documentation is equally important in each stage of the nursing process. While documenting assessment findings is very important, it is equally important to document the interdisciplinary care plan, and the client's care and progress. Computer-assisted documentation guides the nurse's documentation but it should not limit his/her options or choices. Charting by exception is an accepted form of documentation at many facilities.
Nursing Process: Documentation
Client Need: Safe, Effective Care Environment

6. Answer: 4
Rationale: Assessment leads to outcomes planning. The nurse can look at the effectiveness of the assessment, but this is not the focus of the evaluation stage. Nursing diagnoses will lead to a plan, but are not a plan in themselves that can be evaluated. The planning stage includes developing measurable outcomes. These measurable outcomes that are implemented in the implementation stage are evaluated in the nursing process.
Nursing Process: Evaluation
Client Need: Psychosocial and Physiological Integrity

7. Answer: 1
Rationale: When outcomes are not met, the nurse and the client should modify the outcome so that the outcome continues to be measurable and attainable. Outcomes evaluation is not a measure of success or failure for the nurse. If outcomes were not met, it reflects that the team was not able to meet those outcomes, but it is not about the client's or the nurse's success or failure. Outcomes must be attainable for the client in order to maintain the momentum to continue to work toward goals. The ability to modify those outcomes helps both the client and the nurse.
Nursing Process: Evaluation
Client Need: Health Promotion and Maintenance

8. Answer: 3
Rationale: Maintaining confidentiality is a single component of nursing standards but it is not the only component. Client confidentiality is also a legal right. Standards of nursing practice define nursing practice and, in doing so, protect the nurses who meet those standards. Standards of practice help to protect the public by establishing the accepted guidelines of nursing practice. Ethical guidelines help nurses work through nursing dilemmas.

Nursing Process: Evaluation
Client Need: Safe, Effective Care Environment

9. Answer: 2
Rationale: The focus is on health promotion and illness prevention; while this may lead to fewer hospital days, the goal is the highest level of client wellness. The role of educator is of greater importance now than in the past because clients are in the acute care setting for less time. Fewer days and increased number of comorbidities make nursing educators an extremely important part of the healing process. Client teaching must begin at the time of admission, not after discharge. Advocacy assists the client in decision-making. Education may allow the client to make better decisions, but the focus of client education is not decision making.
Nursing Process: Implementation
Client Need: Health Promotion and Maintenance

10. Answer: 4
Rationale: Primary nursing requires little delegation because the nurse provides individualized care to a small number of clients. Team nursing is predominately in hospital care, with a variety of team members who work together to provide client care, and is led by the registered nurse. Case management involves in- and out-of-hospital care coordination, and a variety of members of the healthcare team are coordinated by the registered nurse. Both team nursing and case management require a high degree of delegation and trust in the healthcare team.
Nursing Process: Planning
Client Need: Health Promotion and Maintenance

Chapter 2

Case Study Answers

1. *What alterations in health is Jacob at risk for developing as a middle adult?* Jacob is at risk for alterations in health from obesity, cardiovascular disease, cancer, substance abuse, and physical and psychosocial stressors.

2. *What guidelines are useful in assessing the achievement of significant developmental tasks in the middle adult?* The nurse can use the following guidelines to assess the developmental tasks of the middle adult. Does the middle adult:
   a. Accept the aging body?
   b. Feel comfortable with and respect oneself?
   c. Enjoy the freedom to be independent?
   d. Accept changes in family roles?
   e. Enjoy success and satisfaction from work and/or family roles?
   f. Interact well and share activities with a partner?
   g. Expand or renew previous interests?
   h. Pursue charitable and altruistic activities?
   i. Consider plans for retirement?

j. Have a meaningful philosophy of life?

k. Follow preventive health care practices?

3. *How can the nurse promote healthy behaviors in Jacob?*

Healthy Behaviors in the Middle Adult

- Choose foods from all food groups and eat a variety of foods.
- Choose a diet low in fat (30% or less of total calories), saturated fat (less than 10% of calories), and cholesterol (less than 300 mg daily.)
- Adjust daily calorie intake to maintain healthy weight.
- Choose a diet that each day includes at least three servings of vegetables, two servings of fruits, and six servings of grains.
- Use sugar, salt, and sodium in moderation.
- Increase calcium intake (in perimenopausal women) to 1,200 mg daily.
- Consume high-fiber foods.
- Make exercise a part of life, carrying out regular exercise that is moderately strenuous, is consistent, and avoids overexertion. Exercise for 30 minutes at least 4 to 5 times a week.
- Include exercise as part of any weight reduction program.
- Have an annual vision examination.
- Have an annual dental checkup.

NCLEX Review Question Answers

1. Answer: 1

Rationale: Influenza is an acute illness that lasts for a relatively short time, and is self-limiting. Hemophilia, cancer, and sickle cell disease are chronic illnesses that are associated with genetic makeup.
Nursing Process: Assessment
Client Need: Physiological Integrity

2. Answer: 3

Rationale: Examples of altered responses are the relationship of obesity to hypertension, cigarette smoking to chronic obstructive pulmonary disease, a sedentary lifestyle to heart disease, and a high-stress career to alcoholism.
Nursing Process: Diagnosis
Client Need: Health Promotion and Maintenance

3. Answer: 1

Rationale: Practices that are known to promote health and wellness include exercising moderately and regularly, sleeping seven to eight hours each day, limiting alcohol consumption to a moderate amount and favoring red wine, smoking cessation, keeping sun exposure to a minimum, maintaining recommended sleeping for five to six hours a day is not known to promote health and wellness. Immunizations.
Nursing Process: Assessment
Client Need: Health Promotion and Maintenance

4. Answer: 4

Rationale: Self-preoccupation is characteristic of assuming the sick role stage, and the person focuses on alterations in function that result from the illness. Experiencing symptoms is the first stage of an acute illness. During this stage, a person experiences one or more manifestations that serve as cues that a change in normal health is occurring. The stage of assuming a dependent role begins when a person accepts the diagnosis and planned treatment of the illness. As the severity of the illness increases, so does the dependent role. The final stage of an acute illness is recovery and rehabilitation. This focus makes client education and continuity of care a major goal for nursing.
Nursing Process: Assessment
Client Need: Psychological Integrity

5. Answer: 1

Rationale: The adult years commonly are divided into three stages: the young adult (age 18 to 40), the middle adult (age 40 to 65), and the older adult (over age 65).
Nursing Process: Assessment
Client Need: Health Promotion and Maintenance

6. Answer: 2

Rationale: Cancers of the breast, colon, lung, and reproductive system are common in the middle years. The middle adult is at risk for cancer as a result of increased length of exposure to environmental carcinogens, as well as alcohol and nicotine use.
Nursing Process: Diagnosis
Client Need: Health Promotion and Maintenance

7. Answer: 4

Rationale: Obesity is a frequently-occurring condition in the middle adult years. The most frequently occurring conditions in the older adult are hypertension, arthritis, heart diseases, cancer, sinusitis, and diabetes.
Nursing Process: Diagnosis
Client Need: Health Promotion and Maintenance

8. Answer: 3

Rationale: The developmental tasks of the family with adolescents and young adults focus on transition. The family with infants or preschoolers must adjust to having and supporting the needs of more than two members. The family with school-age children has the developmental tasks of adjusting to the expanded world of children in school and encouraging educational achievement. The family with middle adults has the developmental tasks of maintaining ties with older and younger generations and planning for retirement.
Nursing Process: Diagnosis
Client Need: Psychosocial Integrity

9. Answer: 4

> **Rationale:** From age 18 to 25, the healthy young adult is at the peak of physical development and is at risk for alterations in health from sexually transmitted diseases. Certain diseases occur at a higher rate of incidence in some races and ethnic groups than in others. For example, eye disorders are more prevalent in Chinese Americans. Cardiovascular disorders are uncommon in young adults, but the incidence increases after the age of 40. The middle adult often has a problem maintaining a healthy weight.
> **Nursing Process:** Diagnosis
> **Client Need:** Health Promotion and Maintenance

10. Answer: 2

> **Rationale:** Confronting the inevitability of death is a positive coping skill for clients with chronic illnesses.
> **Nursing Process:** Assessment
> **Client Need:** Psychosocial Integrity

Chapter 3

Case Study Answers

1. *What distractions limited the nurse's ability to assess and care for Mr. Cohen?* Mr. Cohen's friends are a wonderful support system but if they interrupt the nurse's visit they are a distraction. Explaining the importance of focus during the nurse's visit may help both Mr. Cohen and his friends to respect that time. Schedule visits so that they are not during a high visitation time.

Encourage Mr. Cohen to have a support person with him if this would help him with the information. The nurse should make note of the time the client is having lunch, ask if this is his normal lunch time, and avoid visits during this time.

2. *What safety concerns do you see in Mr. Cohen's home setting? Would these be expensive to repair?* Isolation could be a concern. But while Mr. Cohen lives alone, his friends help to prevent social isolation and would find him if he were to fall or have an emergency. There is no expense related to this issue. The extension cord, particularly the electrical cord that is under the rug, increases the risk of fire. It could be expensive to have additional outlets put in, but the nurse needs to check to see if the plugged-in item is necessary, or whether it could be moved to a safer location?

The heavy cookware could be another concern. The client is able to handle the cookware today, but the risk of dropping the heavy cookware when he is in a hurry, tired, or becomes weaker increases the fire safety risk. There is some small-to-moderate expense in replacing the cookware. The real expense may be emotional if this cookware was used by his now-deceased wife.

3. *What can you do to improve Mr. Cohen's safety with regard to his medication administration?* A weekly medication holder designed for the elderly might make it easier for him to get to his medications, and determine whether or not they were taken. The medications can be organized by Mr. Cohen with the assistance of the nurse.

NCLEX Review Question Answers

1. Answer: 1

> **Rationale:** The ability to provide care in a client's home affects the individual, not the community. The number of extended families in a community provides support for the members of the community. Environmental factors such as air and water quality increase or decrease the community members' risk of both acute and chronic illnesses. Access to health care improves preventative care as well as care during acute situations.
> **Nursing Process:** Evaluation
> **Client Need:** Health Promotion and Maintenance

2. Answer: 2

> **Rationale:** Community-based healthcare services often allow clients with early stages of Alzheimer's disease to remain at home while their caregivers work or run errands. These programs are designed around providing for the client's physical and psychosocial needs in a safe environment. Meals on Wheels is a wonderful example but is not a description of community programs. These programs help to promote wellness and early intervention so that, in the long run, they may decrease the need for hospitalization; but that is not the focus of community-based health care.
> **Nursing Process:** Implementation
> **Client Need:** Physical and Psychosocial Integrity

3. Answer: 4

> **Rationale:** The purpose of home health care is to promote, maintain, or restore the level of independence of the client, not to promote their dependence. Clients who require daily nursing care will do best in a more intensive care setting. The largest single source of reimbursement for home health care is Medicare. Clients who do not need inclient care benefit most from the type of assistance and education that home health care provides.
> **Nursing Process:** Assessment
> **Client Need:** Health Promotion and Maintenance

4. Answer: 2

> **Rationale:** While home health care is less expensive per day than a hospital admission, it is not inexpensive. Contact a local home health agency and find out what the cost would be for a registered nurse to do a dressing change or administer and IV antibiotic once a day for one week. Some home healthcare agencies receive donations, endowments, or monies from charities to help provide home health care for clients who

have limited income and no health insurance. Family members can be one referral source for home health care. Friends and family may see needs or issues that the client does not recognize. A physician's order and management of the client's care is legally and ethically required for home health care.
Nursing Process: Planning
Client Need: Health Promotion and Maintenance

5. Answer: 3
Rationale: Evaluation of outcomes established during the hospital stay should occur during that stay. The home health nurse will work with the client to establish outcomes for the home health experience. A referral and physician order must be obtained prior to the initial visit. The initial visit is similar to the first meeting in any other setting. It focuses on assessment and obtaining data that will allow the nurse and client to establish the goals of care. The goal for all clients is to be successful in reaching their maximum level of independence.
Nursing Process: Assessment
Client Need: Health Promotion and Maintenance

6. Answer: 3
Rationale: Deficient knowledge related to a diagnosis of chronic obstructive pulmonary disease AEB questions about oxygen use is a nursing diagnosis that could be used for a home health client but is not an outcome statement. Client will use oxygen statement is not measurable. Client will demonstrate application of oxygen by the second home health visit is a statement that identifies who, the means, and a timeframe for evaluation. Apply oxygen per physician order is not measurable.
Nursing Process: Planning
Client need: Physiological Integrity

7. Answer: 1
Rationale: The nurse must be able to communicate with all members of the healthcare team to coordinate the care of the client. Changes in the plan of care may begin with the client, nurse, or physician but changes in the plan of care must be approved by the physician. Documentation is a legal requirement and is a necessary part of the nursing process. Documentation supports care for the purpose of reimbursement as well. A fax machine may be used in some organizations to share information but it does not help to maintain client confidentiality.
Nursing Process: Planning
Client Need: Safe, Effective Care Environment

8. Answer: 2
Rationale: The client should be independent in the home and have ample support to provide for their health and safety. The nurse can be seen as an extension of the family, visiting on days off, and receiving calls after the discharge. In order to work with the client and family, a positive rapport must be established. Multiple caregivers who share responsibility for the client's care help to reduce the risk of caregiver burnout.
Nursing Process: Planning
Client Need: Safe, Effective Care Environment

9. Answer: 2
Rationale: The client will have many influential people in their lives, including members of their family and friends. Encouraging the client to be in-tune with their bodies and encouraging them to ask questions makes them an active participant in the learning process. Providing the client with information that is currently of concern is much more effective. Involving an individual in the learning process with the client will help to provide support but involving too many people in the process can limit the learning opportunities by creating distractions.
Nursing Process: Implementation
Client Need: Health Promotion and Maintenance

10. Answer: 4
Rationale: A discussion with social services should come only after a discussion with the client and failure to correct the safety issues. Ignoring safety issues is considered nursing negligence. These suggestions do not address the medication issue or identify any underlying issues. By talking with the client the nurse is able to advocate for the client.
Nursing Process: Assessment
Client Need: Safe, Effective Care Environment

Chapter 4

Case Study Answers

1. *Mrs. Elvira's informed consent document includes the surgeon's name, the alternatives and risks of treatments, and the date and time she and her surgeon signed the consent. What is missing?* The type of surgery is missing, which is a right radical mastectomy.

2. *What postoperative complication(s) is Mrs. Elvira at most risk of developing based on her history?* Due to her smoking history, she is at risk for developing pneumonia. Her inactivity places her at risk for a deep vein thrombosis (DVT). The client's aspirin use and herbal diet aids place her at risk for hemorrhage.

3. *What preoperative studies and interventions will Mrs. Elvira undergo to reduce the likelihood of intraoperative and postoperative complications?* She will undergo lab testing such as blood and urine testing to determine her blood count, clotting ability, and creatinine levels. Based on her smoking history, she will be given a chest X-ray. Antiembolism stockings will be placed on her preoperatively.

Pre- and postoperative teaching will include the need for coughing and deep breathing exercises, as well as the importance of mobility.

4. *Prior to discharge, Mrs. Elvira will be instructed to assess her incision site for signs of infection. What are they?* Signs of incision infection include redness, pain, swelling, an increased temperature, and presence of purulent material.

NCLEX Review Question Answers

1. Answer: 1
   Rationale: Outpatient procedures decrease cost to the client, hospital, and insuring agency. Patients undergoing outpatient procedures must cope with the additional stress of needing to learn a great deal of information in a short span of time. Inclient procedures may afford the client and family a longer period of time to learn a great deal of information in a more comfortable span of time. Outpatient surgery provides for less time for pain relief before discharge. Outpatient surgery provides for less interruption in the client's and family's routine.
   Nursing Process: Planning
   Client Need: Psychosocial Integrity

2. Answer: 3
   Rationale: Informed consent does not include the date, time, and location of the planned surgical procedure. This information will be shared with the client as part of their preoperative surgical instructions. Informed consent must include the proposed surgical procedure, alternative treatments available, and the client's right to refuse or withdraw from treatment.
   Nursing Process: Planning
   Client Need: Safe, Effective Care Environment

3. Answer: 3
   Rationale: Fluids for irrigation and intravenous administration must be warmed to prevent hypothermia. The application of warm blankets upon arrival in the surgical area and after sterile drapes are removed will prevent the client from becoming chilled. Warm, humidified air will assist in the prevention of hypothermia. Wet surgical drapes allows cooling of the body through evaporation. Keeping the surgical drapes dry will prevent hypothermia in the surgical client.
   Nursing Process: Implementation
   Client Need: Physiological Integrity

4. Answer 4
   Rationale: There are three stages of anesthesia that clients experience under general anesthesia. They include: induction, maintenance, and emergence.
   Nursing Process: Diagnosis
   Client Need: Physiological Integrity

5. Answer: 4
   Rationale: Administration of an epidural blood patch is an effective method to eliminate a spinal headache. Hydration should be increased in a client suffering from a spinal headache. Intake of caffeine may be increased to help decrease the severity of the headache. The client's head should remain flat because any elevation will increase the intensity of the headache.
   Nursing Process: Implementation
   Client Need: Physiological Integrity

6. Answer: 2
   Rationale: The circulating nurse is responsible for documenting intraoperative nursing activities, medications, blood administration, placement of drains and catheters, and length of the procedure. The surgeon is the physician who performs the procedure. The Certified Registered Nursing Assistant (CRNA) evaluates the client preoperatively, administers the anesthesia and other required medications, transfuses blood or other blood products, infuses intravenous fluids, continuously monitors the client's physiologic status, alerts the surgeon to developing problems and treats them as they arise, and supervises the client's recovery in the Post Anesthesia Care Unit). The role of the scrub person primarily involves technical skills, manual dexterity, and in-depth knowledge of the anatomic and mechanical aspects of a particular surgery. The scrub person handles sutures, instruments, and other equipment that is immediately adjacent to the sterile field.
   Nursing Process: Planning
   Client Need: Safe, Effective Care Environment

7. Answer: 1
   Rationale: Improper positioning can lead to sensory and motor dysfunction, and result in nerve damage. Improper positioning can cause injury to muscles and joints.
   Nursing Process: Evaluation
   Client Need: Physiological Integrity

8. Answer: 3
   Rationale: Postoperative testing must be completed as ordered to assess for any physiologic contraindication to the proposed surgical intervention. Nail polish and contacts should be removed prior to arriving at the hospital. Patients should bring a pair of eyeglasses with a case with them for pre- and postoperative use. The client must adhere to the NPO order as directed by the surgeon and reinforced by means of preoperative teaching.
   Nursing Process: Evaluation
   Client Need: Safe, Effective Care Environment

9. Answer: 1
   Rationale: Nursing care includes keeping the affected extremity at or above heart level, ensuring that the affected area is not rubbed or

massaged, recording bilateral calf or thigh circumferences every shift, and teaching and supporting the client and family.
Nursing Process: Implementation
Client Need: Physiological Integrity

10. Answer: 3

Rationale: The respiratory rate of a client who is experiencing a pulmonary embolism will increase. Other common assessment findings include mild to moderate dyspnea, chest pain, diaphoresis, anxiety, restlessness, rapid pulse, dysrhythmias, cough, and cyanosis.
Nursing Process: Assessment
Client Need: Physiological Integrity

Chapter 5

Case Study Answers

1. *Is a hospice organization available to members of your community? What other community resources would be helpful for this client?*
   a. Public transportation to and from appointments
   b. A medical supply company
   c. Grief counseling or support groups for both the client and her family
   d. Meals on Wheels
   e. Pharmacy delivery

2. *According to Kübler-Ross's stages of coping with loss, in what stage of grieving is the client? At what stage can you anticipate her parents will begin?*
   a. The client is in denial.
   b. While there is no way to know where her parents will begin the grieving process, we could anticipate that they, like the client, may begin in denial based on her understanding of the disease, her age, and her role in the family.

3. *What factors will affect the parents' ability to grieve their upcoming loss?*
   a. The client's age, role in the family, their social support network, spiritual issues, cultural practices, everyday family function, and the actions of the healthcare team.

NCLEX Review Question Answers

1. Answer: 3

Rationale: Asking whether the physician told the client about the testing is a yes or no question, and these types of questions do not encourage the client to express his/her feelings. Asking whether there is someone the nurse can call for the client demonstrates that the nurse is uncomfortable. Asking what is troubling the client does not assume anything; it simply acknowledges what the nurse has observed and asks the client to share his/her feelings. Asking whether the client is upset about tomorrow's testing is again a yes or no question, which does not encourage discussion

and makes assumptions about what is bothering the client.
Nursing Process: Assessment
Client Need: Psychosocial Integrity

2. Answer: 1

Rationale: If the client has cultural needs that don't interfere with the diagnosis and treatment process, it should be supported by the healthcare team. If the nurse has concerns about potential, but not immediate, risks the nurse should ask the supervisor and/or physician before bringing those concerns to the family. Not all cultural issues are religious. If the nurse thinks that the physician will have concerns about the medallions, the nurse can call the physician without alarming the client and family.
Nursing Process: Assessment
Client Need: Psychosocial Integrity

3. Answer: 2

Rationale: An advance directive allows the client to state his/her choices for care and may allow the client to choose a durable power of attorney. A durable power of attorney or healthcare surrogate is the person designated by the client to make decisions if the client is unable to make those decisions. Living wills give directions for care if the client is determined to be in an unrecoverable state and is unable to make decisions. Client's bills of rights explain the rights and responsiblities of the client. These include developing an advance directive and appointing a healthcare surrogate.
Nursing Process: Planning
Client Need: Psychosocial and Physiological Integrity

4. Answer: 4

Rationale: This is not the best answer because it is the nurse who is not allowing the family to burn the candle. While it was based on hospital policy, it seemed to be coming from the nurse. There was also no offer of alternatives. Breaking hospital policy is not the answer. Open flame risks client safety. Open flame even for a minute could cause a fire, expecially with oxygen sources. Hospital policy does not allow for the anyone to have an open flame inside the building. The best response is to ask whether there is anything else they could do that would have similar meaning, because it not only reflects hospital policy but shows caring for the client's family by searching for other comforting alternatives.
Nursing Process: Planning
Client Need: Psychosocial Integrity

5. Answer: 2

Rationale: Assessment is required prior to administering PRN medications.Assessment and repositioning may be all the client requires and the open reassessment allow the nurse to look for more information beyond pain, such as nausea.

While asking the family can be helpful, the nurse should do his/her own assessment. This would only help if the client was actually in pain. If the nurse's assessment shows that the client is having pain and has been medicated without adequate relief, this would be a great option.
Nursing Process: Assessment
Client Need: Safety and Physiological Integrity

6. Answer: 2, 3, and 5
    Rationale: Kubler-Ross would describe the anger stage as denial. Engel's acute stage includes the shock and disbelief that is being expressed by this client. Bowlby's protest stage includes the lack of acceptance. Lindemann's morbid grief reaction is delayed, dysfunctional grief—not anticipatory grief or anxiety about an upcoming loss. Caplan's theory of stress and loss acknowledges the factors of loss and the anticipation of loss throughout the theory.
    Nursing Process: Evaluation
    Client Need: Psychosocial Integrity

7. Answer: 3
    Rationale: Hourly vital signs are unnecessary, although assessments for comfort continue to be important. Repositioning the client as needed for comfort remains vital but moving the client every two hours may take them from a position where he or she is comfortable. Elevating the head of the bed and providing a gentle breeze with a fan can ease the client's breathing. Clients at the end of life often are not hungry. Families may need help to understand this.
    Nursing Process: Implementation
    Client Need: Physiological Integrity

8. Answer: 4
    Rationale: A small amount of morphine will ease breathing and decrease anxiety. Two liters of oxygen via nasal cannula will provide a small amount of oxygen; it may be enough to improve the oxygen saturation and ease breathing. Repositioning the client by raising the head of the bed improves oxygenation. Administration of 100% oxygen via nonrebreather mask may be an eventual act but considering the client's saturation of 92%, it is an overreaction.
    Nursing Process: Implementation
    Client Need: Physiological Integrity

9. Answer: 4
    Rationale: Encouraging sips or ice chips will increase the vomiting. The client should be given nothing by mouth. A side effect of morphine is nausea. This may be causing the client's nausea. Anything given by mouth may contribute to the client's nausea. Giving a medication by mouth with intractible nausea does not provide adequate absorption. Odansetron (Zofran) by IV infusion is the most effective intervention for this client.
    Nursing Process: Implementation
    Client Need: Physiological Integrity

10. Answer: 2
    Rationale: Providing oral care and repositioning are interventions, not evaluations. These reflect an outcome statement such as, "mucous membranes will remain moist and intact during hospital stay." Administration of oxygen is an intervention. Stating that the oxygen was applied and the saturation improved to 92% would be an evaluation of the saturation. Stating that the client is confused, and sister is at bedside is an assessment finding. Stating how the client responded to having the sister at the bedside would be an evaluation statement.
    Nursing Process: Evaluation
    Client Need: Physiological Integrity

Chapter 6

Case Study Answers

1. *How long does Ryan have to have had excessive drinking behaviors to be considered substance dependent?* Three months or more.

2. *What factors affect the rate of alcohol absorption?* Factors such as body mass, food intake, and liver function can affect the rate of alcohol absorption.

3. *What vitamin deficiency is associated with alcoholism?* Thiamine. *How will the nurse assist Ryan in meeting his nutritional needs?* The nurse will perform the following interventions:
    a. Administer vitamins and dietary supplements as ordered by the physician.
    b. Monitor lab work and report significant changes to the physician.
    c. Collaborate with dietitian to determine the number of calories needed to provide adequate nutrition and realistic weight gain.
    d. Teach the importance of adequate nutrition by explaining the food guide pyramid and relating the physical effects of malnutrition on body systems.

4. *The nurse will teach Ryan HALT. What is HALT?* HALT is a method to identifying relapsing behavior. The acronym HALT stands for: hungry, angry, lonely, and tired.

NCLEX Review Question Answers

1. Answer: 1
    Rationale: Dopamine and dopamine receptor sites are intricately involved in the complex workings between the nervous system and abusive substances. Studies show that dopamine D(1) and D(2) receptors sustain the addictive danger of drugs. Recent studies have also shown that the dopamine D(3) receptor is involved in drug-seeking behavior.

2. Answer: 4
    Rationale: Compared to other ethnic groups, Asian Americans report the lowest prevalence of

family history of alcoholism (Ebberhart, Luczak, Avenecy, & Wall, 2003). Caucasians, Hispanics, and African Americans, on the other hand, have insufficient amounts of the enzyme aldehyde dehydrogenase for metabolizing alcohol, and report higher alcoholism rates (Bersamin, Paschall, & Flewelling, 2005).
Nursing Process: Diagnosis
Client Need: Health Maintenance and Promotion

3. Answer: 2
   Rationale: Substance abusers have a low tolerance for frustration and pain.
   Nursing Process: Planning
   Client Need: Psychosocial Integrity

4. Answer: 3
   Rationale: Marijuana use can trigger psychosis in schizophrenic clients and according to recent research, cannabis use may be a risk factor in developing future psychotic symptoms (Ferdinand et al, 2005).
   Nursing Process: Diagnosis
   Client Need: Health Promotion and Maintenance

5. Answer: 1
   Rationale: Methamphetamine is a powerful stimulant drug that is commonly referred to as "speed," "crystal," "crank," "go," and, most recently, "ice." Examples of common opiate brand names include Vicodin®, Percocet®, OxyContin®, and Darvon®. Hallucinogens are called psychedelics and include phencyclidine (PCP), 3,4-methylenediosy-methamphetamine (MDMA), d-lysergic acid diethylamide (LSD), mescaline, dimethyltryptamine (DMT), and psilocybin.
   Nursing Process: Diagnosis
   Client Need: Health Promotion and Maintenance

6. Answer: 2
   Rationale: Tears are not tested for drug content. The body fluids most often tested for drug content are blood and urine, although saliva, perspiration, and even hair can be tested.
   Nursing Process: Assessment
   Client Need: Health Promotion and Maintenance

7. Answer: 3
   Rationale: Ask questions in a nonthreatening, matter-of-fact manner, phrased to avoid implying wrongdoing. The appropriate question from those listed is, "Have you ever been treated in an alcohol or drug abuse clinic?" This is an open-ended, nonthreatening question. The other questions are closed-ended and imply wrongdoing.
   Nursing Process: Assessment
   Client Need: Health Promotion and Maintenance

8. Answer: 2
   Rationale: The CAGE questionnaire is more useful when the client may not recognize he or

she has an alcohol problem, or is uncomfortable acknowledging it. This questionnaire is designed to be a self-report of drinking behavior, or may be administered by a professional. Because self-report tools are not always answered truthfully, all clients who screen positive for drug addiction should be evaluated according to other diagnostic criteria. HALT is a tool used to identify addictive relapse behavior.

9. Answer: 1
   Rational: Nursing interventions employed for a client with substance abuse disorder includes: assessing the client's level of disorientation, providing a private room but never leaving the client alone without monitoring, not accepting the use of defense mechanisms as an attempt to blame others for their actions, and encouraging the client to verbalize anxieties.
   Nursing Process: Implementation
   Client Need: Psychosocial Integrity

10. Answer: 3
    Rationale: Healthcare professionals have a higher risk for opiate abuse than other professionals due to the high accessibility of opiates in their line of work (Trinkoff et al, 2000).
    Nursing Process: Diagnosis
    Client Need: Health Promotion and Maintenance

Chapter 7

Case Study Answers

1. *What is a hurricane?* A hurricane is a type of tropical cyclone. It is a low-pressure system that generally forms in the tropics.

2. *What physical effects of a hurricane is Mrs. Deckman at risk for, regardless of her past medical history?* Common physical effects include asphyxia due to drowning; wounds, bone, joint, and muscle injuries; aggravation of chronic illnesses; stress-related symptoms, upper respiratory infections; gastrointestinal illnesses; clean-up injuries; animal, snake, and insect bites; skin irritations and infections; obstetrical complications; waterborne and insect-borne diseases from contaminated water supplies and insect breeding grounds (Clark, 2003; Smith & Maurer, 2000).

3. *Mrs. Deckman was given a triage level of red after she was taken to a local shelter. What does this mean?* Her age and potential complications of diabetes are the reason for her red triage level. Her blood sugar levels require assessment and monitoring, as does her physical health due to uncontrolled blood sugar levels.

4. *Mrs. Deckman asks the nurse for assistance in developing a disaster box to be used in case of another disaster. What items should the nurse suggest to be kept in the box?*

Mrs. Deckman's disaster box should include the following: a current list of medications, doses, and times of administration; names and phone numbers of significant persons; eyeglass prescriptions; style and serial numbers of medical devices; healthcare policies and numbers; identification; list of allergies; blood type; checkbook; credit cards; insurance agent's name and number; copy of driver's license; 72-hour supply of medications; dentures; eyeglasses; list of special dietary needs; sturdy shoes; and warm clothing, blankets, incontinence briefs, prostheses, hearing aids, hearing aid batteries, extra wheelchair batteries, oxygen, and other assistive devices.

NCLEX Review Question Answers

1. Answer: 3
   Rationale: Anthrax is a chemical nonconventional weapon. Conventional weapons include bombs and guns.
   Nursing Process: Planning
   Client Need: Safe, Effective Care Environment

2. Answer: 4
   Rationale: High resistors of electric current include bone, tendon, and fat. A person who has been struck by lightning does carry an electric charge. The immediate flashover of current around the body results in very little skin breakdown or skin burn. High electrolyte and water content area in the body conduct the greatest electrical current.
   Nursing Process: Planning
   Client Need: Safe, Effective Care Environment

3. Answer: 4
   Rationale: People are exposed to ionizing radiation frequently, but in small doses. Some of the sources of this everyday exposure are outer space, the stars, sun, natural radioactive isotopes, and X-ray machines. These sources create little, if any, ill effects.
   Nursing Process: Planning
   Client Need: Safe, Effective Care Environment

4. Answer: 2
   Rationale: A level II disaster requires mutual aid from surrounding communities and regional efforts. A level I disaster is dealt with effectively by local emergency response personnel and organizations. A level III disaster overwhelms local and regional assets and statewide or federal assistance is required (Mothershead, 2005).
   Nursing Process: Planning
   Client Need: Safe, Effective Care Environment

5. Answer: 2
   Rationale: The pre-disaster stage involves warning, preimpact mobilization, and evacuation if appropriate. The nondisaster stage is the time for planning and preparation because the threat of a disaster is still in the future. The impact stage is the time when the disaster event has occurred and the community experiences the immediate effects. The emergency stage involves the immediate response to the effects of the disaster.
   Nursing Process: Planning
   Client Need: Safe, Effective Care Environment

6. Answer: 2
   Rationale: Those less critical but still in need of transport to emergency centers for care are classified as "yellow." Those requiring the most support and immediate emergency care are classified as "red." Those who are least likely to survive or are already deceased are color-coded as "black."
   Nursing Process: Assessment
   Client Need: Physiological Integrity

7. Answer: 3
   Rationale: The site of the disaster where a weapon was released or where the contamination occurred is called the hot zone. The warm zone is adjacent to the hot zone. Another name for this area is the control zone. This area is where decontamination of victims or triage and emergency treatment take place. The cold zone is considered as the safe zone.
   Nursing Process: Planning
   Client Need: Safe, Effective Care Environment

8. Answer: 1
   Rationale: Nursing diagnoses that may apply during disaster situations include: anxiety, impaired communication, ineffective coping, powerlessness, fear, risk for injury, and risk for post-trauma syndrome.
   Nursing Process: Diagnosis
   Client Need: Psychosocial Integrity

9. Answer: 4
   Rationale: Bone marrow transplant clients are instructed not to eat raw fruits and vegetables due to the risk of contamination and subsequent infection. It is safest for this population of clients to consume processed or canned foods if they can be heated to the proper temperatures.
   Nursing Process: Planning
   Client Need: Safe, Effective Care Environment

10. Answer: 2
    Rationale: Overexertion and exhaustion are major problems during the snow shoveling that follows a snowstorm. The exertion required to shovel heavy snow in the extreme cold may cause a myocardial infarction.
    Nursing Process: Planning
    Client Need: Safe, Effective Care Environment

Chapter 8

Case Study Answers
Case Study 1

1. *Why did the physician order carrier testing for Mrs. Steinman?* Carrier testing is completed on asymptomatic individuals who may be carriers of one

copy of a gene alteration that can be transmitted to future children in an autosomal recessive or x-linked pattern of inheritance.

2. *What type of genetic disorder is Tay Sachs classified as?* Tay Sachs is an autosomal recessive or x-linked disorder.

3. *How can the Steinmans be assured of the accuracy of their genetic testing results?* Test sensitivity refers to how specifically the test identifies (positive test result) individuals who are affected and/or who have the disease phenotype. A test with a high degree of sensitivity has very few false negatives and many true positives. Test specificity is how specifically the test does not identify (negative test result) individuals who are unaffected but do not have the disease phenotype. A test with a high degree of specificity has very few false positives (SACGT, 2000). The laboratory selected for the genetic test should have a CLIA 88 (Clinical Laboratories Improvement Amendments Act of 1988) certification (Javitt et al, 2004).

4. *Who may obtain the results of the Steinmans' genetic testing?* Results of genetic tests should only be communicated directly to the individual who gave the consent. In the majority of cases, results of genetic tests should not be shared with extended family members without the written consent from the test recipient. Healthcare providers are legally liable to maintain that confidence. Exceptions to the individual's privacy may be made only when the individual refuses to inform extended family members, a very high probability of irreversible harm exists for the extended family member, and informing the family member can prevent the harm (NHGRI & NIH, 2005).

Case Study 2

1. *Describe the predictive genetic testing that Ms. Simmons will have performed.* Predictive genetic testing is usually made available to the asymptomatic individual and includes both predispositional and presymptomatic testing. A positive predispositional testing result will indicate there is an increased risk that the individual might eventually develop the disease. Common examples include breast cancer and hereditary nonpolyposis colorectal cancer (HNPCC). A presymptomatic test is performed when development of the disease is certain that the gene alteration is present. These tests are medically indicated when the seriousness and mortality of the disease can be reduced with knowledge of the gene alteration. An example of this would be hereditary hemochromatosis or familial hypercholesterolemia. Life planning and lifestyle choices can be influenced by predictive testing.

2. *Why is it important to discuss and map Ms. Simmons' family tree in relation to breast cancer?* A family history illustrates the interaction of genes and environment for an individual and consequently provides a basis for individualized disease prevention (Guttmacher, Collins, & Carmona, 2004). Although an individual's inheritance risks from their genotype are nonmodifiable, knowledge of an individual's increased risk for chronic disease can influence lifestyle choices, clinical management, and sometimes risk reduction and prevention of the disease. Knowledge of a family history can also guide diagnostic tests and clinical treatment (Guttmacher, et al, 2004). A nurse should know how to take a family history, record the history in a pedigree, and think "genetic." A pedigree is a pictorial representation or diagram of the medical history of a family. A pedigree provides the nurse, genetic counselor, or geneticist with a clear, visual representation of relationships of affected individuals to the immediate and extended family. It can identify other individuals in the family who might benefit from a genetic consultation. It also can identify a single gene alteration pattern of inheritance, a cluster of multifactorial conditions, and result in a referral and/or reproductive risk teaching for the individual and family.

3. *What type of nursing diagnoses will the nurse include in Ms. Simmons' genetic counseling care plan?* The nurse is responsible for comprehensively delivering the standard of care to clients. Nursing diagnoses to consider with Ms. Simmons include:
   - Anticipatory grieving
   - Anxiety
   - Body image disturbance
   - Ineffective coping
   - Decisional conflict
   - Family processes
   - Ineffective health maintenance
   - Deficient knowledge

4. *How can the testing information obtained by Ms. Simmons be used in the care of her extended family members?* The information gained from Ms. Simmons' genetic testing can be used by extended family members to determine their risk of breast cancer. The information provided may assist their relative's genetic counselor in determining their own risk assessment.

NCLEX Review Question Answers

1. Answer: 3
   Rationale: A single human cell contains 46 chromosomes in its nucleus. Cells with more than 47 chromosomes would undergo an alteration that results in a nondisjunction.
   Nursing Process: Assessment
   Client Need: Physiological Integrity

2. Answer: 1
   Rationale: DNA molecules consist of long sequences of nucleotides or bases represented by the letters A, G, T, and C. The order of these sequences (bases) gives the exact instructions for the functioning of that particular cell.

Nursing Process: Assessment
Client Need: Physiological Integrity

3. Answer: 3
Rationale: When an egg or sperm cell is fertilized by a normal gamete that contains 23 copies of all of the chromosomes, a zygote that is trisomic (has three chromosomes instead of the usual two) results. These circumstances produce a condition known as trisomy 21 (Down syndrome).
Nursing Process: Assessment
Client Need: Physiological Integrity

4. Answer: 2
Rationale: Persons who are homozygous for the CCR5 mutation (have two copies of the altered gene) are almost completely resistant to infection with HIV type I. There is no known resistance to the Hepatitis B, Hepatitis C, or Human papilloma virus caused by an altered gene.
Nursing Process: Implementation
Client Need: Health Promotion and Maintenance

5. Answer: 2
Rationale: The sex chromosome, X, is unevenly distributed to males and females. The female has two X chromosomes and the male has only one.
Nursing Process: Implementation
Client Need: Physiological Integrity

6. Answer: 4
Rationale: *Newborn screening* is carried out on large sections of the newborn population and provides a means to identify children who have an increased risk for developing a genetic disease such as phenylketonuria (PKU), sickle cell, or maple syrup urine disease. Carrier testing is completed on asymptomatic individuals who may be carriers of one copy of a gene alteration that can be transmitted to future children in an autosomal recessive or X-linked pattern of inheritance. Predictive genetic testing is usually made available to the asymptomatic individual and includes both predispositional and presymptomatic testing. Pharmacogenetic testing involves predicting or studying the client's response to particular medications.
Nursing Process: Diagnosis
Client Need: Health Promotion and Maintenance

7. Answer: 4
Rationale: Informed consent may be given verbally, although written consent is the standard. The nurse will discuss with the client the risks and benefits of the genetic testing along with the emotional impact the results may have on the client and family. The cost of the testing and its impact on family resources would also be discussed.
Nursing Process: Implementation
Client Need: Safe, Effective Care Environment

8. Answer: 3
Rationale: A woman with a strong family history and/or mutations in the BRCA1 and BRCA2 tumor suppressor genes should begin monthly self breast exams, and have screening clinical breast exams and mammographies at an earlier age than the general population. The client should also consider how sharing the test results could impact the preventative care of other females within the family.
Nursing Process: Evaluation
Client Need: Health Promotion and Maintenance.

9. Answer: 1
Rationale: Mitochondrial DNA is primarily inherited from the mother. Therefore, mitochondrial genes and any diseases due to DNA alterations on those genes are transmitted through the mother in a matrilineal pattern. Mitochondrial DNA is not transmitted through the father or patriarchal lines.
Nursing Process: Assessment
Client Need: Physiological Integrity

10. Answer: 1
Rationale: Survivor guilt would affect adults with negative results of a study when their siblings are positive. In this case, all three family members have tested positive for the sickle cell trait. The nurse may expect the client to feel fear about the diagnosis and its prognosis. The client may feel shame for having the disease and passing it to the child. The client may harbor a negative self-image related to a deformity of their red blood cells.
Nursing Process: Assessment
Client Need: Psychosocial Integrity

Chapter 9

Case Study Answers

Case Study 1

1. *What nerve fibers will be involved in sensing pain from J.S. Browning's injury site?* Pain will be transmitted through small afferent A-delta and even smaller C nerve fibers to the spinal cord.

2. *What form of acute pain will J.S. experience immediately after the injury?* The client will experience acute somatic pain.

3. *What form of chronic pain may J.S. experience for several months after the amputation?* J.S. may experience phantom pain for a few months after the amputation.

4. *What strategies will the nurse employ to assess J.S. Browning's pain tolerance?* The nurse will observe the client's posturing, assess his vital signs and ask the client to describe and rate his pain.

Case Study 2

1. *What factors will influence Mr. Bowen's perceived level of pain?* Mr. Bowen's perceived level of pain will be influenced by his age, culture, past experience

with pain, his emotional status, the meaning the pain has for him, and knowledge related to the source of his pain.

2. *What strategies other than medication administration can be used to lessen Mr. Bowen's perceived level of pain?* The following complementary therapies can be used to lessen Mr. Bowen's pain: acupuncture, biofeedback, hypnotism, relaxation techniques, distraction, and cutaneous stimulation.

3. *What types of medications would you expect this client to be placed on for pain control at home?* The client may be placed on one or more of the following medications based on his pain tolerance and control: nonnarcotic analgesics, nonsteroidal anti-inflammatory drugs (NSAIDs), narcotics, synthetic narcotics, and antidepressants.

4. Mr. Bowen's doctor has discussed placing a transcutaneous electrical nerve stimulation (TENS) unit on the client, explain the unit and its benefit to a client with chronic pain. A TENS unit consists of a low-voltage transmitter that is connected by wires to electrodes placed on the client as directed by the physical therapist. The client experiences a gentle tapping or vibrating sensation over the electrodes. The client can adjust the voltage to achieve maximum pain relief.

NCLEX Review Question Answers

1. Answer: 1
   Rationale: All pain is real. Pain affects the whole body, usually negatively. Pain has sociocultural and spiritual dimensions. Pain may serve as a warning of potential trauma.
   Nursing Process: Assessment
   Client Need: Physiological Integrity

2. Answer: 2
   Rationale: Visceral pain is dull and poorly localized because of the low number of nociceptors. Visceral pain is associated with nausea and vomiting, and is described as cramping, intermittent pain, or colicky pain. Somatic pain arises from nerve receptors that originate in the skin or close to the surface of the body and may be sharp and/or well-localized. Referred pain is pain that is perceived in an area distant from the site of the stimuli. Hyperesthesia is a condition of oversensitivity to tactile and painful stimuli.
   Nursing Process: Diagnosis
   Client Need: Physiological Integrity

3. Answer: 3
   Rationale: A client who is experiencing breakthrough pain will benefit from doses timed in relation to patterns of breakthrough. Changing positions frequently may cause indecent pain, thereby increasing the likelihood or intensity of the breakthrough pain. Providing medications

when the breakthrough pain is expected to reoccur will provide more efficient relief than waiting until the client feels the need for the medication. Prolonging the intervals of medication will require longer periods to obtain relief. The client would benefit from an *increase* in baseline dose of analgesic to prevent breakthrough.
   Nursing Process: Planning
   Client Need: Physiological Integrity

4. Answer: 3
   Rationale: Older adult clients may hesitate to ask for pain medication because they fear narcotic addiction and loss of independence. The perception of pain does not decrease with age. Opioids do not cause excessive respiratory depression in older adults. Pain is not a natural part of aging.
   Nursing Process: Diagnosis
   Client Need: Physiological Integrity

5. Answer: 4
   Rationale: Research about treating pain with analgesics consistently shows no impact on physical assessment findings or diagnosis. Pain is a result, not a cause. Pain is only a symptom of a condition. Very few clients lie about their pain. Narcotic medication is used to treat chronic pain. A common misconception that narcotic medications are too risky to be used to treat chronic pain often deprives clients of the most effective source of pain relief.
   Nursing Process: Assessment
   Client Need: Physiological and Psychological Integrity

6. Answer: 2
   Rationale: Anticonvulsants are useful as initial medications for clients with neuropathic pain, including shingles (herpes zoster). Local anesthetics block the initiation and transmission of nerve impulses in a local area. Narcotics, or opioids, are the pharmacologic treatment of choice for moderate to severe pain. NSAIDs are the treatment of choice for mild to moderate pain.

7. Answer: 1
   Rationale: Administering analgesics before the pain occurs allows the client to spend less time in pain. The client's fears and anxiety about pain will be decreased and their physical activity will increase. Frequent analgesic administration may allow for smaller doses and less analgesic administration.
   Nursing Process: Implementation
   Client Need: Physiological Integrity and Psychosocial Integrity

8. Answer: 3
   Rationale: Exercise and use of electric blankets or heating pads also may accelerate absorption of the transdermal medication. A therapeutic level of the medication will be achieved within 12–24 hours.

The patch should not be applied to the same site consecutively; sites should be altered. The effectiveness of a patch lasts about 72 hours.
Nursing Process: Evaluation
Client Need: Physiological Integrity

9. Answer: 4
   Rationale: A cordotomy is an incision into the anterolateral tracts of the spinal cord to interrupt the transmission of pain. Rhizotomy is a surgical severing of the dorsal spinal roots. A neurectomy is the removal of a nerve. A sympathectomy involves destruction by injection or incision of the ganglia of sympathetic nerves.
   Nursing Process: Implementation
   Client Need: Safe, Effective Care Environment

10. Answer: 4
    Rationale: Clients experiencing pain will demonstrate rapid, shallow breathing patterns, an increase in blood pressure and heart rate, and a dilation of the pupils.
    Nursing Process: Assessment
    Client Need: Physiological Integrity

Chapter 10

Case Study Answers

1. *What is normal pH?* 7.35–7.45
   What would you expect Mr. Johnson's pH to be? Below 7.35

2. *The nurse would expect Mr. Johnson's respirations to be of what quality and depth?* Respirations will increase in rate and depth.

3. *What are the early manifestations of metabolic acidosis?* Fatigue, general malaise, anorexia, nausea, and abdominal pain

4. What are the *vital teaching areas for Mr. Johnson?* Diet, medication management, and alcohol dependency treatment are vital teaching areas.

NCLEX Review Question Answers

1. Answer: 1
   Rationale: Plasma is an intravascular fluid and can be immediately replaced through venous access. Transcellular fluids cannot be immediately replaced. They include urine; digestive secretions; perspiration; and cerebrospinal, pleural, synovial, intraocular, gonadal, and pericardial fluids.
   Nursing Process: Assessment
   Client Need: Physiological Integrity

2. Answer: 1
   Rationale: Osmosis is the process that controls body fluid movement between the intracellular fluid (ICF) and extracellular fluid (ECF) compartments from an area of lower solute concentration to an area of higher solute concentration. Diffusion is the process by which

solute molecules move from an area of high solute concentration to an area of low solute concentration and becomes evenly distributed. Active transport allows molecules to move across cell membranes and epithelial membranes against a concentration gradient. Filtration is the process by which water and dissolved substances (solutes) move from an area of high hydrostatic pressure to an area of low hydrostatic pressure.
Nursing Process: Planning
Client Need: Physiological Integrity

3. Answer: 1
   Rationale: Loss of skin elasticity with aging makes skin turgor assessment findings less accurate in older adults. Tongue turgor is not generally affected by age and is a more accurate indicator of fluid volume deficit. Postural or orthostatic hypotension is a sign of hypovolemia. Rapid weight loss is a good indicator of fluid volume deficit.
   Nursing Process: Assessment
   Client Need: Physiological Integrity

4. Answer: 4
   Rationale: Clients experiencing a fluid volume deficit will have *increased* hematocrit laboratory values as they will be dehydrated. Dehydrated client's lab work will demonstrate an increased potassium level, increased urine specific gravity, and an elevated hemoglobin.
   Nursing Process: Assessment
   Client Need: Physiological Integrity

5. Answer: 2
   Rationale: The infusion rate for a client undergoing a fluid challenge is an initial fluid volume of 200 to 300 mL over 5 to 10 minutes. Too fast of an infusion rate may place the client into overload compromising cardiac and renal functioning.
   Nursing Process: Implementation
   Client Need: Safe, Effective Healthcare Environment

6. Answer: 4
   Rationale: The client's weight should be assessed at the same time every day, using approximately the same clothing and a balanced scale. Client's with fluid volume excess must be assessed for lower extremity edema. Sodium restrictions will be placed on the client's diet. Oral hygiene must be provided every two hours to hydrate oral mucosa.
   Nursing Process: Implementation
   Client Need: Health Promotion and Maintenance

7. Answer: 3
   Rationale: Thirst is the first manifestation of hypernatremia. After thirst, the following symptoms of hypernatremia develop: lethargy, weakness, and irritability.
   Nursing Process: Assessment
   Client Need: Physiological Integrity

8. Answer: 4

> **Rationale:** Although all answer choices are symptoms of hypokalemia, muscle weakness and cramping is an early manifestation of the potassium imbalance.
> **Nursing Process:** Assessment
> **Client Need:** Physiological Integrity

9. Answer: 1

> **Rationale:** Buffers are substances that prevent major changes in pH by removing or releasing hydrogen ions. Hydrogen ions control the acid-base balance of the body. Sodium affects intracellular and intravascular fluid volumes. Calcium is essential to cardiac function and blood clotting. Magnesium controls the sedative effects on the neuromuscular junction.
> **Nursing Process:** Planning
> **Client Need:** Physiological Integrity

10. Answer: 4

> **Rationale:** Deep, rapid respirations that are seen in clients with metabolic acidosis are known as Kussmaul's respirations. Stridor is a high-pitched, harsh inspiratory sound indicative of upper airway obstruction. Paradoxical respiration is breathing in which all or part of the chest wall moves in during inspiration and out during respiration. Trousseau's is a sign that is used to assess deep tendon reflexes, and is not related to respirations.
> **Nursing Process:** Assessment
> **Client Need:** Health Promotion and Maintenance

Chapter 11

Case Study Answers

1. *What type(s) of trauma could Richard potentially experience?* Richard may experience multiple trauma, which involves injuries to more than one organ system. Motor vehicle accidents often result in multiple trauma. He may also experience both blunt and penetrating trauma, depending on how he fell and what he fell on. The accident occurred on a country road, which may be covered with gravel or dirt that may have injured or punctured the skin. Falling into a fence or mailbox post could also result in a penetrating injury.

2. *What method of transportation will most likely be used to transport Richard to the hospital? What trauma level hospital should he be transported to?* Due to the fact that he is in the country and may be some distance away from a hospital, he will most likely be airlifted by helicopter to the trauma center. Unstable clients and those injured in the wilderness or other areas in which ground access is difficult may also be airlifted to the closest trauma center.

3. *What is the highest priority of need in caring for a trauma victim?* Assessment of the airway is the highest priority in the trauma client. If the airway is

not patent and the client is unable to deliver oxygen to vital organs, all other interventions are futile.

4. *What diagnostic studies may be performed on Richard once he reaches the trauma center?* Richard may undergo the following diagnostic studies upon arrival in the trauma center: blood type and crossmatch, blood alcohol level, complete blood count (CBC), arterial blood gases (ABG), urine drug screen, focused assessment by sonography in the trauma department, diagnostic peritoneal lavage (based on FAST finding), and/or a computed tomography (CT) scan and/or magnetic resonance imaging (MRI).

NCLEX Review Question Answers

1. Answer: 1

> **Rationale:** Mechanical energy is the most common type of energy transferred to a host in trauma. The most common mechanical source of injury in all adult age groups is the motor vehicle. Gravitational, thermal, and electrical energy do cause trauma but are not as common of injuries as mechanical energy.
> **Nursing Process:** Assessment
> **Client Need:** Physiological Integrity

2. Answer: 4

> **Rationale:** Minor traumas are classified as an injury to a single part or system of the body and is usually treated in a physician's office or in the hospital emergency department. A fracture of the clavicle, a small second-degree burn, and a laceration requiring sutures are examples of minor trauma. A gun shot wound, stab wound, and a compression injury are multiple traumas, which may involve more than one organ system.
> **Nursing Process:** Assessment
> **Client Need:** Physiological Integrity

3. Answer: 2

> **Rationale:** There is a decreased probability of C-spine injury if the following criteria are met: absence of midline cervical spine tenderness, normal alertness, absence of intoxication, absence of a painful distracting injury, and no focal neurological defects.
> **Nursing Process:** Assessment
> **Client Need:** Physiological Integrity

4. Answer: 1

> **Rationale:** The primary organ systems involved in Multiple Organ Dysfunction Syndrome are the respiratory, renal, hepatic, hematologic, cardiovascular, gastrointestinal, and neurological. The reproductive system is not involved in MODS.
> **Nursing Process:** Planning
> **Client Need:** Health Promotion and Maintenance

5. Answer: 2

> **Rationale:** Vasodilators are not commonly used to treat the client who has experienced trauma. Medications used to treat the client who has

experienced trauma depend on the type and severity of the injuries, as well as the degree of traumatic shock that is present. The following general categories of medications may be used: blood components and crystalloids, inotropic drugs, vasopressors, opioids, and immunizations.
Nursing Process: Planning
Client Need: Safe, Effective Care Environment

6. Answer: 4
Rationale: The incorrect statement is that the person with blood type AB has O antibodies. The person with blood type B has A antibodies, the person with type A has B antibodies, the person with type O has both types of antibodies, and the person with blood type AB has no antibodies.
Nursing Process: Diagnosis
Client Need: Health Promotion and Maintenance

7. Answer: 3
Rationale: Manifestations of shock do not include increased gastric motility. Manifestations of shock include *decreased* gastric motility, tachycardia, decreased oxygen levels, increased carbon dioxide levels, and cerebral hypoxia.
Nursing Process: Assessment
Client Need: Physiological Integrity

8. Answer: 2
Rationale: Septic shock is the leading cause of death in intensive care units. It is one part of a progressive syndrome called systemic inflammatory response syndrome (SIRS). Hypovolemic shock is the most common type of shock. It is caused by a decrease in intravascular volume of 15% or more. Distributive shock includes several types of shock that result from widespread vasodilation and decreased peripheral resistance. Neurogenic shock is the result of an imbalance between parasympathetic and sympathetic stimulation of vascular smooth muscle.
Nursing Process: Planning
Client Need: Physiological Integrity

9. Answer: 2
Rationale: The goal of blood administration is to keep the hematocrit at 30% to 35%. A hematocrit below 30% results in clotting dysfunctions. A hematocrit above 35% results in an increase in solids in the circulating blood volume. Obstructions and thrombus may form if the hematocrit rises above 35%.
Nursing Process: Planning
Client Need: Health Promotion and Maintenance

10. Answer: 1
Rationale: Decreased tissue perfusion is evidenced by the skin becoming pale, cool, and moist; as hemoglobin concentrations decrease, cyanosis occurs. Warm skin is not an indication of decreased tissue perfusion.
Nursing Process: Assessment
Client Need: Physiological Integrity

Chapter 12

Case Study Answers

1. *What questions should the nurse ask Sally about her symptoms?*
The nurse should ask questions such as:
   - Where do you feel the pain?
   - How long have you had it?
   - Has anyone else in your household had the same symptoms?
   - Have you had a fever? If so, what is your temperature?
   - Have you taken anything for the fever or pain? If so, what?
   - Have you had any diarrhea, nausea, or vomiting?
   - What medications are you on?

2. *What testing may be performed to identify the infecting organism?*
Sally should have the following studies performed:
   - WBC cell and differential to determine whether an infectious process is occurring
   - Throat culture to identify the bacteria present in the pustules
   - *Serologic testing* to provide an indirect means of identifying infecting agents by detecting antibodies to the suspected organism

3. *What are the key nursing diagnoses the nurse should create for Sally?* The key nursing diagnoses are risk for infection, anxiety, hyperthermia, and pain.
   a. Risk for infection: The spread of infection is a risk in any facility that houses many people. Sally may spread her infection to those she lives with, or those she is in close contact with.
   b. Risk for anxiety: Sally may experience anxiety related to her manifestations, treatment measures, the prognosis, and expected outcome of the disease. The diagnosis of an infection can be traumatic, and cause feelings of uneasiness, isolation, guilt, apprehension, or depression.
   c. Risk for hyperthermia: Hyperthermia is an expected consequence of the infectious disease process. It can be controlled using antipyretics. It is expected that Sally will have an increase in temperature as a result of the body's response to an infection.
   d. Risk for pain: Pain often accompanies infections as part of the inflammatory process or secondary to delayed healing. Sally may experience increased pain secondary to the pustules on her tonsils.

4. *Sally has been placed on antibiotics. What symptoms should she report to her healthcare provider?* Sally should be instructed to notify her healthcare provider if any of the following occur:
   a. Symptoms do not improve within 24 to 48 hours after antibiotic therapy is instituted, or they worsen.
   b. Signs of antibiotic allergy (itching, rash, difficulty breathing or swallowing, swelling of the face or tongue) occur.

c. Adverse responses, such as gastrointestinal distress, interfere with completion of the prescription.

d. Signs of superinfection (vaginitis, oral candidiasis, or diarrhea) occur.

NCLEX Review Question Answers

1. Answer: 3

   Rationale: Monocytes are the largest of the leukocytes and constitute 2% to 3% of circulating leukocytes. Neutrophils are the most plentiful of the granulocytes, and constitute 55% to 70% of the total number of circulating leukocytes. Eosinophils account for 1% to 4% of the total number of circulating leukocytes. Basophils constitute about 0.5% to 1% of the circulating leukocytes.
   Nursing Process: Diagnosis
   Client Need: Physiological Integrity

2. Answer: 2

   Rationale: The thymus and bone marrow, in which T cells and B cells mature, are considered central lymphoid organs. The spleen, lymph nodes, tonsils, and other peripheral lymphoid tissue are peripheral lymphoid organs.
   Nursing Process: Diagnosis
   Client Need: Physiological Integrity

3. Answer: 4

   Rationale: The vascular response localizes invading bacteria and keeps them from spreading. The cellular response involves the margination and emigration of agent or leukocytes into the damaged tissue. Phagocystosis is a process by which a foreign target cell is engulfed, destroyed, and digested. The specific immune response involves the introduction of antigens into the body.
   Nursing Process: Diagnosis
   Client Need: Physiological Integrity

4. Answer: 4

   Rationale: Vaccines stimulate active immunity by inducing the production of antibodies and antitoxins. Vaccines are suspensions of whole or fractionated bacteria or viruses that have been treated to make them *non*pathogenic. Vaccines are administered to induce an immune response and subsequent immunity. Although vaccine development has been a major factor in improving public health, no vaccine is completely effective or entirely safe.
   Nursing Process: Implementation
   Client Need: Health Promotion and Maintenance

5. Answer: 1

   Rationale: Withhold administration of active immunologic products in the presence of an upper respiratory infection (URI) or other infection. Active immunizations can cause a greater inflammatory reaction in the presence of infections. Oral polio vaccine (OPV); measles, mumps, and rubella (MMR); or any live virus vaccines are not administered to immunosuppressed clients.
   Prior to administering a prescribed vaccine, check the expiration date and manufacturer's instructions. Keep epinephrine 1:1000 readily available for subcutaneous injection when administering immunizations.
   Nursing Process: Implementation
   Client Need: Health Promotion and Maintenance

6. Answer: 3

   Rationale: A client with an infectious process is encouraged to rest, to increase fluid intake, and to eat a well-balanced, nutritious diet.
   Anti-inflammatory medications are administered only when the inflammatory process has become problematic.
   Nursing Process: Evaluation
   Client Need: Health Promotion and Maintenance

7. Answer: 2

   Rationale: Keep the inflamed area dry, and expose it to air as much as possible. This promotes healing and helps prevent infection. Interventions to maintain tissue integrity include: cleaning the inflamed tissue gently, balancing rest with a tolerable degree of mobility, and providing protection and support for inflamed tissue.
   Nursing Process: Implementation
   Client Need: Safe, Effective Care Environment

8. Answer: 1

   Rationale: Urinary tract infection is the most common type of nosocomial infection, which leads to the most frequent cause of gram-negative septicemia in hospitalized clients.
   Pneumonia is the second most common hospital-acquired infection. Bacteremia is associated with intravascular and urinary catheters, yet is not the most common type of nosocomial infection.
   Clostridium difficile-associated diarrhea is also frequently-acquired nosocomial infection, but not the most common.
   Nursing Process: Diagnosis
   Client Need: Safe, Effective Care Environment.

9. Answer: 4

   Rationale: Hepatitis has not been used as a biological weapon. The most likely pathogens to be used as a biological weapon include anthrax, smallpox, botulism, pneumonic plague, and viral hemorrhagic fevers.
   Nursing Process: Diagnosis
   Client Need: Safe, Effective Care Environment

10. Answer: 1

   Rationale: Signs of an opportunistic infections include: loose, watery, and foul-smelling diarrhea; vaginal discharge or itching; fuzzy growth or white plaques in mouth or on tongue; blood in urine; chills; fever; or unusual cough.
   Nursing Process: Assessment
   Client Need: Health Promotion and Maintenance

Chapter 13

Case Study Answers

1. *What are the risk factors for HIV that are specific to this client?* Risk factors include homosexuality, IV drug use, and hemophilia. Gary is a homosexual African-American male, which puts him at risk for AIDS.

2. *How long after exposure would the nurse expect seroconversion to occur in Gary?* Antibodies are produced against the HIV proteins within six weeks to six months postexposure.

3. *What acute symptomology can the nurse expect Gary to experience after seroconversion?* Acute symptomology includes fever, sore throat, arthralgias, myalgias, headache, rash, lymphadenopathy, nausea, vomiting, and abdominal cramps.

4. *How long of an asymptomatic period may Gary experience after an acute phase?* Gary may experience an asymptomatic period that lasts 8–10 years after the acute phase.

5. *What opportunistic infections are most common in the AIDS client?* The AIDS client is at risk for *pneumocystis carnii* pneumonia, tuberculosis (TB), candidiasis, and *mycobacterium avium* complex.

NCLEX Review Question Answers

1. Answer: 2
   Rationale: A client with an altered immune system will experience weight loss or wasting, not weight gain. Symptoms of an alteration in immune system functioning include fatigue and weakness, pale or jaundiced skin, and boggy nasal mucosa.
   Nursing Process: Assessment
   Client Need: Physiological Integrity

2. Answer: 1
   Rationale: The red blood cell count (RBC) is not an indicator of a hypersensitivity or allergen. The information gained from an RBC count is used to determine the oxygen-carrying capability of blood cells. Blood type and crossmatch, Direct Coombs, and complement assay testing can give information on hypersensitivity and allergic reactions.
   Nursing Process: Planning
   Client Need: Health Promotion and Maintenance

3. Answer: 3
   Rationale: Clients who have a hypersensitivity to bee venom must carry a bee sting kit with them at all times. Antihistamines taken daily will not prevent a reaction if stung.
   The use of Nasalirom will not stop a hypersensitivity reaction. Daily use of a steroid will not prevent a hypersensitivity reaction.
   Nursing Process: Evaluation
   Client Need: Health Promotion and Maintenance

4. Answer: 2
   Rationale: If signs or symptoms of a transfusion reaction occurs, stop the transfusion immediately, remove the bag and tubing, flush site with normal saline solution, and call the physician and bloodbank. Correct protocols to follow when administering blood products include monitoring the client for complaints of back pain or chest pain. Infusing the blood through a separate site than any other IV and having two healthcare professionals identifying the blood product prior to transfusion.
   Nursing Process: Implementation
   Client Need: Physiological Integrity

5. Answer: 3
   Rationale: An allograft is a graft taken from a member of the same species, such as a cadaver, and transplanted to a live client. An autograft is a transplant using the client's own tissue. An isograft is a graft in which the graft tissue is taken from the client's identical twin. A xenograft is a tissue transplant from an animal to a human.
   Nursing Process: Diagnosis
   Client Need: Physiological Integrity

6. Answer: 4
   Rationale: Graft-versus-host disease occurs within the first 100 days following a transplant. It is a frequent and potentially fatal complication of bone marrow transplants. Hyperacute tissue rejection occurs immediately within two to three days after transplant. Acute tissue reaction is the most common and treatable rejection episode. Acute tissue rejection occurs between four days to three months after transplant. Chronic tissue rejection occurs four months to years after the transplant.
   Nursing Process: Diagnosis
   Client Need: Physiological Integrity

7. Answer: 2
   Rationale: IV bags and tubing must be changed every 24 hours. Peripheral IV sites require changing every 48–72 hours. Changing tubing and sites reduces bacterial contamination. The client's lab values must be closely monitored and changes reported to the physician. The client must be assessed for signs of an adverse reaction to medications. The nurse should offer supplemental feedings to the client.
   Nursing Process: Implementation
   Client Need: Safe, Effective Healthcare Environment

8. Answer: 1
   Rationale: The CDC classification of AIDS-associated cancers currently includes Karposi's sarcoma, non-Hodgkin's lymphoma, primary lymphoma of the brain, and invasive cervical cancer.
   Nursing Process: Planning
   Client Need: Physiological Integrity

9. Answer: 4

> **Rationale:** The blood culture for HIV provides the most specific diagnosis for HIV but is expensive, cumbersome, and not widely available in the United States. ELISA is the most widely-used screening test for HIV. It tests for HIV antibodies but does not detect the virus. The Western Blot detects HIV antibodies that are present in the blood. A CD4 cell count is used to monitor the progress of the disease.
> **Nursing Process:** Diagnosis
> **Client Need:** Health Promotion and Maintenance

10. Answer: 4

> **Rationale:** Ambulation increases circulation to the blister site, decreases pressure, and helps to maintain muscle tone. The area around the blister should be massaged but not the skin directly over the blister. Do not open and drain the blister. The blister should remain intact and dressed. Avoid the use of heat because it will further dry and damage the skin.
> **Nursing Process:** Implementation
> **Client Need:** Physiological Integrity

Chapter 14

Case Study Answers

1. *What race experiences a higher prevalence of breast cancer?* Breast cancer is more prevalent in white women.

2. *What role does Donna's age play in her cancer?* Hormone changes that occur with the aging process are associated with cancers in postmenopausal women. Women who take estrogen supplements have an increased risk for breast and uterine cancer.

3. *What role does estrogen play in breast cancer?* Estrogen often mediates the cancer of the reproductive organs. Estrogen has been linked to breast cancer.

4. *During the surgical procedure, the axillary lymph nodes are removed for examination. Why is this done?* The lymph nodes are removed to determine metastasis.

5. *How can the nurse assist the client in adjusting to her new body image post-mastectomy?*
   a. Allow the client to discuss the meaning of the loss of her breast.
   b. Observe and evaluate the interaction between the client and her significant others.
   c. Allow for denial but do not participate in it.
   d. Provide a supportive environment.
   e. Allow the client and significant others to express feelings about her altered image.
   f. Put client in touch with a mastectomy support group.
   g. Advise the client to visit a mastectomy prosthetic shop.

NCLEX Review Question Answers

1. Answer: 2

> **Rationale:** The incidence of bladder cancer is four times higher in men than women. The incidence of thyroid cancer is higher in women than in men. Lung cancer is the leading cause of death among both men and women.
> **Nursing Process:** Planning
> **Client Need:** Health Promotion and Maintenance

2. Answer: 3

> **Rationale:** Dysplasia is a loss of DNA control over the differentiation that occurs in response to adverse conditions. Hyperplasia is an increase in the number or density of normal cells. Metaplasia is a change in the normal pattern of differentiation. Anaplasia is the regression of a cell to an immature or undifferentiated cell type.
> **Nursing Process:** Diagnosis
> **Client Need:** Physiological Integrity

3. Answer: 2

> **Rationale:** Malignant cells do not perform typical cellular functions. Malignant cells lose specialization and differentiation abilities. Malignant cells undergo rapid cell division. Malignant cells do not respect other cellular boundaries. Transformation of a malignant cell is irreversible.
> **Nursing Process:** Diagnosis
> **Client Need:** Physiological Integrity

4. Answer: 1

> **Rationale:** Elevated enzyme levels can indicate either hyperplasia of the tissue or cancer. The rapid growth of a tumor causes tissue enzymes to spill into the bloodstream. Proteins narrow down the type of tissue that may be malignant. Increased hormone levels may signify a hormone-secreting malignancy. The presence of a large amount of antigens reflects tumor cells.
> **Nursing Process:** Diagnosis
> **Client Need:** Physiological Integrity

5. Answer: 3

> **Rationale:** Computed tomography reveals subtle differences in tissue densities and provides the greatest accuracy in tumor diagnosis. Ultrasonography is more useful in detecting masses in dense breast tissue. Magnetic resonance imaging is the tool of choice for the screening and follow-up of cranial, head, and neck tumors. Nuclear imaging can identify tumors in various body tissues and can be used to determine metastasis.
> **Nursing Process:** Diagnosis
> **Client Need:** Health Promotion and Maintenance

6. Answer: 3

> **Rationale:** Chemotherapy treatment can result in the loss of taste. It is common to experience alopecia when undergoing chemotherapy. Chemotherapy depresses bone marrow, which

results in an impaired ability to respond to an infection. Reproductive ability is impaired as a consequence of chemotherapy.
Nursing Process: Evaluation
Client Need: Physiological Integrity

7. Answer: 1
   Rationale: Signs that identify anxiety include trembling, restlessness, avoidance of direct eye contact, irritability, hyperactivity, withdrawal, and a worried facial expression.
   Nursing Process: Assessment
   Client Need: Psychosocial Integrity

8. Answer: 2
   Rationale: A client who is willing to look at their wound and participate in wound care accepts their altered body image. Body image concerns are identified by the client refusing visitors, refusing to look at or care for their wound, and denying any change to their physical appearance.
   Nursing Process: Evaluation
   Client Need: Psychosocial Integrity

9. Answer: 2
   Rationale: An alcohol-based mouthwash will irritate sensitive oral mucosa and dry out an already moisture-depleted mouth. Proper oral hygiene includes the use of a soft-tipped toothbrush, soaking dentures in hydrogen peroxide, and the use of waxed dental floss.
   Nursing Process: Implementation
   Client Need: Physiological Integrity

10. Answer: 2
    Rationale: Tumor Lysis Syndrome is characterized by two or more of the following metabolic abnormalities: hyperuricemia, hyperphosphatemia, hyperkalemia, and hyponatremia.
    Nursing Process: Assessment
    Client Need: Physiologic Integrity

Chapter 15

Case Study Answers

1. *Is the area on the back of the client's scalp a recurrence of her basal cell carcinoma? Why or why not?* Based on the description of the lesion, this is probably not a basal cell carcinoma; it is more likely to be a squamous cell carcinoma. The lesion is red, scaly, and rapid-growing with papules. There is no pearly edge or ulceration.

2. *What risk factors increase the client's risk of developing this type of skin disorder?* High levels of exposure to the sun or tanning beds, fair skin and hair, immunosupression, and previous personal or immediate family history of skin cancers

3. *The lesion is located on the back of the client's head and she noticed it a week ago. The lesion is 3 mm in size now. Based on knowledge of this type of lesion,*

has the client waited too long to seek treatment? This is a rapid-growing cancer. While it is best to seek care as soon as possible for any suspected skin cancer, the key is to seek care. The fact that this lesion is on the back of the client's head makes it difficult to know how long it has really been there. It is not a good thing that the lesion bleeds easily, but now that it has been identified it can be treated.

4. *Is there a connection between the reason for the client's admission and the lesion found on the back of her head?* No, there is probably no connection between the admission and the lesion. Bradycardia is not associated with an increased risk of basal or squamous cell carcinoma. If the nurse had not done a thorough skin assessment, the lesion may have been ignored and allowed to grow larger and spread.

NCLEX Review Question Answers

1. Answer: 3
   Rationale: Developing a repositioning schedule for each individual client that provides for turning every one to two hours reestablishes blood flow to potentially compromised skin over boney prominences. Repositioning the client every half hour interrupts the client's ability to rest; he or she may have just become comfortable. Changing the diet order is under the purview of the physician, as is changing the client's ambulation order.
   Nursing Process: Implementation
   Client Need: Physiological Integrity

2. Answer: 4
   Rationale: Exploring the background of the rash will help the nurse and the client to understand how best to approach the client's care. Hot weather and bathing too often can dry out the skin, but neither causes a red rash. Scratching will make it worse, and possibly cause a secondary infection; but this does not help the client understand that information. The client never mentioned changing detergent so assuming this is the problem will not help the client to explore the true nature of the rash.
   Nursing Process: Diagnosis
   Client Need: Physiological Integrity

3. Answer: 3
   Rationale: Edema is best assessed by depressing the skin over the ankle or a bony prominence. A finding of 3+ edema indicates that the edema has caused the extremity to appear distorted, but the depression does not remain visible when the pressure is released. Findings of 1+ and 2+ indicate that the edema does not cause distortion. A finding of 4+ indicates that the edema caused the imprint to remain for some time after the pressure was released.
   Nursing Process: Assessment
   Client Need: Physiological Integrity

4. Answer: 2

Rationale: The fact that the client has lost his natural protection, his hair, and has been exposed to the ultraviolet light of the sun for many hours a day as a construction worker significantly increases his risk of skin cancer. Smoking has a closer link to oral and lung cancer, and a high-fat diet is loosely associated with gastrointestinal cancers. There is no connection between hypothyroidism and skin cancer.

Nursing Process: Diagnosis

Client Need: Health Promotion and Maintenance

5. Answer: 1

Rationale: The tendency to burn does increase the risk of skin cancer, especially if the skin is not protected from the sun with sunscreens or by avoiding the harmful rays. Family history and genetics are strong indicators, but taking measures to protect skin from UVA and UVB rays can counteract that risk. Men, especially those who are more than 50 years old, are at greater risk than women. Exposure to UVA and UVB rays, regardless of a natural tan or one from a tanning bed, increases the risk of skin cancers.

Nursing Process: Diagnosis

Client Need: Health Promotion and Maintenance

6. Answer: 2

Rationale: The sclera of the eye is the best place to see jaundice in a client with dark skin tone. Jaundice can be missed in the mucous membranes of the mouth or the area under the nail. The forearm has too much pigment, which makes it difficult to see the yellow undertone of jaundice.

Nursing Process: Assessment

Client Need: Physiological Integrity

7. Answer: 1

Rationale: Tinea capitis or scalp ringworm is associated with hair loss, pustules, and scales on the scalp. Head lice may cause redness, but the nurse would see white oval-shaped nits in the hair. Seborrhea causes a greasy, flaky scalp. A boil causes a larger, fluid-filled area.

Nursing Process: Assessment

Client Need: Physiological Integrity

8. Answer: 1 and 4

Rationale: Both fungal infections and psoriasis can cause nails to become yellow and thicken. Trauma can cause the nail to appear dark, black-green, or have red splinter hemorrhages. Pseudomonas infection will cause the nail to take on a blackish-green appearance.

Nursing Process: Assessment

Client Need: Physiological Integrity

9. Answer: 3

Rationale: The Tzanct test is used to determine the presence of herpes, but does not differentiate between herpes simplex and herpes zoster.

Anti-infectives are used to control a herpes infection, but antibiotics will not be effective.

Nursing Process: Diagnosis

Client Need: Health Promotion and Maintenance

10. Answer: 1

Rationale: Hypothyroidism is commonly associated with coarse, dry skin because of the metabolic changes of the disease. Oily skin is seen in acne vulgaris. In fever, the nurse would see hot skin which could be dry, as in lacking moisture, but not dry as in flaky. Seborrhea produces a greasy, scaly appearance.

Nursing Process: Assessment

Client Need: Physiological Integrity

Chapter 16

Case Study Answers

1. *What factors place Chrissy at risk for developing malignant melanoma?* She is a naturally fair-skinned person. She is Caucasian and has a significant history of sun exposure and tanning. She is an upper middle-class professional who works indoors and research demonstrates that these individuals have a higher-than-average incidence of developing malignant melanoma.

2. *What is Chrissy's prognosis?* The prognosis for Chrissy will be determined by several variables, including tumor thickness, ulceration, metastasis, site, age, and gender. Younger clients and women have a somewhat better chance of survival.

3. *What treatments are available to Chrissy?* If the tumor is treatable, it is removed through surgical excision. Malignant melanoma is also treated with chemotherapy, immunotherapy, and radiation therapy. Other therapies used with success include biological therapies with interleukin-2, interferon, and therapeutic vaccines that contain melanoma antigens.

4. *How often must Chrissy be seen for a checkup after removal of the lesion?* She should be seen every three months for the first two years, every six months for the next five years, and yearly thereafter.

NCLEX Review Question Answers

1. Answer: 2

Rationale: Nevi, more commonly called *moles,* are flat or raised macules or papules with rounded, well-defined borders. Cysts of the skin are benign, closed sacs in or under the skin surface that are lined with epithelium and contain fluid or a semisolid material. Keloids are elevated, irregularly-shaped, scars that progressively enlarge. Skin tags are soft papules that are on a pedicle.

Nursing Process: Assessment

Client Need: Physiological Integrity

2. Answer: 1
    Rationale: It is not appropriate to teach a client with psoriasis to avoid exposure to the sun. Interventions for psoriasis include: expose the skin to sunlight, but avoid sunburn; avoid trauma to the skin (e.g., do not scrub off scales, and use only an electric razor); avoid exposure to contagious illnesses such as influenza and colds; certain drugs, such as indomethacin (Indocin), lithium, and beta-adrenergic blocking agents, are known to precipitate exacerbations of psoriasis.
    Nursing Process: Implementation
    Client Need: Safe, Effective Care Environment

3. Answer: 4
    Rationale: Erysipelas is an infection of the skin most often caused by group A streptococci. Cellulitis is a localized infection of the dermis and subcutaneous tissue. A carbuncle is a group of infected hair follicles. Furuncles, often called *boils*, are also inflammations of the hair follicle.
    Nursing Process: Assessment
    Client Need: Physiological Integrity

4. Answer: 3
    Rationale: The behavior that indicates the client's understanding about caring for a vaginal *candida albicans* infection is that the client reports bathing more frequently. Other interventions include: avoid wearing tight clothing such as jeans and pantyhose, wearing cotton underwear, and having the sexual partner tested to prevent the spread of infection.
    Nursing Process: Evaluation
    Client Need: Health Promotion and Maintenance

5. Answer: 3
    Rationale: Seborrheic dermatitis is a chronic inflammatory disorder of the skin that involves the scalp, eyebrows, eyelids, ear canals, nasolabial folds, axillae, and trunk. Contact dermatitis is a type of dermatitis that is caused by a hypersensitivity response or chemical irritation. Atopic dermatitis is an inflammatory skin disorder that is also called eczema. Exfoliative dermatitis is an inflammatory skin disorder that is characterized by excessive peeling or shedding of skin.
    Nursing Process: Assessment
    Client Need: Physiological Integrity

6. Answer: 3
    Rationale: Unprotected exposure to UV radiation is a risk factor for developing nonmalignant skin cancer. Other risk factors include: having naturally blonde hair and blue or green eyes; having a family history of skin cancer; and having occupational exposures to coal tar.
    Nursing Process: Assessment
    Client Need: Health Promotion and Maintenance

7. Answer: 2
    Rationale: The skin freezes when the temperature drops to 14° to 24.8° Fahrenheit (210° to 24°C).

Nursing Process: Assessment
Client Need: Physiological Integrity

8. Answer: 4
    Rationale: Laser surgery is used to treat clients with a wide variety of skin disorders, including port wine stains. Chemical destruction is the application of a specific chemical to produce destruction of skin lesions. Chemical destruction is used to treat both benign and premalignant lesions. Sclerotherapy is the removal of benign skin lesions with a sclerosing agent that causes inflammation and tissue fibrosis. Curettage is the removal of lesions with a curette, which is a semisharp cutting instrument.
    Nursing Process: Planning
    Client Need: Safe, Effective Care Environment

9. Answer: 4
    Rationale: A full-thickness graft contains both epidermis and dermis. These layers contain the greatest number of skin elements (sweat glands, sebaceous glands, or hair follicles) and are best able to withstand trauma. A split-thickness graft contains epidermis and only a portion of dermis of the donor site. A common donor site for a skin graft is the anterior thigh. Skin grafting is an effective way to cover wounds that have a good blood supply, are not infected, and in which bleeding can be controlled.
    Nursing Process: Planning
    Client Need: Physiological Integrity

10. Answer: 2
    Rationale: Ovarian, adrenal, or pituitary tumors are causes for hirsutism. Uterine tumors, Cushing's syndrome, and central nervous system disorders are not associated causes of hirsutism.
    Nursing Process: Assessment
    Client Need: Health Promotion and Maintenance

Chapter 17

Case Study Answers

1. *What changes need to be made immediately in the client's care?* The client's IV fluids should be changed to lactated Ringer's solution. She should be intubated to protect her airway, especially in light of the risk of respiratory burn as evidenced by the soot on the nasal mucosa. The client's intake and output should be carefully monitored to determine the adequacy of fluid resuscitation.

2. *To what setting would you expect this client to be transferred when she is stable?* This client will be transferred to either a specific burn unit or a critical care unit.

3. *Why would the client be intubated and placed on a ventilator?* The risk of the client's respiratory system being compromised by burn is a great risk; therefore, the airways should be protected. Intubating the client is a safety measure. The client's respiratory rate and

oxygen saturation reading, as well as the soot around the nares, demonstrates that injury.

4. *Based on the client's injuries, from what type of immediate surgical intervention might she benefit?*
Tracheostomy

NCLEX Review Question Answers

1. Answer: 2
   Rationale: Lactated Ringer's (LR) is the recommended solution during the client's fluid resuscitation. Crystalloid fluids are administered through two large-bore (14- to 16-gauge) catheters, preferably inserted through unburned skin. Warmed Ringer's lactate solution is the intravenous fluid most widely used during the first 24 hours after burn injury, because it most closely approximates the body's extracellular fluid composition. Several formulas may be used to replace fluid loss. Two commonly used formulas are as follows:
   - Parkland formula, in which lactated Ringer's solution is administered 4 mL·kg·% TBSA burn
   - ABLS Consensus formula, in which lactated Ringer's solution is administered 2 to 4 mL·kg·% TBSA burn (Ahrns, 2004). This client weighs 68 kg with a second-degree burn over 40% of the body so use the Parkland calculation: $4 \text{ mL} \times 68 \times 40 = 10880 \text{ mL}$ over 24 hours, with 50% to be infused over the first eight hours and the other 50% over the remaining 16 hours.
   Nursing Process: Implementation
   Client Need: Physiological Integrity

2. Answer: 1
   Rationale: Elevating the head of the bed to at least 30 degrees improves the client's ability to ventilate better. Oxygen should be administered at 100% via mask, not a nasal cannula. Protecting the graft and skin at the burn site and premedicating the client are extremely important, but oxygenation holds a higher priority.
   Nursing Process: Implementation
   Client Need: Physiological Integrity

3. Answer: 3
   Rationale: A variety of tasks can be delegated to unlicensed personnel, but none should involve assessment. Encouraging the client to use the patient-controlled analgesia and spirometer are things that the client has already been taught, so these are just reminders. The first time ambulating requires the nurse to assess how the client tolerates the new activity. Changing the dressing and documenting the change again requires the nurse to assess the client, as does checking urinary output for adequacy of fluid resuscitation.
   Nursing Process: Planning
   Client Need: Physiological Integrity

4. Answer: 4
   Rationale: Wound healing and helping the body to heal are the most important and most common goals of radiation burn treatment. The other statements are true but are not goals of care; instead, they are information only.
   Nursing Process: Implementation
   Client Need: Health Promotion and Maintenance

5. Answer: 1
   Rationale: The client's daily caloric intake dramatically increases by as much as 100% of the normal intake, possibly as high as 4000 to 6000 Kcal per day. Therefore, the nurse must provide 4000 Kcal per 24 hours. The Parkland formula is designed for clients with burns over more than 20% total body surface area, so it may be possible to titrate oxygen down at this point, but it should be humidified to prevent damage to the nasal mucosa. Support garments should be applied no sooner than five to seven days postgraft.
   Nursing Process: Diagnosis
   Client Need: Physiological Integrity

6. Answer: 1
   Rationale: If the nurse does not disconnect the client from the electrical source, he/she will be placing themselves at risk by providing care for the client. Electrical injuries can occur in the hospital, so the nurse cannot assume that the injury happened elsewhere. Clients with electrical burns are at greater risk of spinal injury due to the forceful contraction of the muscles during the electrical injury, but waiting to provide care until after the collar and backboard are in place could cause irreversible brain injury to the client. It is important to monitor for cardiac dysrhythmia and for fluid resuscitation requirements, but they are not the highest priority.
   Nursing Process: Diagnosis
   Client Need: Physiological Integrity

7. Answer: 2
   Rationale: Full thickness burns regardless of size require skin grafting to heal due to the depth of damage and location of cells needed to regenerate tissue. Partial thickness grafting may be performed on smaller wounds as well as third intention healing.
   Nursing Process: Assessment
   Client Need: Physiological Integrity

8. Answer: 3
   Rationale: The American Burn Association provides guidelines for major burns; the client with the electrical burn meets those requirements not only because of the possible voltage but because of the trauma associated with the burn. Other requirements for major burns are those that involve 20% total body surface area in adults

older than 40 years of age, and 10% TBSA full-thickness burns in adults older than 40 years of age. Oxygen saturation rates may normally be below 95% for a given client, so this is not indicative of a burn.
Nursing Process: Assessment
Client Need: Physiological Integrity

9. Answer: See figure.
   Rationale: You should have shaded in the anterior trunk along with either arm or the head and neck.
   Nursing Process: Assessment
   Client Need: Physiological Integrity

Anterior
Anterior head
and neck, 4¹/2%

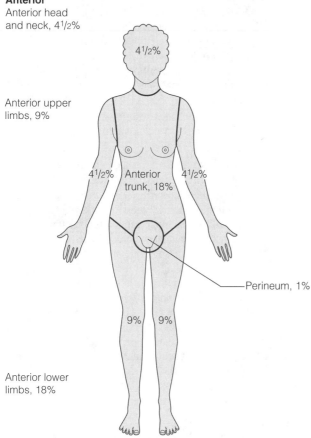

Anterior upper
limbs, 9%

4¹/2% Anterior 4¹/2%
       trunk, 18%

— Perineum, 1%

9% 9%

Anterior lower
limbs, 18%

10. Answer: 2
    Rationale: Hypovolemic shock is the earliest and one of the greatest risks to the burn client, in addition to sepsis. Cardiac collapse due to hypovolemia must be prevented with adequate fluid resuscitation during the first 24 to 36 hours. Compartment syndrome is local damage seen in the extremities that is related to circumferential burns and associated edema. Dysrrhythmias are more commonly associated with electrical burns and clients must be closely monitored. Acute renal failure is associated with hypovolemia; prevent the volume depletion to avoid this complication.
    Nursing Process: Diagnosis
    Client Need: Physiological Integrity

Chapter 18

Case Study Answers

1. *What questions should be included in the client's health history inventory related to her current endocrine issues?* When did the symptoms begin to interfere with the activities of daily living? Has anyone in her family had similar symptoms in the past? How has the client adapted her lifestyle to cope with these symptoms? What support systems does the client feel she has available?

2. *What endocrine-specific diagnostic tests might be used to correctly diagnose Ms. Aummert's health problem?*
   Thyroid stimulating hormone (TSH)
   Thyrozine (T_4)
   Triiodothyronine (T_3)
   Thyroid antibodies
   Radioactive iodine uptake
   Thyroid scan

3. *List the top two physiologic and psychosocial nursing diagnoses for this client.*
   Decreased cardiac output
   Activity intolerance
   Coping
   Anxiety

4. *What possible impediments might the nurse encounter while trying to develop a plan of care for Ms. Aummert?*
   Denial
   Lack of an adequate support system
   Time constraints
   Financial issues

NCLEX Review Question Answers

1. Answer: 3
   Rationale: Thyroid-stimulating hormone (TSH) is produced by the anterior pituitary and directly influences the production of the thyroid hormones. Physical and metabolic growth and control, not psychological development, is influenced by the pituitary. Red blood cell production is controlled by erythropoietin, which is not directly controlled by the pituitary. Blood calcium is regulated by the parathyroid gland with some influence by the thyroid; the pituitary is not responsible for calcium production.
   Nursing Process: Assessment
   Client Need: Physiologic Integrity

2. Answer: 2
   Rationale: Assessment of the neck and the client's ability to swallow may identify enlargement of the thyroid gland. While it is important to assess the abdomen for organomegaly and ascites, this is most likely not the source of the client's health issue. Balance and gait testing may help to identify weakness but this is too general. Assessment of

height and weight is generally important but only in comparison to a previous weight.
Nursing Process: Assessment
Client Need: Physiologic Integrity

3. Answer: 1
Rationale: The pancreas produces insulin, which is responsible for making glucose usable by the body. The pituitary is generally responsible for metabolism but not specifically insulin and carbohydrate metabolism. The thyroid increases metabolism and produces T3, T4, and calcitonin. The parathyroid secretes parathormone and controls phosphate metabolism.
Nursing Process: Assessment
Client Need: Physiologic Integrity

4. Answer: 3
Rationale: The adrenal medulla produces epinephrine and norepinephrine. The pancreas is responsible for the production of insulin and digestive enzymes. The thyroid is responsible for the production of T3, T4, and calcitonin. The adrenal cortex produces corticosteroids.
Nursing Process: Assessment
Client Need: Physiologic Integrity

5. Answer: 3
Rationale: The adrenal cortex secretes corticosteroids. The pituitary gland produces somatotropin, prolactin, thyroid-stimulating hormone, adrenocorticotropic hormone (responsible for glucocorticoids), gonadotropin hormones, and luteinizing hormone. The parathyroid secretes parathyroid hormone (PTH), or parathormone. The adrenal medulla secretes epinephrine and norepinephrine.
Nursing Process: Assessment
Client Need: Physiologic Integrity

6. Answer: 1
Rationale: The pancreas is located behind the stomach between the spleen and the duodenum. The duodenum is not a gland; it is the first segment of the small intestine.The thyroid is located in the neck. The adrenal cortex is found in the abdomen but is located above the kidney.
Nursing Process: Assessment
Client Need: Physiologic Integrity

7. Answer: 3
Rationale: Follicle-stimulating hormone (FSH) stimulates the development of ovarian follicles and induces the secretion of estrogenic female sex hormones. Oxytocin causes contraction of the smooth muscles in the reproductive organs, stimulates the myometrium of the uterus to contract during labor, and induces the production of milk from the breasts. Vasopressin is responsible for decreasing urine production. Luteinizing hormone (LH) induces ovulation and the formation of the corpus luteum from an ovarian follicle.

Nursing Process: Assessment
Client Need: Physiologic Integrity

8. Answer: 2
Rationale: The length of time the client experiences symptoms has little to do with genetics and much more to do with the client's ability to adapt. Many genetic disorders are associated with age of symptom onset. Many genetic disorders are more common in one gender than the other. Immediate family blood connection identifies genetic connection.
Nursing Process: Assessment
Client Need: Physiologic Integrity

9. Answer: 4
Rationale: Assessing the client's medication list for anything that may affect the outcome of the testing is an appropriate safety measure and a nursing responsibility.
Medical diagnosis is outside of the RN's scope of practice. Obtaining consent for the diagnostic testing is the function of the physician or nurse practitioner, not the RN. Providing the client and family with the results of the diagnostic testing is also outside of the RN's scope of practice.
Nursing Process: Implementation
Client Need: Safe, Effective Care Environment

10. Answer: 1
Rationale: Hypocalcemic tetany is assessed with either Trousseau's or Chvostek's sign. Testing for hypercalcemia includes blood and urine testing. Hyperkalemia is most commonly assessed through blood testing and can be seen in some clients' electrocardiograms. Hyperinsulinism would cause a decrease in the client's level of consciousness and would be assessed through blood testing.
Nursing Process: Assessment
Client Need: Physiologic Integrity

Chapter 19

Case Study Answers

1. *How should the nurse explain Addison's disease to Ms. Moss?* Explain to Ms. Moss that Addison's disease is a condition in which the body attacks its own adrenal gland.

2. *What manifestations should the nurse look for during the assessment of Ms. Moss?* Ms. Moss may demonstrate any of the following symptoms: dizziness, confusion, neuromuscular irritabilty, cardiac arrythmias, lethargy, weakness, anorexia, nausea, vomiting, and diarrhea.

3. *What skin changes should the nurse expect Ms. Moss to experience?* Ms. Moss's skin will begin to appear deeply tanned or bronzed.

4. *What diagnostic testing procedures may have been used to diagnose Ms. Moss's condition?* The following

diagnostic studies are used to make a diagnosis of Addison's disease: serum cortisol, blood glucose, serum sodium, serum potassium, blood urea nitrogen (BUN), urinary 17 hydroxycorticoids and 17 ketosteroids, plasma ACTH, (a cortisol) ACTH stimulation test, and a computed tomography (CT) scan.

NCLEX Review Question Answers

1. Answer: 4
   Rationale: The client with hyperthyroidism will experience diarrhea, not constipation. The client with hyperthyroidism will have the following manifestations: increased appetite, decreasing weight, hypermobile bowels, heat intolerance, insomnia, palpitations, increased sweating, and emotional lability.
   Nursing Process: Assessment
   Client Need: Physiologic Integrity

2. Answer: 2
   Rationale: Reducing the client's temperature with aspirin will increase the free thyroid hormone in the body and worsen the crisis. The client's body temperature should be reduced with aspirin-free medication. Their fluids and electrolytes should be replaced and oxygen should be administered due to their increased oxygen needs.
   Nursing Process: Implementation
   Client Need: Safe, Effective Care Envrionment

3. Answer: 2
   Rationale: Clients with hyperthyroidism must learn to keep the environment as distraction-free as possible. Decreasing stress lowers the cardiac output and circulating catecholamines. Clients must learn to balance periods of activity with periods of rest. The client must monitor their weight closely and weigh themselves at the same time every day. Carbohydrates and proteins must be added to the diet.
   Nursing Process: Evaluation
   Client Need: Health Promotion and Maintenance

4. Answer: 2
   Rationale: Estrogen increases thyroid function. Other medications that increase thyroid function include clofibrate, methadone, amiodarone, and birth control pills. Lithium, anabolic steroids, and propanolol may decrease thyroid function.
   Nursing Process: Assessment
   Client Need: Physiologic Integrity

5. Answer: 1
   Rationale: Hashimoto's thyroiditis is more common in women than men. It is an autoimmune disease that causes a goiter. It does have a familial link.
   Nursing Process: Assessment
   Client Need: Health Promotion and Maintenance

6. Answer: 4
   Rationale: Large doses of vitamins A and D must be avoided in clients with hyperthyroidism.

Clients with hyperthyroidism should drink plenty of liquids, be kept well-hydrated, and stay active.
   Nursing Process: Implementation
   Client Need: Physiologic Integrity

7. Answer: 2
   Rationale: Cushing's syndrome is a chronic disorder in which hyperfunction of the adrenal cortex produces excessive amounts of circulating cortisol or ACTH. Cushing's syndrome is more common in women, with the average age of onset between 30 and 50 years and clients undergoing long-term steroid treatment and chemotherapy.
   Nursing Process: Assessment
   Client Need: Health Promotion and Maintenance

8. Answer: 3
   Rationale: Behavior that demonstrates client understanding of treatment for Cushing's syndrome includes restricting fluid intake. Clients who understand health teaching will discuss their altered body image, increase their dietary intake of vitamins A and C, and use bright lighting in their rooms to avoid falls and injury.
   Nursing Process: Evaluation
   Client Need: Health Promotion and Maintenance

9. Answer: 4
   Rationale: The onset of Addison's is slow and symptoms appear after 90% of the gland function is lost. Symptoms may not appear in clients with less than a 90% gland function loss.
   Nursing Process: Assessment
   Client Need: Physiologic Integrity

10. Answer: 3
    Rationale: In diabetes insipidus, the urine exhibits hyperosmolality, not hypoosmolality. The client will experience polyuria, polydipsia, and their urine specific gravity will be low.
    Nursing Process: Assessment
    Client Need: Physiologic Integrity

Chapter 20

Case Study Answers

1. *What type of diabetes would Mr. Brown be diagnosed with and why?* Mr. Brown would be diagnosed with type 2 diabetes. He is being discharged with prescriptions for an oral hypoglycemic. Type 2 diabetes can occur at any age, but it is usually seen in middle-age and older people. Mr. Brown is middle-aged at age 56.

2. *How do oral hypoglycemics regulate blood sugar?* Hypoglycemic agents lower blood sugar by stimulating or increasing insulin secretion, preventing breakdown of glycogen to glucose by the liver, and increasing peripheral uptake of glucose by making cells less resistant to insulin. Some hypoglycemics keep blood sugar low by blocking absorption of carbohydrates in the intestines.

3. *What modifications will Mr. Brown need to make to his diet?* There are no specific diet guidelines for type 2 diabetes mellitus (DM). The general dietary guidelines are to decrease kilocalories, and to consume three meals of equal size that are evenly spaced approximately four to five hours apart, with one or two snacks. The person with type 2 DM should also decrease fat intake.

4. *How should Mr. Brown be taught to manage an episode of hypoglycemia?* When mild hypoglycemia occurs, immediate treatment is necessary. Mr. Brown should take about 15 g of a rapid-acting sugar. This amount of sugar is found, for example, in three glucose tablets, one-half cup of fruit juice or regular soda, eight ounces of skim milk, five Life Savers candies, three large marshmallows, or three teaspoons of sugar or honey. If Mr. Brown continues to experience symptoms of hypoglycemia, the 15/15 rule should be followed: wait 15 minutes, monitor blood glucose, and, if it is low, eat another 15 g of carbohydrate. This procedure can be repeated until the blood glucose levels return to normal. If the symptoms are not relieved or if they get worse, he should call his healthcare provider immediately or go to the nearest emergency room.

NCLEX Review Question Answers

1. Answer: 2
   Rationale: Type 2 diabetes mellitus (DM) is a non-ketonic form of diabetes. Type 1 DM begins most often in childhood, is a ketonic form of diabetes, can be triggered by a virus, and requires an exogenous form of insulin. Type 2 DM can occur at any age, but it is usually seen in middle-age and older people. Type 2 DM requires a diet change, increased exercise, and weight loss. Oral hypoglycemics may be ordered to assist in lowering the blood sugar.
   Nursing Process: Assessment
   Client Need: Health Promotion and Maintenance

2. Answer: 3
   Rationale: Manifestations of type 2 diabetes mellitus (DM) include: blurred vision, fatigue, paresthesias, and skin infections. Type 2 symptoms do not include polyuria, polydipsia, or polyphagia.
   Nursing Process: Assessment
   Client Need: Physiologic Integrity

3. Answer: 3
   Rationale: Normal fasting blood glucose is 100mg/dL.
   A fasting blood glucose of >100 mg/dL is abnormal. A fasting blood glucose of over 200 mg/dL is also abnormal.
   Nursing Process: Assessment
   Client Need: Physiologic Integrity

4. Answer: 4
   Rationale: Syringes for administering U-100 insulin can be purchased in either 0.3 mL (30 U), 0.5 mL (50 U), or 1.0 mL (100 U) sizes.

   Nursing Process: Implementation
   Client Need: Safe, Effective Care Environment

5. Answer: 2
   Rationale: Do not massage the site after administering the insulin injection, because this may interfere with absorption; pressure. Correct insulin administration includes: injecting the needle at 90 degrees, rotating the sites of injection, and do not inject insulin into an area that will be exercised.
   Nursing Process: Implementation
   Client Need: Safe, Effective Care Environment

6. Answer: 1
   Rationale: The use of alcohol places the client at an increased risk for an insulin reaction. Oral hypoglycemics may react with alcohol and cause headache, flushing, and nausea. Light beer is the recommended alcoholic drink because it is lower in alcohol. Alcohol should be consumed with meals and added to the daily food intake.
   Nursing Process: Implementation
   Client Need: Health Promotion and Maintenance

7. Answer: 3
   Rationale: The dawn phenomenon is a rise in blood glucose between 4:00 a.m. and 8:00 a.m. and is not a response to hypoglycemia. This condition occurs in people with both type 1 and type 2 diabetes mellitus (DM). The exact cause is unknown but is believed to be related to nocturnal increases in growth hormone, which decreases peripheral uptake of glucose.
   Nursing Process: Planning
   Client Need: Physiologic Integrity

8. Answer: 2
   Rationale: Hypotension is not a characteristic of diabetic nephropathy. Characteristics of diabetic neuropathy include hypertension, albumin in the urine, edema, and progressive renal insufficiency.
   Nursing Process: Assessment
   Client Need: Physiologic Integrity

9. Answer: 1
   Rationale: Alteration in the peripheral and autonomic nervous systems of diabetic clients include: palsy of the third cranial (oculomotor) nerve; loss of cutaneous sensation, most often located in the chest; pain, weakness, and areflexia in the anterior thigh and medial calf; and compression of the medial nerve, not radial nerve at the wrist.
   Nursing Process: Assessment
   Client Need: Physiologic Integrity

10. Answer: 4
    Rationale: Diabetic foot care includes: bathing the feet daily, patting the feet dry, and drying well between the toes. Tight shoes and clothing must be avoided. The feet must be inspected daily for lesions. The feet should be elevated to facilitate return circulation to the heart and minimize edema.
    Nursing Process: Evaluation
    Client Need: Health Promotion and Maintenance

Chapter 21

Case Study Answers

1. *What additional questions should the nurse ask this client?* Is the pain more intense before or after the client eats? Is the pain associated with positioning? What makes the pain better or worse? What has the client done to relieve the pain? Did those methods work?

2. *Epigastric pain of this type is often associated with what disorders? If the client's pain is more intense between meals and less intense after eating, it is more likely to be what disorder?* These symptoms are commonly associated with gastric or duodenal ulcers, gastroesophageal reflux disease (GERD), and hiatal hernia. Considering that the pain symptoms are more intense between meals, ulcers and GERD are the more likely diagnoses.

3. *What diagnostic studies might be ordered to further assess the client's epigastric pain?* This client would probably be scheduled for an upper GI swallow/series and possibly an endoscopy.

4. *What type of teaching needs does this client have?* The client needs teaching about smaller, frequent meals, as well as removing caffeine and alcohol from his diet. This client also needs education about managing his hypertension.

NCLEX Review Questions Answers

1. Answer: 2
   Rationale: The currently recommended daily intake of carbohydrates is 125 to 175 g. Protein, while important, should not comprise the majority of the daily intake; doing so will lead to obesity. Milk is an excellent source of calcium and vitamins A and D. Vitamin E is fat-soluble.
   Nursing Process: Implementation
   Client Need: Health Promotion and Maintenance

2. Answer: 1
   Rationale: Nutrients from food begin absorption in the duodenum and absorption continues through the small bowel. While the client will absorb nutrients through the remaining small bowel, the amount of loss will determine the body's ability to compensate. Water is absorbed in both the large and small bowel. Vitamin D is produced in the skin with exposure to sunlight. Bile is produced in the liver, stored in the gallbladder, and is delivered to the small bowel. Depending upon the extent of the injury, it may be important to decrease fat intake.
   Nursing Process: Assessment
   Client Need: Health Promotion and Maintenance

3. Answer: 3
   Rationale: Peanut butter is a fairly inexpensive source of protein, very stable, and can be stored without refrigeration in most conditions. It can also be purchased in low-fat and low-sodium varieties. A vegan vegetarian will not eat salmon or dairy products. Italian wedding soup is high in protein but that is due to the meat and a Vegan vegetarian will not eat lamb, beef, or chicken.
   Nursing Process: Implementation
   Client Need: Health Promotion and Maintenance

4. Answer: 2
   Rationale: A midarm muscle circumference of less than 60% of standard indicates not only a lack of subcutaneous tissue but muscle breakdown associated with severe malnutrition. Triceps skin fold thickness 10% below standard and decreased midarm circumference is associated with malnutrition but does not assess the degree. A client that is 10% above their ideal body weight is overnourished, not undernourished.
   Nursing Process: Assessment
   Client Need: Physiologic Integrity

5. Answer: 3
   Rationale: This is a normal assessment finding. All of the other findings are associated with an abnormal finding of cirrhosis, cancer, or other liver disorders.
   Nursing Process: Assessment
   Client Need: Physiologic Integrity

6. Answer: 4
   Rationale: In order to determine that a client's bowel sounds are absent, the nurse must listen for 5 minutes in each quadrant. Bowel sounds are most active in the lower right quadrant and the activity may vary from one quadrant to another. It could take up to 20 minutes to completely assess all quadrants for bowel sounds.
   Nursing Process: Assessment
   Client Need: Physiologic Integrity

7. Answer: 2
   Rationale: When the client becomes dehydrated, the body pulls intracellular fluid to maintain intravascular circulation. This causes the mucous membranes to dry out and become cracked. Cheliosis comes from painful lesions at the corners of the mouth and is often associated with a riboflavin or niacin deficiency. Acute infections produce a variety of symptoms and may include candidiasis, but this infection would cause white cheese-like patches that bleed easily.
   Nursing Process: Assessment
   Client Need: Physiologic Integrity

8. Answer: 4
   Rationale: This sharp pain that stops on inspiration is also called Murphy's sign and is associated with inflammation of the gallbladder. Gastric ulcers are more likely to present as epigastric pain; pancreatitis as upper middle abdominal pain; and appendicitis as lower right quadrant pain.
   Nursing Process: Assessment
   Client Need: Physiologic Integrity

9. Answer: 2

    Rationale: Bowel sounds should be present in the bowel at all times and should occur every 5 to 15 seconds normally. Plaque on the teeth is related to inflammation and poor dental hygiene. Borborygmus relates to hyperactive bowel sounds, diarrhea, or early bowel obstruction. Venous hum is often heard over the liver in cirrhosis or other venous restriction.

    Nursing Process: Assessment

    Client Need: Physiologic Integrity

10. Answer: 2

    Rationale: The nurse should always inspect the abdomen before any other portion of the assessment. Auscultation is the second step in the abdominal assessment since manipulation can cause a change in the presence of bowel activity. Percussion and palpation are the final steps in the abdominal assessment.

    Nursing Process: Assessment

    Client Need: Physiologic Integrity

Chapter 22

Case Study Answers

1. *What psychosocial factors may have contributed to Ms. Spencer's eating disorder?* Ms. Spencer may have an underlying depression or impulsivity disorder that manifests in an eating disorder. Up to half of the clients with a binge-eating disorder suffer from depression, alcohol abuse, and impulsivity.

2. *What diagnostic studies may be ordered to assess Ms. Spencer's nutritional status?* Ms. Spencer may be ordered a complete blood count (CBC) and a chemistry panel to assess her nutritional status due to her eating disorder.

3. *What treatments are instituted for clients with a binge-eating disorder?* Ms. Spencer's treatment will focus on establishing healthy eating patterns, psychological therapy, and may include prescribing an antidepressant or selective serotonin inhibitor (SSI).

4. *What role can Ms. Spencer's family play in assisting her to be successful with her treatment regimen?* The family can monitor her food intake and record it in a log. Ms. Spencer's family can assist in preparing well-balanced meals. Her family can also participate in counseling and educational nutritional sessions to foster healthy eating habits.

NCLEX Review Question Answers

1. Answer: 4

    Rationale: A BMI of 30 kg/m^2 or greater is defined as obese. A BMI of below 30 kg/m^2 is not considered obese.

    Nursing Process: Assessment

    Client Need: Health Promotion and Maintenance

2. Answer: 1

    Rationale: Physical inactivity is the most important factor that contributes to obesity. Obesity as a purely genetic condition is rare. Culture does play a role in one's dietary preferences but it is not the most important factor that causes obesity.

    Psychological factors such as low self-esteem do play a role in obesity, but do not have as great an impact as physical inactivity.

    Nursing Process: Evaluation

    Client Need: Health Promotion and Maintenance

3. Answer: 2

    Rationale: High HDL cholesterol is not a factor in metabolic syndrome. Metabolic syndrome includes three or more of the following factors: increased waist circumference, hypertension, increased blood triglycerides, increased fasting blood glucose levels, and low HDL cholesterol.

    Nursing Process: Assessment

    Client Need: Physiologic Integrity

4. Answer: 4

    Rationale: Orlistat or Xenical's adverse effects include oily stools, flatulence, and fecal urgency. Sibutramine (meridian) increases both the pulse rate and blood pressure, potentially limiting its appropriateness for use in clients with hypertension, CHD, or heart failure. Acutrim and Dexatrim are bulk producing medications giving a feeling of fullness. They may cause flatulence and diarrhea.

    Nursing Process: Assessment

    Client Need: Physiologic Integrity

5. Answer: 2

    Rationale: The Roux-en-Y procedure creates a small pouch for the stomach to restrict food intake. The biliopancreatic diversion involves removing a portion of the stomach and bypassing the jejunum and duodenum. An adjustable gastric banding creates a restricted stomach by placing a silicone rubber band across the proximal stomach. The vertical banded gastroplasty uses both staples and a band to create a small stomach pouch.

    Nursing Process: Assessment

    Client Need: Physiologic Integrity

6. Answer: 2

    Rationale: Nursing interventions to assist a client in weight reduction include setting a goal of losing 1–2 pounds per week. Identifying cues to eating, planning a well-balanced menu, and monitoring laboratory values are also key nursing interventions to be used for client weight reduction. Setting a goal to lose 3–4 pounds per week is an inappropriate and unrealistic goal.

    Nursing Process: Implementation

    Client Need: Health Promotion and Maintenance

7. Answer: 1

    Rationale: The nurse must assess the client for risk factors that contribute to malnutrition such as

a recent acute infection, weight loss of greater than 20% of usual weight, an inability to eat for more than five days, and poverty or homelessness.
Nursing Process: Assessment
Client Need: Physiologic Integrity

8. Answer: 2
    Rationale: Parental nutrition solutions must always be administered using an infusion pump to ensure a correct rate of infusion. If the nurse finds parental nutrition being infused through gravity, it must be corrected by being immediately placed onto an infusion pump. Parental nutrition is infused through a central line. The only solutions that may be mixed with parental nutrition is intralipids. The client should remain afebrile during parental nutrition therapy.
    Nursing Process: Implementation
    Client Need: Safe, Effective Care Environment

9. Answer: 1
    Rationale: Serving sizes for the newly-diagnosed client with anorexia must begin small and gradually increase over time. Clients may find normal-sized portions overwhelming. Proper home care includes weighing the client at least weekly at the same time of the day, adding vitamin supplements to the diet, and not allowing the client to use the bathroom unattended after meals.
    Nursing Process: Evaluation
    Client Need: Health Promotion and Maintenance

10. Answer: 3
    Rationale: Dumping syndrome can be caused by meals high in simple carbohydrates. Fats, proteins, and fiber in the diet do not cause dumping syndrome.
    Nursing Process: Planning
    Client Need: Health Promotion and Maintenance

Chapter 23

Case Study Answers

1. *What role does Mr. Hess's age, smoking history, and Excedrin use play in his peptic ulcer disease?* Duodenal ulcers are the most common peptic ulcer disease. They usually develop between the ages of 30 and 55, and are more common in men than in women. Ulcers are also more common in people who smoke and who are chronic users of NSAIDs.

2. *Why might Mr. Hess be screened for* H. pylori *infection?* H. pylori infection is found in about 70% of people who have peptic ulcer disease; this organism is unique in colonizing the stomach. *H. pylori* contributes to gastric epithelial cell damage without producing immunity to the infection. This is possibly related to the increased gastric acid production that is associated with *H. pylori* infection.

3. *What symptoms of peptic ulcer disease must the nurse assess Mr. Hess for?* The nurse should assess Mr. Hess for pain that is described as gnawing,

burning, aching, or hunger-like and is experienced in the epigastric region, sometimes radiating to the back. Mr. Hess may report heartburn or regurgitation and may vomit. The nurse must assess for signs of bleeding such as weakness, fatigue, dizziness, and orthostatic hypotension. Mr. Hess should be assessed for feelings of epigastric fullness, accentuated ulcer symptoms, and nausea which would indicate a gastric outlet obstruction.

4. *Describe the most lethal complication of peptic ulcer disease and its symptomology.* The most lethal complication of peptic ulcer disease is perforation of the ulcer through the mucosal wall. When an ulcer perforates, the client has immediate, severe upper abdominal pain that radiates throughout the abdomen and possibly to the shoulder. The abdomen becomes rigid and board-like, with absent bowel sounds. Signs of shock may be present, including diaphoresis, tachycardia, and rapid, shallow respirations.

NCLEX Review Question Answers

1. Answer: 4
    Rationale: Client health practices that demonstrate understanding of stomatitis prevention include: limiting the ingestion of highly spiced, acidic foods; brushing and flossing regularly; using a non-drying mouth rinse to cleanse the oral mucosa; and visiting the dentist to ensure proper-fitting dentures.
    Nursing Process: Evaluation
    Client Need: Health Promotion and Maintenance

2. Answer: 2
    Rationale: The upper lip is not a common site for oral cancers to initially form. The common sites for oral cancers to form include the tongue, lower lip, and the floor of the mouth. Most early cancers present as inflamed areas with irregular, ill-defined borders.
    Nursing Process: Assessment
    Client Need: Health Promotion and Maintenance

3. Answer: 4
    Rationale: The Trendelenberg position is not appropriate because it will keep oral secretions in the back of the throat and impede the airway. In order to maintain an open airway after surgery for oral cancer, place the client in Fowler's position, turn the client every 2 hours, and have the client cough and deep-breathe.
    Nursing Process: Implementation
    Client Need: Physiologic Integrity

4. Answer: 3
    Rationale: If the client will not be able to verbally communicate with the staff after surgery, have a tablet with pens or a picture menu ready at the bedside for the client to use for communication. Recording questions preoperatively does not allow for all of the situations and questions that may

arise after the surgery. Having a spokesperson available at all times for the client is not feasible. Providing cell phone numbers of staff will not aid a client who cannot speak into the phone.
Nursing Process: Planning
Client Need: Safe, Effective Care Environment

5. Answer: 1
   Rationale: A barium enema is performed to diagnose diseases of the colon. Diagnostic studies that may be performed for gastroesophageal reflux disease (GERD) include a 24-hour ambulatory pH monitoring, barium swallow, and upper endoscopy.
   Nursing Process: Planning
   Client Need: Health Promotion and Maintenance

6. Answer: 1
   Rationale: There are two types of esophageal tumors, adenocarcinoma and squamous cell carcinoma. Over the past two decades, the incidence of squamous cell tumors of the esophagus has been decreasing. Basal cell and status cell are not causes of esophageal cancer.
   Nursing Process: Assessment
   Client Need: Health Promotion and Maintenance

7. Answer: 1
   Rationale: Hyperkalemia is not a complication of vomiting. Potential complications of vomiting include dehydration, hypokalemia, metabolic alkalosis (from loss of hydrochloric acid from the stomach), aspiration with resulting pneumonia, and rupture or tears of the esophagus.
   Nursing Process: Planning
   Client Need: Health Promotion and Maintenance

8. Answer: 4
   Rationale: Ginger, an aromatic root that is frequently used in cooking, may also be helpful in relieving nausea and vomiting, particularly when due to motion sickness. Anise, catmint and sage are not known to relieve nausea and vomiting due to motion sickness.
   Nursing Process: Implementation
   Client Need: Health Promotion and Maintenance

9. Answer: 3
   Rationale: Hematochezia is defined as frankly bloody stools. Vomiting blood is known as hematemesis. Melena is defined as black tarry stools. Frothy white vomitus may occur with an empty stomach.
   Nursing Process: Assessment
   Client Need: Physiologic Integrity

10. Answer: 2
    Rationale: To prevent dumping syndrome, liquids and solids should not be mixed at meal time but consumed separately. The client must eat smaller, more frequent meals throughout the day. Protein must be increased in the diet, while sugars should be decreased.
    Nursing Process: Evaluation
    Client Need: Health Promotion and Maintenance

Chapter 24

Case Study Answers

1. *What role does Mr. Wales's past medical history play in his current episode of chronic pancreatitis?* Mr. Wales's history of alcoholism could have been a factor in causing his previous acute pancreatitis episode. His history of acute pancreatitis injures the pancreas, and makes it more susceptible to a recurrent infection. Mr. Wales's continued alcohol use increases his risk for developing chronic pancreatitis.

2. *What symptoms will Mr. Wales experience?* Mr. Wales will likely present with the following manifestations: gastric and left upper abdominal pain, nausea, vomiting, weight loss, flatulence, constipation, and steatorrhea.

3. *What complications from chronic pancreatitis must be assessed by the nurse?* Mr. Wales must be assessed for manifestations of malabsorption such as abscess formation, stricture, and diabetes mellitus.

4. *Describe discharge teaching that must occur with Mr. Wales.* Mr. Wales and his family must be taught how to prevent additional attacks of pancreatitis. The nurse should cover the following topics in teaching Mr. Wales:
   a. Alcohol use must be stopped. Continued alcohol use will cause further inflammation and destruction of pancreatic tissue.
   b. Smoking and stress should be avoided. Stress stimulates the pancreas.
   c. Pancreatic enzyme supplements must be taken as ordered.
   d. A low-fat diet must be followed.
   e. Mr. Wales should report any symptoms of infection to his healthcare provider immediately. Symptoms of infection include fever, pain, malaise, and a rapid pulse.

NCLEX Review Question Answers

1. Answer: 1
   Rationale: Eighty-one percent of gallstones consist primarily of cholesterol. The remaining 20% is a mixture of bile components.
   Nursing Process: Planning
   Client Need: Health Promotion and Maintenance

2. Answer: 4
   Rationale: Diarrhea is not a manifestation of acute cholecystitis. Manifestations of acute cholecystitis include anorexia, nausea, vomiting, fever, and right upper quadrant pain. Intestinal obstruction may develop due to the development of large gallstones.
   Nursing Process: Assessment
   Client Need: Physiologic Integrity

3. Answer: 2

Rationale: To reduce the risk of cholelithiasis, clients should be instructed to follow a low-fat, low-cholesterol diet; discuss the use of cholesterol-lowering medications with their physician; and increase their physical and daily activity levels. Instructing the client to increase their intake of carbohydrates is not appropriate teaching to reduce the risk of cholelithiasis.

Nursing Process: Implementation

Client Need: Health Promotion and Maintenance

4. Answer: 3

Rationale: Jaundice is first noticeable in the sclera of the eyes and then the skin. Nailbeds, skin, and oral mucosa are darker hued tissue and jaundice is hard to discern in these tissues.

Nursing Process: Assessment

Client Need: Physiologic Integrity

5. Answer: 1

Rationale: Clients with abnormal liver function studies and impaired consciousness with mental status changes are experiencing portal systemic encephalopathy. Portal systemic encephalopathy is the accumulation of toxic waste products in the blood as blood bypasses the congested liver and is not filtered. Ascites is the accumulation of fluid within the peritoneal cavity. Hepatorenal syndrome is an acute renal failure caused by the disruption of blood flow to the kidneys. Splenomegaly is the enlargement of the spleen.

Nursing Process: Diagnosis

Client Need: Physiologic Integrity

6. Answer: 1

Rationale: Hepatitis A and B are preventable, because vaccines are available. No vaccine is available for hepatitis Delta, C, and E.

Nursing Process: Planning

Client Need: Health Promotion and Maintenance

7. Answer: 3

Rationale: The client who states that they must use a condom during sexual activity demonstrates knowledge about the transmission and care for the hepatitis C viral infection. Hepatitis C is usually asymptomatic. Hepatitis C does not produce a lasting immunity to reinfection. Hepatitis B is spread through blood born contact.

Nursing Process: Evaluation

Client Need: Health Promotion and Maintenance

8. Answer: 4

Rationale: Asterixis is a muscle tremor that affects the upper extremities, tongue, and feet. The eyes are not affected by the tremor.

Nursing Process: Assessment

Client Need: Physiologic Integrity

9. Answer: 4

Rationale: Altered body image related to bruising is not an appropriate diagnosis for the client with liver trauma. Nursing diagnoses for clients with liver trauma include: deficient fluid volume related to hemorrhage; risk for infection related to wound or abdominal contamination; and ineffective protection related to impaired coagulation.

Nursing Process: Diagnosis

Client Need: Physiologic Integrity

10. Answer: 2

Rationale: Following a low-fat diet is not a risk factor for pancreatic cancer. Risk factors for developing pancreatic cancer include smoking, exposure to industrial chemicals or environmental toxins, chronic pancreatitis, diabetes mellitus, and a high fat diet.

Nursing Process: Assessment

Client Need: Health Promotion and Maintenance

Chapter 25

Case Study Answers

1. *What is the condition Mr. Parsons is describing when he mentions feeling as if he will pass out while bearing down during a bowel movement?* Valsalva's maneuver. Valsalva's maneuver stimulates the parasympathetic nervous system and slows the heart. The client may report feeling as if they are going to pass out.

2. *What could result from frequent bouts of constipation?* External hemorrhoids result from frequent bouts of constipation due to the client attempting to discharge fecal material.

3. *What radiographic study may be performed to assess Mr. Parsons's large bowel function?* Barium enema.

4. *Would you screen a client who describes bouts of constipation for depression or an anxiety disorder?* Clients with a depressive disorder often report constipation.

NCLEX Review Question Answers

1. Answer: 1

Rationale: The ileum is the terminal end of the small intestine. The cecum, colon, and rectum are all structures of the large bowel.

Nursing Process: Diagnosis

Client Need: Physiologic Integrity

2. Answer: 4

Rationale: Triglycerides enter the small bowel as fat globules and are coated by bile salts and emulsified pancreatic amylase acts on starches in the small intestine. Pancreatic enzymes in the small intestine break down proteins.

Triglycerides break down dextrin in the small intestine.
Nursing Process: Diagnosis
Client Need: Physiologic Integrity

3. Answer: 2
Rationale: Almost all food products and water, vitamins, and electrolytes are absorbed in the small bowel. The large intestine receives indigestible fibers, water, and bacteria.
Nursing Process: Diagnosis
Client Need: Physiologic Integrity

4. Answer: 1
Rationale: Stool specimen examination does not include assessment for odor. Stool specimen examination includes assessment for volume, water, color, blood, pus, mucous, fat, WBC, unabsorbed fat, and parasites.
Nursing Process: Assessment
Client Need: Health Promotion and Maintenance

5. Answer: 3
Rationale: Sexual history will not impact bowel function. Asking questions about the client's sexual history is inappropriate. Asking questions about travel, lifestyle stressors, and allergies will help to determine a cause for abnormal bowel function.
Nursing Process: Assessment
Client Need: Health Promotion and Maintenance

6. Answer: 2
Rationale: In order to completely palpate and auscultate the abdomen, the client should be in the supine position. The client will need to stand to assess for hernias and placed in the Sims' position for a rectal exam. Lithotomy position is used to examine the perineal area. It is not conducive to performing an abdominal examination as the legs would hamper examination of the abdomen
Nursing Process: Assessment
Client Need: Physiologic Integrity

7. Answer: 4
Rationale: Dullness is an abnormal finding and is heard when the bowel is displaced with fluid, tumors, or filled with a fecal mass. The abdomen should be concave in appearance. Gurgling or clicking sound heard upon auscultation is a normal finding. Tympany heard over gas-filled bowels upon palpation is a normal finding
Nursing Process: Assessment
Client Need: Physiologic Integrity

8. Answer: 1
Rationale: Right lower quadrant rebound tenderness is indicative of acute appendicitis. Right upper quadrant pain is associated with acute cholecystitis. Upper middle quadrant pain is indicative of acute pancreatitis. Left lower quadrant pain is a sign of acute diverticulitis.
Nursing Process: Assessment
Client Need: Health Promotion and Maintenance

9. Answer: 1
Rationale: Anal fissures are not caused by hemorrhoids. Anal fissures are caused by large, hard stools or diarrhea.
Nursing Process: Diagnosis
Client Need: Physiologic Integrity

10. Answer: 2
Rationale: To assess the anus, lubricate a gloved finger, slowly insert it into the anus, and point it toward the umbilicus. Pointing the finger toward the rectal floor, the right lung, or the heart places the finger in the wrong direction causing pain, discomfort, and the inabilty to feel structures being examined.
Nursing Process: Assessment
Client Need: Safe, Effective Care Environment

Chapter 26

Case Study Answers

1. *What is a positive McBurney's sign?* A positive McBurney's sign is rebound tenderness after pressure is applied to the right lower abdominal quadrant.

2. *What are the possible complications of untreated appendicitis?* Potential complications of untreated appendicitis include local peritonitis, abscess, or generalized peritonitis.

3. *What diagnostic studies will Ms. Bowman undergo?* The nurse should expect the following diagnostic studies to be performed: CBC, chemistry profile, urinalysis, ultrasound, and WBC with differential.

4. *Ms. Bowman undergoes an appendectomy. What should the nurse's postoperative teaching include?* Teaching topics should include wound care instructions, symptoms of infection that need to be reported to the healthcare provider, activity limitations, and when the client may return to work.

NCLEX Review Question Answers

1. Answer: 4
Rationale: Stimulants will increase diarrhea. Common antidiarrheal medications include opium and some of its derivatives, absorbants, and demulcents.
Nursing Process: Planning
Client Need: Health Promotion and Maintenance

2. Answer: 2
Rationale: Managing diarrhea involves teaching the client to eat small, frequent meals, drink electrolyte solutions such as Gatorade, limit food intake during acute episodes, and avoid foods high in fiber, milk products, and caffeine.
Nursing Process: Implementation
Client Need: Health Promotion and Maintenance

3. Answer: 3
Rationale: The client would demonstrate understanding of teaching about managing

constipation by following a diet high in fiber including prunes. Additional fluids should be added to the diet and a form of daily exercise should be practiced. Drinking a glass of warm water before breakfast helps stimulate peristalsis. Drinking a glass of ice cold water can slow peristalsis.
Nursing Process: Evaluation
Client Need: Health Promotion and Maintenance

4. Answer: 1
Rationale: Abdominal ultrasound is the most effective diagnostic study for diagnosing acute appendicitis. A CT scan can identify an enlarged appendix but not as well as an ultrasound. An MRI is used to identify tissue injury. Fluroscopy identified bony structures.
Nursing Process: Assessment
Client Need: Safe, Effective Care Environment

5. Answer: 1
Rationale: Urine output of less than 30 mL/hr may indicate hypovolemia.
Nursing Process: Assessment
Client Need: Physiologic Integrity

6. Answer: 4
Rationale: Salmonellosis is a food poisoning caused by ingesting raw or improperly cooked meat, eggs, and dairy products. Symptoms of salmonellosis develop 8 to 48 hours after ingestion. Shigellosis is caused by the shigella organism and is transferred via the fecal-oral route through contaminated food. Its incubation period is 1–4 days. Traveler's diarrhea develops when traveling to another country and is caused by a difference in climate, sanitation standards, food, or drink. Cholera is diarrhea caused by *Vibrio cholerae* found in contaminated food and water.
Nursing Process: Assessment
Client Need: Health Promotion and Maintenance

7. Answer: 3
Rationale: Amebiasis is an infection that affects the cecum, appendix, ascending colon, sigmoid colon, and rectum. Giardiasis is a protozoal infection of the proximal small intestine. Helminths are parasitic worms capable of causing bowel infections. Coccidiosis secretes an enterotoxin that causes watery diarrhea.
Nursing Process: Assessment
Client Need: Health Promotion and Maintenance

8. Answer: 2
Rationale: The client with IBD must increase their fluid intake to 2–3 quarts of liquids per day. The client should add nutritional supplements such as Ensure and vitamins to their diet. The client must adhere to their prescribed medication regimen as ordered by their physician. The participation in an ostomy support group can be of great benefit to the client as they learn to manage IBD.

Nursing Process: Evaluation
Client Need: Health Promotion and Maintenance

9. Answer: 4
Rationale: Clients with celiac sprue are placed on gluten-free diets. The client must add calories and protein to their diet to correct nutritional deficits. Fats and lactose must be avoided.
Nursing Process: Implementation
Client Need: Health Promotion and Maintenance

10. Answer: 3
Rationale: Painful rectal bleeding is not a symptom of intestinal polyps. Clients with polyps manifest the following symptoms: intermittent painless rectal bleeding, abdominal cramping, diarrhea, and a mucous discharge.
Nursing Process: Assessment
Client Need: Physiologic Integrity

11. Answer: 3
Rationale: Most recurrences of colorectal cancer occur within the first four years. Adding calcium and folic acid supplements can prevent colorectal cancer. Colorectal cancer often produces no symptoms until it is advanced. Colorectal cancer is always treated by a surgical resection.
Nursing Process: Planning
Client Need: Health Promotion and Maintenance

12. Answer: 3
Rationale: A transverse loop colostomy involves placing a portion of the colon onto the abdomen and securing it by a bridge or plastic rod. A sigmoid colostomy is the most common permanent colostomy performed. A double barrel colostomy involves the creation of two separate stomas. The Hartman procedure is the most common temporary colostomy procedure performed.
Nursing Process: Planning
Client Need: Health Promotion and Maintenance

13. Answer: 2
Rationale: Umbilical hernias are congenital and are detected in infancy. Inguinal, ventral, and incisional hernias or acquired hernias are usually caused by weaknesses in the fascia or musculature.
Nursing Process: Assessment
Client Need: Physiologic Integrity

14. Answer: 1
Rationale: Vomiting is not often seen in large bowel obstructions. If it does occur it is a late manifestation. Clients with a large bowel obstruction will complain of colicky abdominal pain and constipation. The abdomen may become distended.
Nursing Process: Assessment
Client Need: Physiologic Integrity

15. Answer: 4
Rationale: Diverticuli may occur anywhere in the gastrointestinal tract except for the rectum.
Nursing Process: Assessment
Client Need: Physiologic Integrity

Chapter 27

Case Study Answers

1. *Explain the functions of the kidney.* Functions of the kidney are to form urine; balance solute and water transport; excrete metabolic waste products; conserve nutrients; regulate acid–base balance; and secrete hormones to help regulate blood pressure, erythrocyte production, and calcium metabolism.

2. *What could tenderness and pain on percussion of the costovertebral angle suggest?* Tenderness and pain on percussion of the costovertebral angle suggest glomerulonephritis or glomerulonephrosis.

3. *What could pallor of the skin and mucous membranes indicate?* Pallor of the skin and mucous membranes may indicate kidney disease with resulting anemia.

NCLEX Review Question Answers

1. Answer: 4
   Rationale: The kidney is not supported by the inner renal fascia. The kidney is supported by three layers of connective tissue: the outer renal fascia, the middle adipose capsule, and the inner renal capsule.
   Nursing Process: Assessment
   Client Need: Physiologic Integrity

2. Answer: 1
   Rationale: The functions of the kidney are to: form urine; balance solute and water transport; excrete metabolic waste products; conserve nutrients; regulate acid–base balance; and secrete hormones to help regulate blood pressure, erythrocyte production, and calcium metabolism.
   Nursing Process: Assessment
   Client Need: Physiologic Integrity

3. Answer: 1
   Rationale: Glomerular filtration is a passive, nonselective process in which hydrostatic pressure forces fluid and solutes through a membrane. The amount of fluid filtered from the blood into the capsule per minute is called the glomerular filtration rate (GFR). Three factors influence this rate: the total surface area available for filtration, the permeability of the filtration membrane, and the net filtration pressure. The glomerulus is a far more efficient filter than most capillary beds, because the filtration membrane of the glomerulus is much more permeable to water and solutes than other capillary membranes.
   Nursing Process: Assessment
   Client Need: Physiologic Integrity

4. Answer: 1
   Rationale: Urine is composed, by volume, of about 95% water and 5% solutes. The largest component of urine by weight is urea. Other solutes that are normally excreted in the urine include sodium, potassium, phosphate, sulfate, creatinine, uric acid, calcium, magnesium, and bicarbonate.
   Nursing Process: Assessment
   Client Need: Physiologic Integrity

5. Answer: 2
   Rationale: Vitamin D is necessary for the absorption of calcium and phosphate by the small intestine. The stimulus for the production of erythropoietin by the kidneys is decreased oxygen delivery to kidney cells. Erythropoietin stimulates the bone marrow to produce red blood cells in response to tissue hypoxia. Hormones that are either activated or synthesized by the kidneys include the active form of vitamin D, erythropoietin, and natriuretic hormone.
   Nursing Process: Assessment
   Client Need: Physiologic Integrity

6. Answer: 1
   Rationale: The layers of the bladder wall (from internal to external) are the epithelial mucosa lining the inside, the connective tissue submucosa, the smooth muscle layer, and the fibrous outer layer. The muscle layer, called the detrusor muscle, consists of fibers arranged in inner and outer longitudinal layers and in a middle circular layer. This arrangement allows the bladder to expand or contract according to the amount of urine it holds.
   Nursing Process: Assessment
   Client Need: Physiologic Integrity

7. Answer: 2
   Rationale: In males, the bladder lies immediately in front of the rectum; in females, the bladder lies in front of the vagina and the uterus. The urinary bladder is posterior to the symphysis pubis and serves as a storage site for urine. Openings for the ureters and the urethra are inside the bladder. The size of the bladder varies with the amount of urine it contains. In healthy adults, the bladder holds about 300 to 500 mL of urine before internal pressure rises and signals the need to empty the bladder through micturition (also called urination or voiding). However, the bladder can hold more than twice that amount if necessary.
   Nursing Process: Assessment
   Client Need: Physiologic Integrity

8. Answer: 4
   Rationale: Oliguria means voiding scant amounts of urine. Polyuria means voiding excessive amounts of urine. Hematuria means blood in the urine. Nocturia means excessive urination at night.
   Nursing Process: Assessment
   Client Need: Physiologic Integrity

9. Answer: 4
   Rationale: The ketone level should be negative. The color of urine should be light straw to amber yellow. The pH range is 4.5–8.0. WBCs should be 3–4.
   Nursing Process: Assessment
   Client Need: Physiologic Integrity

10. Answer: 2

    Rationale: Urinary incontinence is not a normal outcome of aging. Common age-related urinary system changes include: urinary retention, urinary frequency, urgency, and nocturia. Larger amounts of residual urine present after voiding.
    Nursing Process: Assessment
    Client Need: Physiologic Integrity

Chapter 28

Case Study Answers

1. *Explain cystitis.* Cystitis, inflammation of the urinary bladder, is the most common urinary tract infection (UTI). The infection tends to remain superficial, and involves the bladder mucosa. The mucosa becomes hyperemic (red) and may hemorrhage. The inflammatory response causes pus to form.

2. *What can occur if cystitis is left untreated?* Typical presenting symptoms of cystitis include dysuria (painful or difficult urination), urinary frequency and urgency (a sudden, compelling need to urinate), and nocturia (voiding two or more times at night). In addition, the urine may have a foul odor and appear cloudy (pyuria) or bloody (hematuria) because of mucus, excess white blood cells in the urine, and bleeding of the inflamed bladder wall. Suprapubic pain and tenderness also may be present.

3. *Why does cystitis occur more frequently in adult females?* Cystitis occurs most frequently in adult females because of colonization of the bladder by bacteria normally found in the lower gastrointestinal tract. These bacteria gain entry by ascending the short, straight female urethra. In addition to the risk factors, personal hygiene practices and voluntary urinary retention can contribute to the risk for urinary tract infection (UTI) in women.

NCLEX Review Question Answers

1. Answer: 4

    Rationale: Most community-acquired UTIs are caused by *Escherichia coli,* a common gram-negative enteral bacteria. More than 8 million people are treated annually for UTI. Community-acquired UTIs are common in young women, and unusual in men under the age of 50. Catheter-associated UTIs often involve other gram-negative bacteria such as *Proteus, Klebsiella, Seratia,* and *Pseudomonas.*
    Nursing Process: Assessment
    Client Need: Physiologic Integrity

2. Answer: 1

    Rationale: The urinary tract is normally sterile above the urethra. Adequate urine volume, a free flow from the kidneys through the urinary meatus, and complete bladder emptying are the most important mechanisms for maintaining sterility. Pathogens that enter and contaminate the distal urethra are washed out during voiding. Other defenses for maintaining sterile urine include the normal acidity and bacteriostatic properties of the bladder and urethral cells.
    Nursing Process: Evaluation
    Client Need: Physiologic Integrity

3. Answer: 3

    Rationale: A long, straight urethra is not a risk factor for UTIs. Risk factors for UTIs in the female include a short, straight urethra; the proximity of the urinary meatus to the vagina and anus; sexual intercourse; use of diaphragm and spermicidal compounds for birth control; and pregnancy. Risk factors that are common to both females and males are aging, urinary tract obstruction, neurogenic bladder dysfunction, and vesicouretal reflux.
    Nursing Process: Assessment
    Client Need: Physiologic Integrity

4. Answer: 2

    Rationale: Stress incontinence is the loss of urine associated with increased intraabdominal pressure during sneezing, coughing, and lifting. The quantity of urine lost is usually small. Urge incontinence is the involuntary loss of urine associated with a strong urge to void. Overflow incontinence is the inability to empty the bladder, which results in overdistention and frequent loss of small amounts of urine. Functional incontinence is the type of incontinence that results from physical, environmental, or psychosocial causes.
    Nursing Process: Assessment
    Client Need: Physiologic Integrity

5. Answer: 1

    Rationale: Urinary anti-infectives should not be taken with milk products because they interfere with absorption. Health education for the client and family with urinary anti-infectives includes taking the drug with meals or food to reduce gastric effects; however, avoid milk products because they may interfere with absorption. These drugs are used along with hygiene practices to prevent recurrent UTI. The client should take as directed, even when no symptoms are present. The client should drink six to eight glasses of water or fluid per day while taking these drugs. Trimethoprim (Proloprim, Trimpex) should not be taken during pregnancy. The client should contact their physician before attempting to become pregnant. The client should contact their doctor if they develop any of the following: chest pain, difficulty breathing, cough, chills, and fever; numbness and tingling or weakness of the extremities; and rash or pruritus (itching). If the client is taking an oral suspension of nitrofurantoin (Furadantin, Nitrofan), they should rinse their mouth thoroughly after each dose to avoid staining the teeth. Nitrofurantoin turns the urine brown. This is not harmful and subsides when the drug is discontinued. If the client is taking trimethoprim (Proloprim, Trimpex) along

with phenytoin (Dilantin) or a related anticonvulsant, they should contact their doctor if they become sedated or begin to stagger.
Nursing Process: Assessment
Client Need: Physiologic Integrity

6. Answer: 1
   Rationale: The client with urolithiasis should receive the following information: increase fluid intake to 2500 to 3500 mL per day not increasing fluid intake to 3550 to 4550 mL per day; collect and strain all urine, saving any stones; report stone passage to the physician and bring the stone in for analysis; and report any changes in the amount or character of urine output to physician.
   Nursing Process: Planning
   Client Need: Physiologic Integrity

7. Answer: 2
   Rationale: The incidence of bladder cancer is about four times higher in men than it is in women, and about twice as high in whites as it is in blacks. An estimated 63,210 new cases of bladder cancer were diagnosed in the United States in 2005, and 13,180 people died as a result of the disease. Most people who develop bladder cancer are over age 60. Two major factors are implicated in the development of bladder cancer: the presence of carcinogens in the urine and chronic inflammation or infection of the bladder mucosa. Cigarette smoking is the primary risk factor for bladder cancer. The risk in smokers is twice that of nonsmokers.
   Nursing Process: Evaluation
   Client Need: Physiologic Integrity

8. Answer: 2
   Rationale: Because alkaline urine promotes formation of calcium stones and urinary tract infections, the diet may be modified to lower the pH of the urine. Foods that high in oxalate include asparagus, beer and colas, beets, cabbage, celery, chocolate and cocoa, fruits, green beans, nuts, tea, and tomatoes. Foods that affect urinary pH and foods that are high in various stone components are as follows: foods high in calcium include beans and lentils, chocolate and cocoa, dried fruits, canned or smoked fish except tuna, flour, and milk and milk products; purine-rich foods include goose, organ meats, sardines and herring, and venison; purine-moderate foods include beef, chicken, crab, pork, salmon, and veal; acidifying foods include cheese, cranberries, eggs, grapes, meat and poultry, plums and prunes, tomatoes, and whole grains; and alkalinizing foods include green vegetables, fruit (except as noted above), legumes, milk and milk products, and rhubarb.
   Nursing Process: Evaluation
   Client Need: Physiologic Integrity

9. Answer: 4
   Rationale: An opening of no more than 3 to 4 mm wider than the outside of the stoma is too wide.

The bag should be applied with an opening no more than 1 to 2 mm wider than outside of the stoma. Allow no wrinkles or creases where the bag contacts the skin. All supplies should be gathered: a clean, disposable pouch; liquid skin barrier or barrier ring; 4-by-4 gauze squares; stoma guide; adhesive solvent; clean gloves; and a clean washcloth. Assess knowledge, learning needs, and ability and willingness to assist with procedure. Explain the procedure as needed. Use standard precautions. Remove old pouch, pulling gently away from skin. Warm water or adhesive solvent may be used to loosen the seal if necessary. Assess stoma. Normally the stoma is bright red and appears moist. Report a dark purple, black, or very pale stoma to the physician. Slight bleeding with cleansing is normal, especially in the immediate postoperative period. Prevent urine flow during cleaning by placing a rolled gauze square or tampon over the stoma opening. Cleanse skin around the stoma with soap and water, rinse, and pat or air dry. Use the stoma guide to determine correct size for the bag opening and/or protective ring seal. Trim the bag or seal as needed. Apply skin barrier; allow to dry. Connect bag to the urine-collection device. Dispose of old pouch, used supplies, and gloves appropriately. Wash hands. Chart the procedure, including stoma appearance and response of the client.
Nursing Process: Implementation
Client Need: Physiologic Integrity

10. Answer: 4
    Rationale: Pelvic muscle exercises (Kegel exercises) should be performed more than two times a day. The client should maintain a generous fluid intake. Reduce or eliminate fluid intake after the evening meal to reduce nocturia. The client should wear comfortable clothing that is easy to remove for toileting. The client should maintain good hygiene, but do not bathe more often than necessary; frequent bathing and feminine hygiene sprays or douches may dry perineal tissues, increasing the risk of UTI or UI. The client should reduce consumption of caffeine-containing beverages (coffee, tea, colas), citrus juices, and artificially-sweetened beverages that contain NutraSweet. The client should use behavioral techniques such as scheduled toileting, habit training, and bladder training to reduce the frequency of incontinence.
    Nursing Process: Planning
    Client Need: Physiologic Integrity

Chapter 29

Case Study Answers

1. *"Why didn't my husband have any signs or symptoms until the last few days?"* Renal tumors are often silent, with few manifestations. The classic triad of symptoms, which are gross hematuria, flank pain,

and a palpable abdominal mass, is seen in only about 10% of people with renal cell carcinoma. Hematuria, often microscopic, is the most consistent symptom. Systemic manifestations include fever without infection, fatigue, and weight loss.

2. *"What tests might the physician order to determine if Brent has a renal tumor?"* Hematuria is often the only initial manifestation of renal cancer; its presence indicates a need for further diagnostic studies, including:
   - *Renal ultrasonography* to detect renal masses and differentiate cystic kidney disease from renal carcinoma
   - *CT scan* to determine tumor density, local extension of the tumor, and regional lymph node or vascular involvement
   - *IVP* and *MRI* may be done to evaluate renal structure and function.
   - *Renal angiography, aortography,* and *inferior venacavography* may be used to evaluate the extent of vascular involvement prior to surgery.
   - Chest X-ray, bone scan, and liver function studies to identify potential metastases

3. *"What is the treatment of choice for a renal tumor?"* *Radical nephrectomy* is the treatment of choice for kidney tumors. In a radical nephrectomy, the adrenal gland, upper ureter, fat, and fascia that surround the kidney, as well as the entire kidney, are removed. Regional lymph nodes may also be resected. Although nephrectomy can be done using a laparoscopic approach, laparotomy is primarily used for radical nephrectomy. No effective treatment is available for advanced renal carcinoma with metastases. Biologic therapies such as interferon or interleukin-2 have been used, but rarely achieve a durable effect. No chemotherapy drug consistently causes tumor regression in more than 20% of clients (Kasper et al, 2005).

NCLEX Review Question Answers

1. Answer: 3
   Rationale: Functional congenital kidney disorders are usually identified in childhood or adolescence. If function is not affected, congenital malformations may be detected only coincidentally. Congenital kidney disorders can affect the form and/or function of the kidney. Malformations include agenesis, hypoplasia, alterations in kidney position, and horseshoe kidney. Abnormal kidney position affects the ureters and urine flow, potentially leading to urinary stasis, increased risk of urinary tract infection (UTI), and lithiasis, or stone formation.
   Nursing Process: Assessment
   Client Need: Physiologic Integrity

2. Answer: 1
   Rationale: The progression to end stage renal disease tends to occur more rapidly in men than in women. Polycystic kidney disease is slowly

progressive. Symptoms usually develop by age 40 to 50. Common manifestations include flank pain, microscopic or gross hematuria (blood in the urine), proteinuria (proteins in the urine), and polyuria and nocturia, because the kidney's concentrating ability is impaired. Urinary tract infection and renal calculi are common, because cysts interfere with normal urine drainage. Most clients develop hypertension from disruption of renal vessels. The kidneys become palpable, enlarged, and knobby. Symptoms of renal insufficiency and chronic renal failure typically develop by age 60 to 70. The progression to end-stage renal disease tends to occur more rapidly in men than in women.
   Nursing Process: Evaluation
   Client Need: Physiologic Integrity

3. Answer: 2
   Rationale: As renal function declines, the elimination of water, solutes, and metabolic wastes are impaired. Accumulation of these wastes in the body leads to uremic symptoms. Instituted early in the course of chronic renal failure (CRF), dietary modifications can slow the progress of nephron destruction, reduce uremic symptoms, and help prevent complications. Sodium is restricted to 2 g per day initially. Unlike carbohydrates and fats, the body is unable to store excess proteins. Unused dietary proteins are degraded into urea and other nitrogenous wastes, which are then eliminated by the kidneys. Protein-rich foods also contain inorganic ions such as hydrogen ion, phosphate, and sulfites that are eliminated by the kidneys. Research has shown that restricting dietary protein intake slows the progression of CRF and reduces uremic symptoms (Kasper et al, 2005). A daily protein intake of 0.6 g/kg of body weight, or approximately 40 g/day for an average male client, provides the amino acids necessary for tissue repair. Proteins should be of high biologic value, rich in the essential amino acids. Water and sodium intake is regulated to maintain the extracellular fluid volume at normal levels. Water intake of 1 to 2 L per day is generally recommended to maintain water balance. More stringent water and sodium restrictions may be necessary as renal failure progresses. When the glomerular filtration rate (GFR) falls to less than 10 to 20 mL/min, potassium and phosphorus intake is also restricted. Potassium intake is limited to less than 60 to 70 mEq/day (normal intake is about 100 mEq/day) (Tierney et al., 2005). The client is cautioned to avoid using salt substitutes, which typically contain high levels of potassium chloride.
   Nursing Process: Planning
   Client Need: Physiologic Integrity

4. Answer: 4
   Rationale: Serum triglyceride levels increase with peritoneal dialysis. For the client who is not a candidate for renal transplantation or who has

had a transplant failure, dialysis is life-sustaining. Hemodialysis for ESRD typically is done three times a week for a total of 9 to 12 hours. Clients on long-term dialysis have a higher risk for complications and death than the general population.
Nursing Process: Planning
Client Need: Physiologic Integrity

5. Answer: 4
    Rationale: Risk factors for acute renal failure (ARF) include: major trauma or surgery, infection, hemorrhage, severe heart failure, severe liver disease, and lower urinary tract obstruction. Drugs and radiologic contrast media that are toxic to the kidney (*nephrotoxic*) also increase the risk for ARF. Older adults develop ARF more frequently due to their higher incidence of serious illness, hypotension, major surgeries, diagnostic procedures, and treatment with nephrotoxic drugs. The older adult also may have some degree of preexisting renal insufficiency associated with aging.
    Nursing Process: Assessment
    Client Need: Physiologic Integrity

6. Answer: 2
    Rationale: In end-stage renal disease (ESRD), the final stage of chronic renal failure (CRF), the glomerular filtration rate (GFR) is less than 5% of normal and renal replacement therapy is necessary to sustain life. The course of CRF is variable, and progresses over a period of months to many years. Chronic renal failure often is not identified until its final, uremic stage is reached. Chronic renal failure affects both the pharmacokinetic and pharmacodynamic effects of drug therapy.
    Nursing Process: Evaluation
    Client Need: Physiologic Integrity

7. Answer: 1
    Rationale: The donor kidney is placed in the lower abdominal cavity of the recipient, and the renal artery, vein, and ureter are anastomosed. Kidney transplant improves both survival and quality of life for the client with end-stage renal disease (ESRD). Most transplanted kidneys are obtained from cadavers. Hypertension is a possible complication of kidney transplant.
    Nursing Process: Evaluation
    Client Need: Physiologic Integrity

8. Answer: 1
    Rationale: Diabetes mellitus and systemic lupus erythematosus are common causes of secondary glomerulonephritis. Glomerular disorders and diseases are the leading cause of chronic renal failure in the United States. Hematuria, proteinuria, and hypertension often are early manifestations of glomerular disorders. Acute poststreptococcal glomerulonephritis (also called acute proliferative glomerulonephritis) is the most common primary glomerular disorder.

Nursing Process: Assessment
Client Need: Physiologic Integrity

9. Answer: 2
    Rationale: Chronic renal failure is the end stage of long-term kidney disease. It is irreversible; renal replacement therapies (transplant or dialysis) are necessary to sustain life. Acute renal failure has an abrupt onset and often is reversible with prompt treatment. Both acute and chronic renal failures are characterized by azotemia, which is the accumulation of nitrogenous (protein) waste products in the blood. The cause of renal failure may be a primary kidney disorder, or renal failure may be secondary to a systemic disease or other urologic defects. Renal failure is a condition in which the kidneys are unable to remove accumulated metabolites from the blood, which leads to altered fluid, electrolyte, and acid–base balance.
    Nursing Process: Assessment
    Client Need: Physiologic Integrity

10. Answer: 1
    Rationale: Intrarenal (or intrinsic) causes of acute renal failure have the greatest effect on renal function because the functional unit of the kidney, the nephron, is damaged. The course of acute renal failure due to acute tubular necrosis (ATN) typically includes three phases: initiation, maintenance, and recovery.
    Nursing Process: Assessment
    Client Need: Physiologic Integrity

Chapter 30

Case Study Answers

1. *What is an ECG?* The electrocardiogram (ECG) is a graphic record of the heart's activity. The electrocardiogram converts the electrical impulses it receives into a series of waveforms that represent cardiac depolarization and repolarization. ECG waveforms and patterns are examined to detect dysrhythmias as well as myocardial damage, the effects of drugs, and electrolyte imbalances.

2. *How are ECG waveforms recorded?* ECG waveforms are recorded by a heated stylus on heat-sensitive paper. The paper is marked at standard intervals that represent time and voltage or amplitude. Each small box is 1 mm^2. The recording speed of the standard ECG is 25 mm/second, so each small box represents 0.04 second. Five small boxes horizontally and vertically make one large box, equivalent to 0.20 second. Five large boxes represent 1 full second. Measured vertically, each small box represents 0.1 millivolt (mV).

3. *What is a standard 12-lead ECG?* A standard 12-lead ECG provides a simultaneous recording of six limb leads and six precordial leads. The limb leads provide information about the heart in the frontal plane and include three bipolar leads (I, II, III) and three unipolar leads (aV_R, aV_L, and aV_F). The bipolar limb leads

measure electrical activity between a negative lead on one extremity and a positive lead on another. The unipolar limb leads (called augmented leads) measure the electrical activity between a single positive electrode on a limb (right arm [R], left arm [L], or left leg [F for foot]), and the center of the heart.

4. *The cardiac cycle is depicted as a series of waveforms: the P, Q, R, S, and T waves. Explain each wave.* The *P wave* represents atrial depolarization and contraction. The impulse is from the sinus node. The P wave precedes the QRS complex and is normally smooth, round, and upright. P waves may be absent when the SA node is not acting as the pacemaker. Atrial repolarization occurs during ventricular depolarization and usually is not seen on the ECG. The *PR interval* represents the time required for the sinus impulse to travel to the AV node and into the Purkinje fibers. This interval is measured from the beginning of P wave to the beginning of QRS complex. If no Q wave is seen, the beginning of the R wave is used. The PR interval is normally 0.12 to 0.20 second (up to 0.24 second is considered normal in clients over age 65). PR intervals greater than 0.20 second indicate a delay in conduction from the SA node to the ventricles. The *QRS complex* represents ventricular depolarization and contraction. The QRS complex includes three separate waves: the Q wave is the first negative deflection, the R wave is the positive or upright deflection, and the S wave is the first negative deflection after the R wave. Not all QRS complexes have all three waves; nevertheless, the complex is called a QRS complex. The normal duration of a QRS complex is from 0.06 to 0.10 second. QRS complexes greater than 0.10 second indicate delays in transmitting the impulse through the ventricular conduction system. The *ST segment* signifies the beginning of ventricular repolarization. The ST segment, the period from the end of the QRS complex to the beginning of the T wave, should be isoelectric. An abnormal ST segment is displaced (elevated or depressed) from the isoelectric line. The *T wave* represents ventricular repolarization. It normally has a smooth, rounded shape that is usually less than 10 mm tall. It usually points in the same direction as the QRS complex. Abnormalities of the T wave may indicate myocardial ischemia or injury, or electrolyte imbalances. The *QT interval* is measured from the beginning of the QRS complex to the end of the T wave. It represents the total time of ventricular depolarization and repolarization. Its duration varies with gender, age, and heart rate; usually, it is 0.32 to 0.44 second long. Prolonged QT intervals indicate a prolonged relative refractory period and a greater risk of dysrhythmias. Shortened QT intervals may result from medications or electrolyte imbalances. The *U wave* is not normally seen. It is thought to signify repolarization of the terminal Purkinje fibers. If present, the U wave follows the same direction as the T wave. It is most commonly seen in hypokalemia.

NCLEX Review Question Answers

1. Answer: 4

   Rationale: Two-thirds of the heart mass lies to the left of the sternum; the upper base lies beneath the second rib, and the pointed apex is approximate with the fifth intercostal space, midpoint to the clavicle. The heart, a muscular pump, beats an average of 70 times per minute, or once every 0.86 seconds, every minute of a person's life. The heart is a hollow, cone-shaped organ approximately the size of an adult's fist, and weighs less than 1 lb. The heart is located in the mediastinum of the thoracic cavity, between the vertebral column and the sternum, and is flanked laterally by the lungs.
   Nursing Process: Assessment
   Client Need: Physiologic Integrity

2. Answer: 3

   Rationale: The heart wall consists of three layers of tissue: the epicardium, the myocardium, and the endocardium. The epicardium covers the entire heart and great vessels, and then folds over to form the parietal layer that lines the pericardium and adheres to the heart surface. The myocardium, which is the middle layer of the heart wall, consists of specialized cardiac muscle cells (myofibrils) that provide the bulk of contractile heart muscle. The endocardium, which is the innermost layer, is a thin membrane composed of three layers; the innermost layer is made up of smooth endothelial cells that line the inside of the heart's chambers and great vessels. The pericardium encases the heart and anchors it to surrounding structures, forming the pericardial sac. The snug fit of the pericardium prevents the heart from overfilling with blood. The outermost layer is the parietal pericardium, and the visceral pericardium (or epicardium) adheres to the heart surface. The small space between the visceral and parietal layers of the pericardium is called the pericardial cavity. A serous lubricating fluid produced in this space cushions the heart as it beats.
   Nursing Process: Assessment
   Client Need: Physiologic Integrity

3. Answer: 2

   Rationale: The right ventricle receives deoxygenated blood from the right atrium and pumps it through the pulmonary artery to the pulmonary capillary bed for oxygenation. The right atrium receives deoxygenated blood from the veins of the body. The left atrium receives freshly oxygenated blood from the lungs through the pulmonary veins. The superior vena cava returns blood from the body area above the diaphragm, the inferior vena cava returns blood from the body below the diaphragm, and the coronary sinus drains blood from the heart.
   Nursing Process: Evaluation
   Client Need: Physiologic Integrity

4. Answer: 2

Rationale: The greater the volume, the greater the stretch of the cardiac muscle fibers, and the greater the force with which the fibers contract to accomplish emptying. This principle is called Starling's law of the heart. The other choices in the question do not exist.

Nursing Process: Assessment
Client Need: Physiologic Integrity

5. Answer: 3

Rationale: The SA node acts as the normal "pacemaker" of the heart, usually generating an impulse 60 to 100 times per minute. The sinoatrial (SA) node is located at the junction of the superior vena cava and right atrium. The cellular action potential serves as the basis for electrocardiography (ECG), a diagnostic test of cardiac function. The electrical stimulus increases the permeability of the cell membrane, which creates an action potential (electrical potential).

Nursing Process: Assessment
Client Need: Physiologic Integrity

6. Answer: 1

Rationale: The recording speed of the standard ECG is 25 mm/second. The electrocardiograph converts the electrical impulses it receives into a series of waveforms that represent cardiac depolarization and repolarization. ECG waveforms and patterns are examined to detect dysrhythmias as well as myocardial damage, the effects of drugs, and electrolyte imbalances. Placement of electrodes on different parts of the body allows different views of this electrical activity.

Nursing Process: Evaluation
Client Need: Physiologic Integrity

7. Answer: 2

Rationale: The ST segment signifies the beginning of ventricular repolarization. The *T wave* represents ventricular repolarization. The PR interval represents the time required for the sinus impulse to travel to the AV node and into the Purkinje fibers. The P wave represents atrial depolarization and contraction.

Nursing Process: Assessment
Client Need: Physiologic Integrity

8. Answer: 2

Rationale: Echocardiograms are conducted in conjunction with Dopplers and color flow imaging to produce audio and graphic data about the motion, wall thickness, and chamber size of the heart; and of blood flow and velocity. A cardiac catheterization with either coronary angiography or coronary arteriography may be performed to identify coronary artery disease (CAD) or cardiac valvular disease, to determine pulmonary artery or heart chamber pressures, to obtain a myocardial biopsy, to evaluate artificial valves, or to do an angioplasty or stent of an area of CAD.

A transesophageal echocardiogram (TEE) allows visualization of structures adjacent to the esophagus to visualize cardiac and extracardiac structures, including mitral valve and aortic valve pathology, left atrium intracardiac thrombosus, acute dissection of the aorta, endocarditis, and ventricular function during and after surgery. Pericardiocentesis is a procedure that removes fluid from the pericardial sac for diagnostic or therapeutic purposes. It may also be an emergency procedure to treat cardiac tamponade.

Nursing Process: Assessment
Client Need: Physiologic Integrity

9. Answer: 3

Rationale: Stroke volume ranges from 60 to 100 mL/beat and averages about 70 mL/beat in an adult. Multiplying the stroke volume by the heart rate determines the cardiac output: $CO \times HR = SV$.

Nursing Process: Assessment
Client Need: Physiologic Integrity

10. Answer: 3

Rationale: If a splitting of S_2 is heard, that is an abnormal assessment finding. The following are normal assessment findings: no splitting of S_2 should be heard; S_1 is loudest at the apex of the heart; S_2 immediately follows S_1 and is loudest at the base of the heart; and no extra heart sounds are present.

Nursing Process: Assessment
Client Need: Physiologic Integrity

Chapter 31

Case Study Answers

1. *What are modifiable and nonmodifiable risk factors for coronary heart disease (CHD)?* Age is a nonmodifiable risk factor for CHD. Over 50% of heart attack victims are 65 or older; 80% of deaths due to myocardial infarction occur in this age group. *Gender* and *genetic factors* also are nonmodifiable risk factors for CHD. Men are affected by CHD at an earlier age than women. A family history of CHD in a male first-degree relative younger than age 55 or a female first-degree relative younger than 65 years is identified as a risk factor for CHD (National Cholesterol Education Program [NCEP], 2002). Modifiable risk factors include lifestyle factors and pathologic conditions that predispose the client to developing CHD. Disease conditions that contribute to CHD include hypertension, diabetes mellitus, and hyperlipidemia. Although these conditions are not a matter of choice, they are modifiable risk factors that can often be controlled through medication, weight control, diet, and exercise. Behavioral or lifestyle factors can be controlled or completely eliminated. Lifestyle changes require significant commitment by the client; ongoing support from the healthcare team is vital for success.

2. What are abnormal blood lipids? *Hyperlipidemia* is an abnormally high level of blood lipids and lipoproteins. Lipoproteins carry cholesterol in the blood. Low-density lipoproteins (LDLs) are the primary carriers of cholesterol. High levels of LDL (memory cue: LDLs = **l**ess **d**esirable **l**ipoproteins) promote atherosclerosis because LDL deposits cholesterol on artery walls. Table 31–3 in your text lists desirable and high-risk levels for total and LDL cholesterol. In contrast, high-density lipoproteins (HDLs = **h**ighly **d**esirable **l**ipoproteins) help clear cholesterol from the arteries, and transport it to the liver for excretion. HDL levels above 35 mg/dL have a protective effect, reducing the risk of CHD; in contrast, HDL levels lower than 35 mg/dL are associated with an increased risk for CHD. Triglycerides, which are compounds of fatty acids bound to glycerol and used for fat storage by the body, are carried on very low-density lipoprotein (VLDL) molecules. Elevated triglycerides also contribute to the risk for CHD.

3. *What are characteristics of metabolic syndrome?* Characteristics of metabolic syndrome include:
   - Abdominal obesity
   - Abnormal blood lipids (low HDL, high triglycerides)
   - Hypertension
   - Elevated fasting blood glucose
   - Clotting tendency
   - Inflammatory factors

4. *How is CPR performed?* The procedure for CPR is as follows:
   1. Assess for responsiveness; shake the client and shout.
   2. Call for help. Dial 911 (if outside the healthcare facility) or initiate the institutional code or cardiac arrest procedure.
   3. Open the airway using the head-tilt, chin-lift maneuvers. Simultaneously press down on the forehead with one hand while lifting the chin upward with the other.
   4. Check for breathing; look and listen. Inspect the chest for rise and fall with respirations; listen and feel for air movement through the nose or mouth. This step should take no more than 10 seconds.
   5. If not breathing, begin rescue breathing using a pocket mask, mouth shield, or bag-valve mask (see part *B* of the figure). Administer two breaths (1 second per breath), observing for rise of the chest with each breath.
   6. Check the carotid or femoral artery for a pulse [leq] 10 sec.).
   7. If a pulse is present, continue rescue breathing, administering 8 to 10 breaths per minute, until help arrives or spontaneous respirations resume. Recheck the carotid pulse every 2 minutes.
   8. If no pulse is present, analyze rhythm and defibrillate or, if there is unwitnessed cardiac arrest or an AED is unavailable, initiate external cardiac compressions. Place on a firm surface. Position the heel of one hand in the center of the chest between the nipples (child and adult), with the other hand on top and the fingers either interlocked or extended.
   9. Initiate hard and fast cardiac compressions, pressing straight down to depress the sternum 1.5 to 2 inches, keeping the elbows locked and positioning the shoulders directly over the hands (part *D* of the figure). Release pressure completely between compressions but do not lift the hands from the chest.
   10. Compress the chest at a rate of approximately 100 times per minute. With one- or two-rescuer CPR, provide 2 breaths after each 30 compressions. Assess the pulse after 5 complete cycles of 30 compressions and 2 breaths; continue CPR until help arrives.

NCLEX Review Question Answers

1. Answer: 2
   Rationale: Coronary heart disease (CHD) may be asymptomatic. CHD is caused by impaired blood flow to the myocardium. CHD affects 13.2 million people in the United States and causes more than 500,000 deaths annually. Accumulation of atherosclerotic plaque in the coronary arteries is the usual cause of CHD.
   Nursing Process: Evaluation
   Client Need: Physiologic Integrity

2. Answer: 3
   Rationale: Dietary recommendations to reduce total cholesterol, LDL levels, and CHD risk include: adjusting calories to attain/maintain desirable body weight; make total fat consumption 25%–35% of total calories, with saturated fat at less than 7% of total calories and monounsaturated fat of up to 20% of total calories; make carbohydrates 50–60% of total calories and primarily complex carbohydrates, such as whole grains, fruits, and vegetables; consume 20–30 g/day of dietary fiber; and make protein about 15% of total calories.
   Nursing Process: Planning
   Client Need: Physiologic Integrity

3. Answer: 3
   Rationale: High HDL is not a characteristic of metabolic syndrome. Characteristics of metabolic syndrome include abdominal obesity, abnormal blood lipids (low HDL, high triglycerides), hypertension, elevated fasting blood glucose, clotting tendency, and inflammatory factors.
   Nursing Process: Assessment
   Client Need: Physiologic Integrity

4. Answer: 3
   Rationale: The client should keep sublingual tablets in their original amber glass bottle to protect them from heat, light, and moisture. They should replace their supply every six months. If the first nitrate dose does not relieve angina within 5

minutes, they should take a second dose. After five more minutes, they may take a third dose if needed. If the pain is unrelieved or lasts for 20 minutes or longer, they should seek medical assistance immediately. The client should carry a supply of nitroglycerin tablets. They should dissolve sublingual nitroglycerin tablets under the tongue or between the upper lip and gum. The client should not eat, drink, or smoke until the tablet is completely dissolved. They should rotate ointment or transdermal patch application sites. They should apply to a hairless area and spread ointment evenly without rubbing or massaging. They should remove the patch or residual ointment at bedtime daily, and apply a fresh dose in the morning.
Nursing Process: Planning
Client Need: Physiologic Integrity

5. Answer: 1
   Rationale: Primary electrical disorders are cardiac causes of sudden cardiac death. Choking, cerebral hemorrhage, and pulmonary embolism are noncardiac causes of sudden cardiac death.
   Nursing Process: Assessment
   Client Need: Physiologic Integrity

6. Answer: 3
   Rationale: Cardiopulmonary resuscitation: Assess for responsiveness; shake the client and shout. Open the airway using the head-tilt, chin-lift maneuvers. Check the carotid or femoral artery for a pulse (≤ 10 sec.). With one- or two-rescuer CPR, provide 2 breaths after each 30 compressions. Assess the pulse after 5 complete cycles of 30 compressions and 2 breaths; continue CPR until help arrives.
   Nursing Process: Implementation
   Client Need: Physiologic Integrity

7. Answer: 4
   Rationale: Ischemia, which is deficient blood flow to tissue, may be caused by partial obstruction of a coronary artery, coronary artery spasm, or a thrombus. Angina pectoris, or angina, is chest pain that results from reduced coronary blood flow, which causes a temporary imbalance between myocardial blood supply and demand. Aberrant (abnormal) impulses may originate outside normal conduction pathways, and cause ectopic beats. The AV nodal delay allows the atria to contract, and delivers an extra bolus of blood to the ventricles before they contract (the atrial kick).
   Nursing Process: Assessment
   Client Need: Physiologic Integrity

8. Answer: 3
   Rationale: Supraventricular dysrhythmias arise in the sinus node or the atria. A P wave *may be* present; the QRS appears normal, and a T wave *may be* seen. The normal sinus rate is 60 to 100 beats per minute. Each complex includes a P wave, QRS, and T wave. Junctional dysrhythmias arise in tissue just above or just below the AV node. The P wave may be inverted, and may precede, follow, or be buried in

the QRS complex. The QRS usually appears normal and is followed by a T wave. Ventricular dysrhythmias arise in ventricular myocardium. They do not reset the sinus node or activate the atria. QRS complexes are wide and bizarre.
   Nursing Process: Assessment
   Client Need: Physiologic Integrity

9. Answer: 2
   Rationale: Myocardial infarction usually affects the *left* ventricle because it is the major "workhorse" of the heart; its muscle mass and oxygen demands are greater. Myocardial infarction (MI) occurs when blood flow to a portion of cardiac muscle is completely blocked, which results in prolonged tissue ischemia and irreversible cell damage. MIs are described by the damaged area of the heart. Risk factors for MI are the same as those for coronary heart disease: age, gender, heredity, race, smoking, obesity, hyperlipidemia, hypertension, diabetes, sedentary lifestyle, diet, and others.
   Nursing Process: Assessment
   Client Need: Physiologic Integrity

10. Answer: 4
   Rationale: Risk factors for coronary heart disease (CHD) are frequently classified as nonmodifiable, or factors that cannot be changed, and modifiable, which are factors that can be changed. Modifiable risk factors include lifestyle factors and pathologic conditions that predispose the client to developing CHD. Disease conditions that contribute to CHD include hypertension, diabetes mellitus, and hyperlipidemia. Although these conditions are not a matter of choice, they are modifiable risk factors that can often be controlled through medication, weight control, diet, and exercise. Behavioral or lifestyle factors can be controlled or completely eliminated. Lifestyle changes require significant commitment by the client; ongoing support from the healthcare team is vital for success. Age is a nonmodifiable risk factor. Over 50% of heart attack victims are 65 or older; 80% of deaths due to myocardial infarction occur in this age group. Gender and genetic factors also are nonmodifiable risk factors for CHD. Men are affected by CHD at an earlier age than women. A family history of CHD in a male first-degree relative younger than age 55 or a female first-degree relative younger than 65 years is identified as a risk factor for CHD (National Cholesterol Education Program [NCEP], 2002).
   Nursing Process: Assessment
   Client Need: Physiologic Integrity

Chapter 32

Case Study Answers

1. *"What is heart failure?"* Heart failure is common in older adults, and affects nearly 10% of people over the age of 75 years. Aging affects cardiac function. In heart failure, diastolic filling is impaired by

decreased ventricular compliance. With aging, the heart is less responsive to sympathetic nervous system stimulation. As a result, maximal heart rate, cardiac reserve, and exercise tolerance are reduced. Concurrent health problems such as arthritis that affect stamina or mobility often contribute to a more sedentary lifestyle, which further decreases the heart's ability to respond to increased stress.

2. *"What are the causes of heart failure?"* Causes of impaired myocardial function include: coronary heart disease, cardiomyopathies, rheumatic fever, and infective endocarditis. Causes of increased cardiac workload include: hypertension, valve disorders, anemias, and congenital heart defects. Causes of acute noncardiac conditions include: volume overload, hyperthyroidism, fever and infection, and massive pulmonary embolus.

3. *"What are the stages of heart failure?"* The stages of heart failure are as follows:
    Stage A: Clients at high risk for developing heart failure, but without structural heart disease or symptoms of heart failure (clients with hypertension, CHD, diabetes, obesity, metabolic syndrome, or who have a family history of cardiomyopathy, or who are taking cardiotoxic drugs);
    Stage B: Clients with structural heart disease but no manifestations of heart failure (clients with previous MI, asymptomatic valve disease, or left ventricular dysfunction);
    Stage C: Clients with structural heart disease and current or prior symptoms of heart failure (shortness of breath, fatigue, decreased exercise tolerance); and
    Stage D: Refractory heart failure (clients with manifestations of heart failure at rest despite aggressive treatment).

4. *"What are the complications of heart failure?"* The compensatory mechanisms initiated in heart failure can lead to complications in other body systems. Congestive hepatomegaly and splenomegaly caused by engorgement of the portal venous system result in increased abdominal pressure, ascites, and gastrointestinal problems. With prolonged right-sided heart failure, liver function may be impaired. Myocardial distention can precipitate dysrhythmias, which further impairs cardiac output. Pleural effusions and other pulmonary problems may develop. Major complications of severe heart failure are cardiogenic shock and acute pulmonary edema, a medical emergency described in the next section of this chapter.

NCLEX Review Question Answers

1. Answer: 4
    Rationale: As left ventricular function fails, cardiac output falls. Pressures in the left ventricle and atrium increase as the amount of blood that remains in the ventricle after systole increases.

These increased pressures impair filling, which causes congestion and increased pressures in the pulmonary vascular system. Increased pressures in this normally low-pressure system increase fluid movement from the blood vessels into interstitial tissues and the alveoli. Left-sided heart failure also can lead to right-sided failure as pressures in the pulmonary vascular system increase with congestion behind the failing left ventricle.
    Nursing Process: Assessment
    Client Need: Physiologic Integrity

2. Answer: 3
    Rationale: Clients with structural heart disease and current or prior symptoms of heart failure (shortness of breath, fatigue, decreased exercise tolerance) are in stage C of heart failure. Clients at high risk for developing heart failure, but without structural heart disease or symptoms of heart failure (clients with hypertension, CHD, diabetes, obesity, metabolic syndrome, or who have a family history of cardiomyopathy, or who are taking cardiotoxic drugs) are in stage A of heart failure. Clients with structural heart disease but no manifestations of heart failure (clients with previous MI, asymptomatic valve disease, or left ventricular dysfunction) are in stage B of heart failure. Refractory heart failure (clients with manifestations of heart failure at rest despite aggressive treatment) are in stage D of heart failure.
    Nursing Process: Assessment
    Client Need: Physiologic Integrity

3. Answer: 1
    Rationale: An advantage of a prosthetic heart valve is the long-term durability. Disadvantages of prosthetic heart valves include: lifetime anticoagulation; audible click; and infections are harder to treat.
    Nursing Process: Planning
    Client Need: Physiologic Integrity

4. Answer: 4
    Rationale: Withhold digitalis and notify the physician if heart rate is below 60 BPM and/or manifestations of decreased cardiac output are noted. Assess apical pulse before administering. Record apical rate on the client's medication record. Assess potassium, magnesium, calcium, and serum digoxin levels before giving digitalis. Hypokalemia can precipitate toxicity even when the serum digitalis level is in the "normal" range. Evaluate ECG for scooped (spoon-shaped) ST segment, AV block, bradycardia, and other dysrhythmias (especially PVCs and atrial tachycardias).
    Nursing Process: Implementation
    Client Need: Physiologic Integrity

5. Answer: 4
    Rationale: Home activity guidelines for a client with heart failure include: use laxatives or stool softeners; eat six small meals a day; do not lift

heavy objects; and begin a graded exercise program. Space your meals and activities. Avoid straining. Avoid constipation and straining during bowel movements. Plan to walk twice a day at a comfortable, slow pace for the first couple of weeks at home, and then gradually increase the distance and pace.
Nursing Process: Planning
Client Need: Health Promotion and Maintenance

6. Answer: 3
Rationale: Encourage the client to notify their dentist and other healthcare providers about MVP before (not after) dental or any invasive procedure. Teach the client about infective endocarditis risk and prevention with prophylactic antibiotics. Discuss symptoms of progressive mitral regurgitation, and the need to report these to the cardiologist. Teach the client about MVP, including heart valve anatomy, physiology, and function, common manifestations of MVP, and treatment rationale. Instruct the client to keep a weekly record of symptoms and their frequency for one month.
Nursing Process: Evaluation
Client Need: Physiologic Integrity

7. Answer: 4
Rationale: Diet restrictions for valvular disease are done to *reduce* fluid retention and symptoms of heart failure. Managing valvular disease includes: notifying all healthcare providers about valve disease or surgery to facilitate prescription of prophylactic antibiotics before invasive procedures or dental work and adequate rest to prevent fatigue. The client with valvular disease should; immediately report to the healthcare provider increasing severity of symptoms, especially of worsening heart failure or pulmonary edema; signs of transient ischemic attacks or other embolic events; and evidence of bleeding, such as joint pain, easy bruising, black and tarry stools, bleeding gums, or blood in the urine or sputum.
Nursing Process: Evaluation
Client Need: Physiologic Integrity

8. Answer: 2
Rationale: Stress the relationship between effective *diabetes* management and reduced risk of heart failure. Teach clients about coronary heart disease (CHD), the primary underlying cause of heart failure. Discuss CHD risk factors, and ways to reduce those risk factors. Routinely screen clients for elevated blood pressure, and refer clients to a primary care provider as indicated. Discuss the importance of effectively managing hypertension to reduce the future risk for heart failure.
Nursing Process: Assessment
Client Need: Health Promotion and Maintenance

9. Answer: 1
Rationale: In cardiogenic pulmonary edema, the contractility of the *left* (not the right) ventricle is

severely impaired. Pulmonary edema is a medical emergency. Immediate treatment for acute pulmonary edema focuses on restoring effective gas exchange and reducing fluid and pressure in the pulmonary vascular system. The client often is restless and highly anxious, although severe hypoxia may cause confusion or lethargy.
Nursing Process: Evaluation
Client Need: Physiologic Integrity

10. Answer: 3
Rationale: The peak incidence of rheumatic fever is in children ages 5 to 15, not in adults ages 18 to 35. Rheumatic heart disease frequently damages the heart valves and is a major cause of mitral and aortic valve disorders. Rheumatic fever is a systemic inflammatory disease caused by an abnormal immune response to pharyngeal infection by group A beta-hemolytic streptococci. Rheumatic fever and rheumatic heart disease remain significant public health problems in many developing countries.
Nursing Process: Evaluation
Client Need: Health Promotion and Maintenance

Chapter 33

Case Study Answers

1. *List the normal values of a CBC.*
Hemoglobin (Hb): women: 12–16 g/dl; men: 13.5–18 g/dl
Hematocrit (Hct): women: 38%–47%; men: 40%–54%
Total RBC count: women: 4–5×10^6/µl; men: 4.5–6×10^6/µ
Red cell indices: MCV = 82–98 fl; MCH = 27–33 pg; MCHC 32%–36%
Total WBC count: 4000–11,000/µl (4–11×10^9/L)
WBC differential: neutrophils: 50%–70%
Platelets: 150,000–400,000/µl (15–400×10^9/L)

2. *What are the factors that influence arterial blood pressure?*
Blood flow, peripheral vascular resistance, and blood pressure, all of which influence arterial circulation, are in turn influenced by various factors:
• The sympathetic and parasympathetic nervous systems are the primary mechanisms that regulate blood pressure. Stimulation of the sympathetic nervous system exerts a major effect on peripheral resistance by causing vasoconstriction of the arterioles, thereby increasing blood pressure. Parasympathetic stimulation causes vasodilation of the arterioles, which lowers blood pressure.
• Baroreceptors and chemoreceptors in the aortic arch, carotid sinus, and other large vessels are sensitive to pressure and chemical changes and cause reflex sympathetic stimulation, which results in vasoconstriction, increased heart rate, and increased blood pressure.

- The kidneys help maintain blood pressure by excreting or conserving sodium and water. When blood pressure decreases, the kidneys initiate the renin-angiotensin mechanism. This stimulates vasoconstriction, which results in the release of the hormone aldosterone from the adrenal cortex, increasing sodium ion reabsorption and water retention. In addition, pituitary release of antidiuretic hormone (ADH) promotes renal reabsorption of water. The net result is an increase in blood volume and a consequent increase in cardiac output and blood pressure.
- Temperatures may also affect peripheral resistance: cold causes vasoconstriction, whereas warmth produces vasodilation. Many chemicals, hormones, and drugs influence blood pressure by affecting cardiac output and/or peripheral vascular resistance. For example, epinephrine causes vasoconstriction and increased heart rate; prostaglandins dilate blood vessel diameter (by relaxing vascular smooth muscle); endothelin, a chemical released by the inner lining of vessels, is a potent vasoconstrictor; nicotine causes vasoconstriction; and alcohol and histamine cause vasodilation.
- Dietary factors, such as intake of salt, saturated fats, and cholesterol elevate blood pressure by affecting blood volume and vessel diameter.
- Race, gender, age, weight, time of day, position, exercise, and emotional state may also affect blood pressure. These factors influence the arterial pressure. Systemic venous pressure, though it is much lower, is also influenced by such factors as blood volume, venous tone, and right atrial pressure.

3. *Explain PVR and MAP.* Peripheral vascular resistance (PVR) refers to the opposing forces or impedance to blood flow as the arterial channels become more and more distant from the heart. Peripheral vascular resistance is determined by three factors:
- Blood viscosity: The greater the viscosity, or thickness, of the blood, the greater its resistance to moving and flowing.
- Length of the vessel: The longer the vessel, the greater the resistance to blood flow.
- Diameter of the vessel: The smaller the diameter of a vessel, the greater the friction against the walls of the vessel and, thus, the greater the impedance to blood flow.

Blood pressure is the force exerted against the walls of the arteries by the blood as it is pumped from the heart. Blood pressure is most accurately referred to as mean arterial pressure (MAP). The highest pressure exerted against the arterial walls at the peak of ventricular contraction (systole) is called the systolic blood pressure. The lowest pressure exerted during ventricular relaxation (diastole) is the diastolic blood pressure.

Mean arterial blood pressure is regulated mainly by cardiac output (CO) and peripheral vascular resistance (PVR), as represented in this formula: $MAP = CO \times PVR$. For clinical use, the MAP may be estimated by calculating the diastolic blood pressure plus one-third of the pulse pressure (the difference between the systolic and diastolic blood pressure).

NCLEX Review Question Answers

1. Answer: 2
   Rationale: Red blood cells (RBCs) have a lifespan of about 120, not 10, days. The red blood cell is shaped like a biconcave disk. Abnormal numbers of RBCs, changes in their size and shape, or altered hemoglobin content or structure can adversely affect health. RBCs are the most common type of blood cell.
   Nursing Process: Assessment
   Client Need: Physiologic Integrity

2. Answer: 4
   Rationale: An excess of platelets is thrombocytosis, not thrombocytopenia. Thrombocytopenia is a deficit of platelets. Platelets remain in the spleen for about eight hours before entering the circulation. Platelets live up to 10 days in circulation. There are about 250,000 to 400,000 platelets in each milliliter of blood.
   Nursing Process: Assessment
   Client Need: Physiologic Integrity

3. Answer: 2
   Rationale: Height of a blood vessel is not one of the three factors that determine peripheral vascular resistance. Peripheral vascular resistance is determined by three factors: blood viscosity, in which the greater the viscosity, or thickness, of the blood, the greater its resistance to moving and flowing; length of the vessel, in which the longer the vessel, the greater the resistance to blood flow; and the diameter of the vessel, in which the smaller the diameter of a vessel, the greater the friction against the walls of the vessel and, thus, the greater the impedance to blood flow.
   Nursing Process: Assessment
   Client Need: Physiologic Integrity

4. Answer: 1
   Rationale: The organs of the lymphatic system are the lymph nodes, the spleen, the thymus, the tonsils, and the Peyer's patches of the small intestine. The spleen is in the upper left quadrant of the abdomen under the thorax. The main function of the spleen is to filter the blood by breaking down old red blood cells. The spleen also synthesizes lymphocytes, stores platelets for blood clotting, and serves as a reservoir of blood.
   Nursing Process: Assessment
   Client Need: Physiologic Integrity

5. Answer: 1

Rationale: All blood vessel walls have three layers: the tunica intima, the tunica media, and the tunica adventitia. The tiniest vessels do not include all these layers. The smaller arterioles are less elastic than arteries but contain more smooth muscle. Veins have a thicker tunica adventitia than do arteries. The tunica adventitia, or outermost layer, is made of connective tissue and serves to protect and anchor the vessel.

Nursing Process: Assessment
Client Need: Physiologic Integrity

6. Answer: 1

Rationale: Mean arterial blood pressure is regulated mainly by cardiac output (CO) and peripheral vascular resistance (PVR), as represented in this formula: $MAP = CO \times PVR$. For clinical use, the MAP may be estimated by calculating the diastolic blood pressure plus one-third of the pulse pressure (the difference between the systolic and diastolic blood pressure).

Nursing Process: Assessment
Client Need: Physiologic Integrity

7. Answer: 4

Rationale: Lymph nodes should not be enlarged or painful. A weak and thready pulse, often with tachycardia, reflects decreased cardiac output. Capillary refill that takes more than two seconds reflects circulatory compromise, such as hypovolemia or anemia. A bruit heard over the aorta suggests an aneurysm.

Nursing Process: Assessment
Client Need: Physiologic Integrity

8. Answer: 3

Rationale: Edema can be graded on a scale of from 1+ to 4+:
1+ (–2 mm depression): no visible change in the leg; slight pitting
2+ (–4 mm depression): no marked change in the shape of the leg; pitting slightly deeper
3+ (–6 mm depression): leg visibly swollen; pitting deep
4+ (–8 mm depression): leg very swollen; pitting very deep

Nursing Process: Assessment
Client Need: Physiologic Integrity

9. Answer: 4

Rationale: Describe the pulses as increased, normal, diminished, or absent. Scales that range from 0 to 4+ are sometimes used as follows:
0 = Absent
1+ = Diminished
2+ = Normal
3+ = Increased
4+ = Bounding

Nursing Process: Assessment
Client Need: Physiologic Integrity

10. Answer: 3

Rationale: Blood in the veins (not arteries) travels at a much lower pressure than blood in the arteries. Veins have thinner walls, a larger lumen, and greater capacity, and many are supplied with valves that help blood flow against gravity back to the heart. Blood pressure is the force exerted against the walls of the arteries by the blood as it is pumped from the heart. The highest pressure exerted against the arterial walls at the peak of ventricular contraction (systole) is called the systolic blood pressure.

Nursing Process: Assessment
Client Need: Physiologic Integrity

Chapter 34

Case Study Answers

1. *List the types of anemias.* The different types of anemias include: iron-deficiency anemia, vitamin B_{12} deficiency anemia, folic acid deficiency anemia, sickle cell anemia, thalassemia, and aplastic anemia.

2. *What are the dietary sources of heme and nonheme iron?* Sources of heme iron include: beef, pork loin, chicken, turkey, egg yolk, veal, clams, and oysters. Sources of nonheme iron include: dried fruits, bran flakes, brown rice, greens, whole-grain breads, oatmeal, and dried beans.

3. *What is the classification, characteristics, manifestations, and treatments for acute lymphoblastic leukemia (ALL).*
   Classification: acute lymphoblastic leukemia (ALL)
   Characteristics: primarily affects children and young adults; leukemic cells may infiltrate CNS
   Manifestations: recurrent infections, bleeding, pallor, bone pain, weight loss, sore throat, fatigue, night sweats, and weakness
   Treatment: chemotherapy; bone marrow transplant (BMT), or stem cell transplant (SCT)

NCLEX Review Questions Answers

1. Answer: 3

Rationale: The amount of oxygen that reaches the tissues does not depend on the number of white blood cells. The amount of oxygen that reaches the tissues depends on available oxygen in the alveoli, the diffusing surface and capacity of the lungs, the number of red blood cells and the amount and type of hemoglobin they contain, and the ability of the cardiovascular system to transport blood and oxygen to the tissues.

Nursing Process: Assessment
Client Need: Physiologic Integrity

2. Answer: 3

Rationale: The body cannot synthesize hemoglobin without iron. Iron deficiency anemia

is the most common type of anemia. Iron deficiency anemia results in fewer numbers of RBCs, microcytic and hypochromic RBCs, as well as malformed RBCs (poikilocytosis). Inadequate dietary iron intake also contributes to anemia in the older adult.
Nursing Process: Evaluation
Client Need: Physiologic Integrity

3. Answer: 4
   Rationale: Dried fruit is not a source of heme iron. Sources of heme iron include: beef, pork loin, chicken, turkey, egg yolk, veal, clams, and oysters.
   Nursing Process: Planning
   Client Need: Health Promotion and Maintenance

4. Answer: 2
   Rationale: The caregiver should provide medications for pain or nausea 30 minutes before meals, if prescribed. The caregiver should also provide rest periods before meals, liquids with different textures and tastes, and mouth care before and after meals.
   Nursing Process: Evaluation
   Client Need: Physiologic Integrity

5. Answer: 3
   Rationale: The Ann Arbor Staging System is used to assess the extent and severity of lymphomas. In stage III, there is involvement of lymph node regions or structures on both sides of the diaphragm. The other stages are:
   Stage I: involvement of a single lymph node region or lymphoid structure (e.g., spleen, thymus, lymphoid tonsillar tissue)
   Stage II: involvement of two or more lymph node regions on the same side of the diaphragm
   Stage III$_1$: limited to upper abdomen (spleen, splenic, celiac, or portal nodes)
   Stage III$_2$: involvement of lower abdominal nodes (para-aortic, iliac, or mesenteric)
   Stage IV: involvement of an extranodal site (not proximal or contiguous with an involved node) such as the liver, lung or pleura, bone or bone marrow, or skin.
   The presence or absence of systemic symptoms is indicated by either an A (no systemic symptoms) or B (systemic symptoms of fever, night sweats, and weight loss).
   Nursing Process: Assessment
   Client Need: Physiologic Integrity

6. Answer: 3
   Rationale: Teach measures to prevent or relieve nausea and vomiting, which include: eating soda crackers and sucking on hard candy; eating soft, bland foods that are cold or at room temperature; avoiding unpleasant odors, and getting fresh air. Crackers and hard candy often relieve queasiness. The other measures enhance appetite and promotes nutritional intake.
   Nursing Process: Planning
   Client Need: Health Promotion and Maintenance

7. Answer: 2
   Rationale: In aplastic anemia, the bone marrow fails to produce all three types of blood cells, which leads to pancytopenia. Manifestations of aplastic anemia include fatigue, pallor, progressive weakness, exertional dyspnea, headache, and ultimately tachycardia and heart failure. Aplastic anemia also may occur with viral infections such as mononucleosis, hepatitis C, and HIV disease. Aplastic anemia is rare.
   Nursing Process: Planning
   Client Need: Physiologic Integrity

8. Answer: 2
   Rationale: In relative polycythemia, the hematocrit is *elevated* because of increased cell concentration. In primary polycythemia, RBC production is increased. In relative polycythemia, the total RBC count is normal. Secondary polycythemia occurs when erythropoietin levels are elevated.
   Nursing Process: Evaluation
   Client Need: Physiologic Integrity

9. Answer: 1
   Rationale: Restrict visitors with colds, flu, or infections. Provide oral hygiene after every meal. Ensure meticulous handwashing among all people in contact with the client. Maintain protective isolation as indicated. These precautions minimize exposure to bacterial, viral, and fungal pathogens. Infection is the major cause of death in clients with leukemia. Mucous membranes are especially susceptible to breakdown and infection as a result of tissue damage from chemotherapy or radiation.
   Nursing Process: Implementation
   Client Need: Physiologic Integrity

10. Answer: 2
    Rationale: Non-Hodgkin's lymphoma is *more* common than Hodgkin's disease. Non-Hodgkin's lymphomas tend to arise in peripheral lymph nodes and spread early to tissues throughout the body. Non-Hodgkin's lymphoma is a diverse group of lymphoid tissue malignancies that do not contain Reed-Sternberg cells. Older adults are more often affected, and it occurs more frequently in men than in women.
    Nursing Process: Evaluation
    Client Need: Physiologic Integrity

Chapter 35

Case Study Answers

1. *Discuss the manifestations of primary hypertension.*
   The early stages of primary hypertension typically are asymptomatic, marked only by elevated blood pressure. Blood pressure elevations are initially transient but eventually become permanent. When symptoms do appear, they are usually vague. Headache, usually in the back of the head and neck,

may be present on awakening, and subside during the day. Other symptoms result from target organ damage, and may include nocturia, confusion, nausea and vomiting, and visual disturbances. Examination of the retina of the eye may reveal narrowed arterioles, hemorrhages, exudates, and *papilledema* (swelling of the optic nerve).

2. *Explain the complications of primary hypertension.* Sustained hypertension affects the cardiovascular, neurologic, and renal systems. The rate of atherosclerosis accelerates, which increases the risk for coronary heart disease and stroke. The workload of the left ventricle increases, which leads to ventricular hypertrophy. This increases the risk for coronary heart disease, dysrhythmias, and heart failure. The diastolic blood pressure is a significant cardiovascular risk factor until age 50; the systolic pressure then becomes the more important factor that contributes to cardiovascular risk (NHLBI, 2004). Most deaths due to hypertension result from coronary heart disease and acute myocardial infarction or heart failure (Kasper et al, 2005). Accelerated atherosclerosis associated with hypertension increases the risk for cerebral infarction (stroke). Increased pressure in the cerebral vessels can lead to development of microaneurysms and an increased risk for cerebral hemorrhage. *Hypertensive encephalopathy*, a syndrome characterized by extremely high blood pressure, altered level of consciousness, increased intracranial pressure, papilledema, and seizures, may develop. Its etiology is unclear. Hypertension also can lead to nephrosclerosis and renal insufficiency. Proteinuria and microscopic hematuria develop, as well as signs of chronic renal failure. African Americans experience hypertensive kidney disease more frequently than whites. Renal failure causes about 10% of deaths that are attributed to hypertension (Kasper et al, 2005).

3. *Summarize the lifestyle modifications that Elizabeth should be following.* Elizabeth should maintain a normal body weight, and lose weight if overweight. Dietary modifications include eating a diet rich in fruits, vegetables, and low-fat dairy products. Reduce sodium, cholesterol, and total and saturated fat intake. Limit alcohol intake to no more than 1 oz of ethanol (1/2 oz for women and lighter weight people) per day. Engage in aerobic exercise for 30 minutes most days of the week (five to six days). Stop smoking, and use stress management techniques such as relaxation therapy.

NCLEX Review Question Answers

1. Answer: 2
   Rationale: The systolic blood pressure is felt as the peripheral pulse and heard as the Korotkoff's sounds during blood pressure measurement. In healthy adults the average systolic pressure is less than 120 mmHg. During diastole, or cardiac relaxation and filling, elastic arterial walls maintain a minimum pressure, which is the diastolic blood pressure, to maintain blood flow through the capillary beds. The average diastolic pressure in a healthy adult is less than 80 mmHg. The difference between the systolic and diastolic pressure, normally about 40 mmHg, is known as the pulse pressure. The mean arterial pressure (MAP) is the average pressure in the arterial circulation throughout the cardiac cycle.
   Nursing Process: Assessment
   Client Need: Physiologic Integrity

2. Answer: 3
   Rationale: The mean arterial pressure (MAP) is the average pressure in the arterial circulation throughout the cardiac cycle. It can be calculated using the formula [systolic BP + 2 (diastolic BP)] / 3.
   Nursing Process: Assessment
   Client Need: Physiologic Integrity

3. Answer: 1
   Rationale: Primary hypertension is thought to develop from complex interactions among factors that regulate cardiac output and systemic vascular resistance. These interactions may include: excess sympathetic nervous system with overstimulation of α- and β-adrenergic receptors, which results in vaso*constriction* and *increased* cardiac output; altered function of the renin-angiotensin-aldosterone system and its responsiveness to factors such as sodium intake and overall fluid volume; other chemical mediators of vasomotor tone and blood volume such as atrial natriuretic peptide (factor) also play a role by affecting vasomotor tone and sodium and water excretion; and the interaction between insulin resistance, hyperinsulinemia, and endothelial function may be a primary cause of hypertension.
   Nursing Process: Assessment
   Client Need: Physiologic Integrity

4. Answer: 4
   Rationale: A number of risk factors have been identified for primary hypertension; age is one of those risk factors. Secondary hypertension is elevated blood pressure that results from an identifiable underlying process. The pathophysiology of selected causes of high blood pressure are kidney disease, Cushing's syndrome, and pregnancy.
   Nursing Process: Assessment
   Client Need: Physiologic Integrity

5. Answer: 1
   Rationale: Implement interventions to reduce the risk of aneurysm rupture: maintain bed rest with legs flat (not elevated); maintain a calm environment and implement measures to reduce psychologic stress; instruct client to prevent straining during defecation and avoid holding the

breath while moving; and administer beta blockers and antihypertensives as prescribed.
Nursing Process: Implementation
Client Need: Physiologic Integrity

6. Answer: 3
Rationale: Raynaud's disease has been called "the *blue-white-red* disease" because affected digits initially turn blue as blood flow is reduced due to vasospasm, then white as circulation is more severely limited, and finally very red as the fingers are warmed and the spasm resolves. Raynaud's disease primarily affects young women between the ages of 20 and 40. Raynaud's disease is characterized by episodes of intense vasospasm in the small arteries and arterioles of the fingers and sometimes the toes. Raynaud's disease has no identifiable cause; Raynaud's phenomenon occurs secondarily to another disease (such as collagen vascular diseases like scleroderma and rheumatoid arthritis), other known causes of vasospasm, or long-term exposure to cold or machinery.
Nursing Process: Assessment
Client Need: Physiologic Integrity

7. Answer: 2
Rationale: Prevention of venous thrombosis is an important component of nursing care for all at-risk clients. Avoid placing pillows under the knees and positions in which the hips and knees are sharply flexed. Position clients to promote venous blood flow from the lower extremities, with the feet elevated and the knees slightly bent. The client should use a recliner chair or foot stool when sitting. Ambulate clients as soon as possible, and maintain a regular schedule of ambulation throughout the day. Teach ankle flexion and extension exercises, and frequently remind clients to perform them.
Nursing Process: Evaluation
Client Need: Physiologic Integrity

8. Answer: 2
Rationale: Elastic compression stockings compress the veins and promote venous return from the lower extremities. During ambulation, the stockings enhance the blood-pumping action of the muscles. Because elastic stockings inhibit blood flow through small superficial vessels, they should be removed at least once each day for at least 30 minutes. Complications of varicose veins include venous insufficiency and stasis ulcers. Prolonged standing, the force of gravity, lack of leg exercise, and incompetent venous valves all weaken the muscle-pumping mechanism, which reduces venous blood return to the heart. Varicose veins may be asymptomatic, but most cause manifestations such as severe aching leg pain, leg fatigue, leg heaviness, itching, or feelings of heat in the legs.
Nursing Process: Planning
Client Need: Physiologic Integrity

9. Answer: 1
Rationale: Obesity is a modifiable risk factor for hypertension. Age, race, and family history are nonmodifiable risk factors.
Nursing Process: Planning
Client Need: Physiologic Integrity

10. Answer: 2
Rationale: Per the DASH diet recommendations, three to four servings of grains per day is inadequate; DASH recommendations include seven to eight servings of grains per day. Correct client statements regarding the DASH diet include four to five servings of fruit per day; four to five servings of vegetables per day; and two to three servings of low-fat dairy products per day.
Nursing Process: Evaluation
Client Need: Physiologic Integrity

Chapter 36

Case Study Answers

1. *"What are the factors that affect ventilation and respiration?"* Many factors affect ventilation and respiration. Those discussed here include changes in volume and capacity; air pressures; oxygen, carbon dioxide and hydrogen ion concentrations in the blood; airway resistance, lung compliance, and elasticity; and alveolar surface tension.

2. *"Where are the sinuses and what is the purpose of having sinuses?"* The nasal cavity is surrounded by paranasal sinuses, located in the frontal, sphenoid, ethmoid, and maxillary bones. Sinuses lighten the skull, assist in speech, and produce mucus that drains into the nasal cavities to help trap debris.

3. *"What is the difference between IRV and ERV?"* Inspiratory reserve volume (IRV) is the amount of air (approximately 2100 to 3100 mL) that can be inhaled forcibly over the tidal volume. Expiratory reserve volume (ERV) is the approximately 1000 mL of air that can be forced out over the tidal volume.

4. *"What is bradypnea, tachypnea, and apnea?"* Damage to the brainstem from a stroke or head injury may result in either tachypnea or bradypnea (low respiratory rate). Bradypnea is seen with some circulatory disorders, lung disorders, and as a side effect of some medications. Tachypnea (rapid respiratory rate) is seen in atelectasis (collapse of lung tissue following obstruction of the bronchus or bronchioles), pneumonia, asthma, pleural effusion, pneumothorax, congestive heart failure, anxiety, and in response to pain. Apnea, cessation of breathing that lasts from a few seconds to a few minutes, may occur following a stroke or head trauma, as a side effect of some medications, or following airway obstruction.

NCLEX Review Questions Answers

1. Answer: 2

Rationale: The nasopharynx serves only as a passageway for air. The oropharynx lies behind the oral cavity and extends from the soft palate to the level of the hyoid bone. It serves as a passageway for both air and food. The external nose is given structure by the nasal, frontal, and maxillary bones as well as plates of hyaline cartilage. The nasal hairs filter the air as it enters the nares. Sinuses lighten the skull, assist in speech, and produce mucus that drains into the nasal cavities to help trap debris.
Nursing Process: Assessment
Client Need: Physiologic Integrity

2. Answer: 2

Rationale: The left lung is smaller and has two lobes, whereas the right lung has three lobes. The laryngopharynx extends from the hyoid bone to the larynx. The parietal pleura lines the thoracic wall and mediastinum. During expiration, carbon dioxide is expelled.
Nursing Process: Planning
Client Need: Physiologic Integrity

3. Answer: 1

Rationale: There are 12 pairs of ribs that all articulate with the thoracic vertebrae. Anteriorly, the first seven ribs articulate with the body of the sternum. The eighth, ninth, and tenth ribs articulate with the cartilage immediately above the ribs. The eleventh and twelfth ribs are called floating ribs, because they are unattached.
Nursing Process: Assessment
Client Need: Physiologic Integrity

4. Answer: 1

Rationale: Tidal volume (TV) is the amount of air (approximately 500 mL) moved in and out of the lungs with each normal, quiet breath. Inspiratory reserve volume (IRV) is the amount of air (approximately 2100 to 3100 mL) that can be inhaled forcibly over the tidal volume. Expiratory reserve volume (ERV) is the approximately 1000 mL of air that can be forced out over the tidal volume. The residual volume is the volume of air (approximately 1100 mL) that remains in the lungs after a forced expiration.
Nursing Process: Assessment
Client Need: Physiologic Integrity

5. Answer: 3

Rationale: During expiration, the inspiratory muscles relax, the diaphragm rises, the ribs descend, and the lungs recoil. During inspiration, the diaphragm contracts and flattens out to increase the vertical diameter of the thoracic cavity. Expiration is primarily a passive process that occurs as a result of the elasticity of the lungs. A single inspiration lasts for about 1 to 1.5 seconds, whereas an expiration lasts for about 2 to 3 seconds.

Nursing Process: Evaluation
Client Need: Physiologic Integrity

6. Answer: 3

Rationale: A bronchoscopy is a direct visualization of the larynx, trachea, and bronchi. The bronchoscopy is not used to visualize the pharynx. Arterial blood gases are conducted to evaluate alterations in acid–base balances. Pulse oximetry is used to evaluate or monitor the oxygen saturation of the blood. A thoracentesis, when done for diagnostic purposes, is conducted to obtain a specimen of pleural fluid.
Nursing Process: Evaluation
Client Need: Physiologic Integrity

7. Answer: 1

Rationale: Dullness is heard in clients with atelectasis, lobar pneumonia, and pleural effusion. Retraction of intercostal spaces may be seen in asthma, not pneumothorax. Bulging of intercostal spaces may be seen in pneumothorax, not asthma. Bilateral chest expansion is decreased (not increased) in emphysema.
Nursing Process: Assessment
Client Need: Physiologic Integrity

8. Answer: 4

Rationale: Carbon dioxide is not dissociated from hemoglobin during transport. Carbon dioxide is transported in three forms: dissolved in plasma, bound to hemoglobin, and as bicarbonate ions in the plasma (the largest amount is in this form).
Nursing Process: Assessment
Client Need: Physiologic Integrity

9. Answer: 3

Rationale: The lower respiratory tract includes the pleura. The upper respiratory tract includes the nose, trachea, and sinuses.
Nursing Process: Assessment
Client Need: Physiologic Integrity

10. Answer: 1

Rationale: The upper respiratory tract includes the larynx. The lower respiratory tract includes the lungs, bronchi, and rib cage.
Nursing Process: Assessment
Client Need: Physiologic Integrity

Chapter 37

Case Study Answers

1. *Explain the pathophysiology of sleep apnea.* During sleep, skeletal muscle tone decreases (except the diaphragm). The most significant decrease occurs during rapid eye movement (REM) sleep (Porth, 2005). Loss of normal pharyngeal muscle tone permits the pharynx to collapse during inspiration as pressure within the airways becomes negative in relation to atmospheric pressure. The tongue is also pulled against the posterior pharyngeal wall by gravity during sleep, which causes further obstruction. Obesity or skeletal or soft-tissue changes that decrease inspiratory tone, such as a relatively large tongue in a relatively small oropharynx, contribute to the problem. Airflow obstruction causes the oxygen saturation, PO_2, and pH to fall, and the PCO_2 to rise. This progressive asphyxia causes brief arousal from sleep, which restores airway patency and airflow. Sleep can be severely fragmented as these episodes may occur hundreds of times each night.

2. *List the manifestations of obstructive sleep apnea.*
   - Loud, cyclic snoring
   - Periods of apnea that last 15 to 120 seconds during sleep
   - Gasping or choking during sleep
   - Restlessness and thrashing during sleep
   - Daytime fatigue and sleepiness
   - Morning headache
   - Personality changes and depression
   - Intellectual impairment
   - Impotence
   - Hypertension

3. *Review the complications of obstructive sleep apnea.* Recurrent episodes of apnea and arousal during sleep have secondary physiologic effects. Sleep fragmentation and loss of slow-wave sleep are thought to contribute to neurologic and behavior problems such as excessive daytime sleepiness, impaired intellect, memory loss, and personality changes. Recurrent nocturnal asphyxia and negative intrathoracic pressure due to airway obstruction increase the workload of the heart. People with coronary heart disease may develop myocardial ischemia and angina. Dysrhythmias such as significant bradycardia and dangerous tachydysrhythmias may develop. Left ventricular function may be impaired and heart failure may occur. Systemic blood pressure remains high during sleep and may contribute to systemic hypertension that affects more than 50% of people with obstructive sleep apnea (Kasper et al., 2005). Pulmonary hypertension also may develop. Sudden cardiac death is believed to be a potential fatal complication of obstructive sleep apnea. Obstructive sleep apnea is a common condition in people who are morbidly obese. When these clients undergo gastric bypass surgery to treat their obesity, sleep apnea places them at significant risk for postoperative respiratory complications. Not only does the obesity interfere with chest movement and ventilation, it increases metabolic demands and carbon monoxide production. Anesthetic and analgesics used during surgery and in the postoperative period can lead to hypoxemia due to muscle relaxation and depression of the respiratory drive (Deutzer, 2005).

4. *Review the treatments for obstructive sleep apnea.* Mild to moderate obstructive sleep apnea may be treated by weight reduction, alcohol abstinence, improving nasal patency, and avoiding the supine position for sleep. Although weight reduction often cures the disorder, maintaining optimal weight is difficult. Oral appliances designed to keep the mandible and tongue forward also may be prescribed. Nasal continuous positive airway pressure (CPAP) is the treatment of choice for obstructive sleep apnea. Positive pressure generated by an air compressor and administered through a tight-fitting nasal mask splints the pharyngeal airway, which prevents collapse and obstruction. With proper training, this device is well-tolerated by the client. Nasal airways can become dry and irritated with CPAP, so an in-line humidifier or a room humidifier is recommended. A newer device, the BiPaP ventilator, delivers higher pressures during inhalation and lower pressures during expiration, which provides less resistance to exhaling.

NCLEX Review Question Answers

1. Answer: 2
   Rationale: The client should blow the nose with *both* nostrils open to prevent infected matter from being forced into the eustachian tubes. The client should use disposable tissues to cover the mouth and nose while coughing or sneezing to reduce airborne spread of the virus. The client should wash hands frequently, especially after coughing or sneezing, to limit viral transmission. The client should limit use of nasal decongestants to every four hours for only a few days at a time to prevent rebound effect.
   Nursing Process: Evaluation
   Client Need: Physiologic Integrity

2. Answer: 4
   Rationale: Influenza types A, B, and C are found in humans.
   Nursing Process: Assessment
   Client Need: Physiologic Integrity

3. Answer: 2
   Rationale: White, not yellow, exudate is present on the tonsils. The tonsils appear bright red and edematous. Pressing on a tonsil may produce purulent drainage. The uvula may also be reddened and swollen.
   Nursing Process: Evaluation
   Client Need: Physiologic Integrity

4. Answer: 1
   Rationale: Infectious mononucleosis is caused by the Epstein-Barr virus. The other viruses do not cause mononucleosis.
   Nursing Process: Assessment
   Client Need: Physiologic Integrity

5. Answer: 3
   Rationale: Teaching about home care following polypectomy is the primary nursing responsibility for the client with nasal polyps. The client should

avoid blowing the nose for 24 to 48 hours after nasal packing is removed—to prevent complications. The client should apply ice or cold compresses to the nose to decrease swelling, promote comfort, and prevent bleeding. The client should avoid straining during bowel movements, vigorous coughing, and strenuous exercise. Encourage the client to rest for two to three days after surgery to reduce the risk of bleeding.
Nursing Process: Planning
Client Need: Health Promotion and Maintenance

6. Answer: 1
Rationale: Water sports are contraindicated with a permanent tracheostomy. The client should increase fluid intake to maintain mucosal moisture and loosen secretions. The client should shield the stoma with a stoma guard, such as a gauze square on a tie around the neck, to prevent particulate matter from entering the lower respiratory tract. The client should use a humidifier or vaporizer to add humidity to inspired air.
Nursing Process: Evaluation
Client Need: Health Promotion and Maintenance

7. Answer: 4
Rationale: Emergency care for epistaxis includes pinching the nares or bridge of the nose, sitting upright and leaning forward, and applying ice to the nose.
Nursing Process: Implementation
Client Need: Physiologic Integrity

8. Answer: 1
Rationale: Tobacco use is the major risk factor for laryngeal cancer. Alcohol consumption is a significant cofactor that increases the risk, but is not a major risk factor. Other risk factors include poor nutrition, human papillomavirus infection, exposure to asbestos and other occupational pollutants, and race. But none of these other risk factors are as significant as tobacco use.
Nursing Process: Planning
Client Need: Health Promotion and Maintenance

9. Answer: 3
Rationale: Polyps are usually bilateral and have a stem-like base, which makes them fairly moveable. Polyps form in areas of dependent mucous membrane, which presents as pale, edematous masses that are covered with mucous membrane. Nasal polyps are benign grape-like growths of the mucous membrane that lines the nose. Polyps may be asymptomatic, although large polyps may cause nasal obstruction, rhinorrhea, and loss of sense of smell.
Nursing Process: Planning
Client Need: Physiologic Integrity

10. Answer: 2
Rationale: Effective sleep apnea management depends on the client's willingness to participate in care. Provide teaching about the following topics:

the importance of using CPAP continuously at night; discuss the relationship of alcohol and sedatives to sleep apnea; refer to an alcohol treatment program or Alcoholics Anonymous as indicated; discuss the relationship between obesity and sleep apnea; and maintain moist mucous membranes by having an adequate fluid intake. CPAP is used continuously throughout the night not intermittently. Using the CPAP intermittently would not be effective for the client's condition.
Nursing Process: Planning
Client Need: Health Promotion and Maintenance

Chapter 38

Case Study Answers

1. *What are the manifestations of acute bronchitis?* Acute bronchitis is typically heralded by a nonproductive cough that later becomes productive. The cough often occurs in paroxysms, and may be aggravated by cold, dry, or dusty air. Chest pain, often substernal, is common. Other manifestations include moderate fever and general malaise.

2. *How is acute bronchitis diagnosed?* The diagnosis of acute bronchitis typically is based on the history and clinical presentation. A chest X-ray may be ordered to rule out pneumonia, because the presenting manifestations can be similar. Other diagnostic testing is rarely indicated.

3. *How is acute bronchitis treated?* Treatment is based on symptoms and includes rest, increased fluid intake, and the use of aspirin or acetaminophen to relieve fever and malaise. Many physicians prescribe a broad-spectrum antibiotic such as erythromycin or penicillin, because approximately 50% of acute bronchitis is bacterial in origin. An expectorant cough medication is recommended for use during the day and a cough suppressant is recommended for use at night to facilitate rest.

NCLEX Review Question Answers

1. Answer: 2
Rationale: The most common causative organism for community-acquired pneumonia is *Streptococcus pneumoniae* (also called pneumococcus), a gram-positive bacterium. Inflammation of the lung parenchyma (the respiratory bronchioles and alveoli) is known as pneumonia. Bacteria, viruses, fungi, protozoa, and other microbes can lead to infectious pneumonia. Noninfectious causes include aspiration of gastric contents and inhalation of toxic or irritating gases.
Nursing Process: Evaluation
Client Need: Physiologic Integrity

2. Answer: 4
Rationale: The incubation period for SARS is generally 2 to 7 days, although it may be as long

as 10 days in some people. Fever higher than 100.4°F (38°C) is typically the initial manifestation of the disease. The primary population affected by SARS is previously healthy adults from age 25 to 70 years. The infective agent responsible for SARS is a coronavirus not previously identified in humans.
Nursing Process: Evaluation
Client Need: Physiologic Integrity

3. Answer: 3
    Rationale: A previously-healed tuberculosis lesion may be reactivated. Primary or secondary tuberculosis lesions may affect other body systems such as the kidneys, genitalia, bone, and brain. Worldwide, TB continues to be a significant health problem. *Mycobacterium tuberculosis* is a relatively slow-growing, slender, rod-shaped, acid-fast organism with a waxy outer capsule that increases its resistance to destruction.
    Nursing Process: Planning
    Client Need: Physiologic Integrity

4. Answer: 4
    Rationale: Tuberculosis is not spread by touching inanimate objects, so no special precautions are required for eating utensils, clothing, books, or other objects used. Client teaching for ways to limit transmitting the disease to others includes: always cough and expectorate into tissues; dispose of tissues properly, and place them in a closed bag; and wear a mask if you are sneezing or unable to control respiratory secretions.
    Nursing Process: Planning
    Client Need: Health Promotion and Maintenance

5. Answer: 3
    Rationale: Histoplasmosis, an infectious disease caused by *Histoplasma capsulatum*, is the most common fungal lung infection in the United States. The organism is found in the soil and is linked to exposure to bird droppings and bats. Initial chest X-rays are nonspecific; later ones show areas of calcification. Infection occurs when the spores are inhaled and reach the alveoli.
    Nursing Process: Evaluation
    Client Need: Physiologic Integrity

6. Answer: 2
    Rationale: Preprocedure fasting or sedation is not required for a thoracentesis. Verify the presence of a signed informed consent for the procedure. Position the client upright and leaning forward with arms and head supported on an anchored overbed table. Administer a cough suppressant if indicated.
    Nursing Process: Implementation
    Client Need: Physiologic Integrity

7. Answer: 1
    Rationale: The nursing care of a client with chest tubes includes keeping the collection apparatus *below* the level of the chest. Additional proper nursing care includes: checking tubes frequently for kinks or loops; taping all connections and securing the chest tube to the chest wall; and assessing respiratory status at least every four hours.
    Nursing Process: Implementation
    Client Need: Physiologic Integrity

8. Answer: 1
    Rationale: A negative response to a tuberculin test is less than 5 mm. A test result of 5 to 9 mm is a negative response, but one that does not rule out infection. This test result is positive for people who are in close contact with a client with infective TB, have an abnormal chest x-ray, have HIV infection or are immunocompromised, or have an organ transplant. A test result of 10 to 15 mm is positive for people with the following risk factors: birth in a high-incidence country; African American, Hispanic, and Asian Americans who live in poverty areas; injection drug use; residence in a long-term care facility, correctional institution, residential care setting, homeless shelter; and medical risk factors (e.g., malnutrition, diabetes, others).
    A test result of greater than 15 mm is positive for all people.
    Nursing Process: Assessment
    Client Need: Physiologic Integrity

9. Answer: 1
    Rationale: Hemothorax, or blood in the pleural space, usually occurs as a result of chest trauma, surgery, or diagnostic procedures. Spontaneous pneumothorax develops when an air-filled bleb, or blister, on the lung surface ruptures. Accumulation of air in the pleural space is called pneumothorax. Pleural effusion is collection of excess fluid in the pleural space.
    Nursing Process: Assessment
    Client Need: Physiologic Integrity

10. Answer: 2
    Rationale: The pleural space normally contains only about 10 to 20 mL of serous fluid.
    Nursing Process: Assessment
    Client Need: Physiologic Integrity

Chapter 39

Case Study Answers

1. *Summarize the triggers of asthma.* Childhood asthma (which may continue into adulthood) is most often linked to inhalation of allergens such as pollen, animal dander, or household dust. Clients with allergic asthma often have a history of other allergies. Environmental pollutants, such as tobacco smoke and irritant gases (e.g., sulfur dioxide, nitrogen dioxide, and ozone) can provoke asthma. Exposure to secondhand smoke as a child is associated with a higher risk for and increased severity of asthma.

Agents found in the workplace, such as noxious fumes and gases, chemicals, and dusts may cause occupational asthma. Respiratory infections, viral infections in particular, are a common internal stimulus for an asthmatic attack. Exercise-induced asthma attacks also are common, and affect 40% to 90% of people with bronchial asthma (Porth, 2005). Loss of heat or water from the bronchial surface may contribute to exercise-induced asthma. Exercising in cold, dry air increases the risk of an asthma attack in susceptible people. Emotional stress is a significant etiologic factor for attacks in as many as half of clients with asthma. Common pharmacologic triggers include aspirin and other NSAIDs, sulfites (which are used as preservatives in wine, beer, fresh fruits, and salad), and beta-blockers.

2. *List the manifestations of acute asthma.* The manifestations of acute asthma are as follows:
   - Chest tightness
   - Cough
   - Dyspnea
   - Wheezing
   - Tachypnea and tachycardia
   - Anxiety and apprehension

3. *Explain how to use a metered-dose inhaler and a dry powder inhaler.*
   Proper use of a metered-dose inhaler is as follows:
   - Firmly insert a charged metered-dose inhaler (MDI) canister into the mouthpiece unit or spacer (if used)
   - Remove mouthpiece cap. Shake canister vigorously for 3 to 5 seconds.
   - Exhale slowly and completely.
   - Hold the canister upside down, place the mouthpiece in the mouth, and close lips around it, if a spacer is being used. When no spacer is used, hold the mouthpiece directly in front of the mouth.
   - Press and hold the canister down while inhaling deeply and slowly for 3 to 5 seconds (see figure).
   - Hold breath for 10 seconds, release pressure on the container, remove from mouth, and exhale. Wait 20 to 30 seconds before repeating the procedure for a second puff.
   - Rinse the mouth after using the inhaler to minimize systemic absorption and drying the mucous membranes.
   - Rinse the inhaler mouthpiece and spacer after use; store in a clean location.
   Proper use of a dry powder inhaler is as follows:
   - Keep the inhaler and medication in a clean, dry location. Do not refrigerate or store in a humid place such as the bathroom.
   - Remove the cap and hold the inhaler upright. Inspect to be sure that the mechanism is clean and the mouthpiece is clear.
   - If necessary, load the dose into the inhaler and follow the manufacturer's directions.
   - Hold the inhaler level with the mouthpiece end facing down.

   - Breathe slowly and completely. Tilt head back slightly.
   - Place the mouthpiece in the mouth with the teeth over the mouthpiece. Seal the lips around the mouthpiece. Do not block the inhaler with the tongue.
   - Breathe in rapidly and deeply through the mouth over 2 to 3 seconds to activate the flow of medication.
   - Remove the inhaler from the mouth and hold breath for 10 seconds.
   - Exhale slowly through pursed lips to allow the medication to enter distal airways. In order to prevent clogging, never exhale into the inhaler mouthpiece.
   - Rinse mouth or brush teeth after using the inhaler to avoid a bad taste from the medication. This will also prevent a yeast infection if a corticosteroid medication is being used.
   - Store the inhaler in a clean, sealed plastic bag; do not wash the inhaler unless directed to do so by the manufacturer. The mouthpiece should be cleaned weekly using a dry cloth.

4. *Discuss preventive measures for asthma.* Asthma attacks often can be prevented by avoiding allergens and environmental triggers. Modifying the home environment by controlling dust, removing carpets, covering mattresses and pillows to reduce dust mite populations, and installing air filtration systems may be useful. Pets may need to be removed from the household. Eliminating all tobacco smoke in the home is vital. Wearing a mask that retains humidity and warm air while exercising in cold weather may help prevent attacks of exercise-induced asthma. Early treatment of respiratory infections is vital to prevent asthma exacerbations.

NCLEX Review Question Answers

1. Answer: 1
   Rationale: Airways within the lungs contain crisscrossing (not vertical) strips of smooth muscle that control their diameter. Asthma is a chronic inflammatory disorder of the airways characterized by recurrent episodes of wheezing, breathlessness, chest tightness, and coughing. Common triggers for an acute asthma attack include exposure to allergens, respiratory tract infection, exercise, inhaled irritants, and emotional upsets. The frequency of attacks and severity of symptoms vary greatly from person to person.
   Nursing Process: Assessment
   Client Need: Physiologic Integrity

2. Answer: 3
   Rationale: Emphysema, not chronic bronchitis, is insidious in onset. Chronic bronchitis is a disorder of excessive bronchial mucus secretion. It is characterized by a productive cough that lasts

three or more months in two consecutive years. Cigarette smoke is the major factor implicated in the development of chronic bronchitis. Chronic bronchitis affected an estimated 8.6 million Americans in 2003.
Nursing Process: Assessment
Client Need: Physiologic Integrity

3. Answer: 1
   Rationale: The hallmark pathophysiologic effects of cystic fibrosis (CF) include: excess mucus production in the respiratory tract with impaired ability to clear secretions and progressive chronic obstructive pulmonary disease (COPD); pancreatic enzyme deficiency and impaired digestion; and abnormal elevation of sodium and chloride concentrations in sweat. Secretions in affected organs become thick and viscous, obstructing glands and ducts.
   Nursing Process: Assessment
   Client Need: Physiologic Integrity

4. Answer: 2
   Rationale: Atelectasis may be acute *or* chronic. The most common cause of atelectasis is obstruction of the bronchus that ventilates a segment of lung tissue. It is a state of partial or total lung collapse and airlessness. The primary therapy for atelectasis is prevention.
   Nursing Process: Assessment
   Client Need: Physiologic Integrity

5. Answer: 1
   Rationale: Inhalation using a metered-dose inhaler (MDI) should be for only 3 to 5 seconds; 5 to 7 seconds is too long. Other client teaching for using a metered-dose inhaler includes: firmly insert a charged metered-dose inhaler (MDI) canister into the mouthpiece unit or spacer (if used) remove mouthpiece cap and shake canister vigorously for 3 to 5 seconds; exhale slowly and completely; hold the canister upside down, place the mouthpiece in the mouth, and close lips around it if a spacer is being used; when no spacer is used, hold the mouthpiece directly in front of the mouth; press and hold the canister down while inhaling deeply and slowly for 3 to 5 seconds; hold breath for 10 seconds, release pressure on the container, remove from mouth, and exhale; wait 20 to 30 seconds before repeating the procedure for a second puff; rinse the mouth after using the inhaler to minimize systemic absorption and drying the mucous membranes; and rinse the inhaler mouthpiece and spacer after use and store in a clean location.
   Nursing Process: Implementation
   Client Need: Physiologic Integrity

6. Answer: 2
   Rationale: When using a dry powder inhaler, the inhaler should be held with the mouthpiece end facing down, not up. Other client teaching for

using a dry powder inhaler includes: keep the inhaler and medication in a clean, dry location; do not refrigerate or store in a humid place such as the bathroom; remove the cap and hold the inhaler upright; inspect the inhaler to be sure that the mechanism is clean and the mouthpiece is clear; if necessary, load the dose into the inhaler and follow manufacturer's directions; hold the inhaler level with the mouthpiece end facing down; breathe slowly and completely; tilt the head back slightly; place the mouthpiece in the mouth with the teeth over the mouthpiece; seal the lips around the mouthpiece; do not block the inhaler with the tongue; breathe in rapidly and deeply through the mouth over 2 to 3 seconds to activate the flow of medication; remove the inhaler from the mouth and hold breath for 10 seconds; exhale slowly through pursed lips to allow the medication to enter distal airways; never exhale into the inhaler mouthpiece to prevent clogging; rinse mouth or brush teeth after using the inhaler to avoid a bad taste from the medication and to prevent a yeast infection if a corticosteroid medication is being used; store the inhaler in a clean, sealed plastic bag; do not wash the inhaler unless directed to do so by the manufacturer; and clean the mouthpiece weekly using a dry cloth.
Nursing Process: Evaluation
Client Need: Physiologic Integrity

7. Answer: 1
   Rationale: Widespread use of tobacco among the male population of the industrialized world began during World War I (not World War II). At one time, tobacco was thought to have medicinal qualities effective against all common diseases. Tobacco is now recognized as the leading cause of preventable illness in the world. The link between tobacco use and lung cancer was reported as early as 1912.
   Nursing Process: Assessment
   Client Need: Physiologic Integrity

8. Answer: 2
   Rationale: Pursed-lip and diaphragmatic breathing techniques help minimize air trapping and fatigue. Pursed-lip breathing helps maintain open airways by maintaining positive pressures longer during exhalation. Diaphragmatic or abdominal breathing helps conserve energy by using the larger and more efficient muscles of respiration.
   Nursing Process: Implementation
   Client Need: Physiologic Integrity

9. Answer: 3
   Rationale: Elevate head of bed to at least 30 degrees at all times. Additional nursing care of a client with chronic obstructive pulmonary disease (COPD) includes: increase fluid intake to at least 2500 mL per day and provide a bedside humidifier; teach "huff" coughing technique; and assess respiratory status and level of

consciousness every 1 to 2 hours until stable, then at least every 4 hours.
Nursing Process: Assessment
Client Need: Physiologic Integrity

10. Answer: 4
Rationale: Bradypnea is not a common manifestation of pulmonary embolism. Common manifestations of pulmonary embolism include: dyspnea and shortness of breath; chest pain; anxiety and apprehension; cough; tachycardia and tachypnea; crackles (rales); and low-grade fever.
Nursing Process: Assessment
Client Need: Physiologic Integrity

Chapter 40

Case Study Answers

1. *Bones are classified by which shapes?* Bones are classified by the following shapes:
   - Long bones are longer than they are wide. They have a midportion, or shaft, called a diaphysis, and two broad ends, called epiphyses. The diaphysis is compact bone and contains the marrow cavity, which is lined with endosteum. Each epiphysis is spongy bone covered by a thin layer of compact bone. Long bones include the bones of the arms and legs, fingers, and toes.
   - Short bones, also called cuboid bones, are spongy bone covered by compact bone. They include the bones of the wrist and ankle.
   - Flat bones are thin and flat, and most are curved. Their disc-like structure consists of a layer of spongy bone between two thin layers of compact bone. Flat bones include most bones of the skull, the sternum, and the ribs.
   - Irregular bones are of various shapes and sizes and, like flat bones, are plates of compact bone with spongy bone between. Irregular bones include the vertebrae, the scapulae, and the bones of the pelvic girdle.

2. *Summarize bone remodeling in adults.* Although the bones of adults do not normally increase in length and size, constant remodeling of bones, as well as repair of damaged bone tissue, occurs throughout life. In the bone remodeling process, bone resorption and bone deposit occur at all periosteal and endosteal surfaces. Hormones and forces that put stress on the bones regulate this process, which involves a combined action of the osteocytes, osteoclasts, and osteoblasts. Bones that are in use, and are therefore subjected to stress, increase their osteoblastic activity to increase ossification (the development of bone). Bones that are inactive undergo increased osteoclast activity and bone resorption. The hormonal stimulus for bone remodeling is controlled by a negative feedback mechanism that regulates blood calcium levels. This stimulus involves the interaction of parathyroid hormone (PTH) from the parathyroid glands and

calcitonin from the thyroid gland. When blood levels of calcium decrease, PTH is released; PTH then stimulates osteoclast activity and bone resorption so that calcium is released from the bone matrix. As a result, blood levels of calcium rise, and the stimulus for PTH release ends. Rising blood calcium levels stimulate the secretion of calcitonin, inhibit bone resorption, and cause the deposit of calcium salts in the bone matrix. Thus, bones are necessary to regulate blood calcium levels. Calcium ions are necessary for the transmission of nerve impulses, the release of neurotransmitters, muscle contraction, blood clotting, glandular secretion, and cell division. Of the body's 1200 to 1400 g of calcium, over 99% is present as bone minerals. Bone remodeling is also regulated by the response of bones to gravitational pull and to mechanical stress from the pull of muscles. Although the exact mechanism is not fully understood, it is known that bones that undergo increased stress are heavier and larger. This finding supports Wolff's law, which states that bone develops and remodels itself to resist the stresses placed on it.

3. *What are the different types of joints?* Fibrous joints permit little or no movement, because the articulating bones are joined either by short connective tissue fibers that bind the bones together, as with the sutures of the skull, or by short cords of fibrous tissue called ligaments that permit slight give but no true movement. Some cartilaginous joints, such as the sternocostal joints of the rib cage, are composed of hyaline cartilage growths that fuse together the articulating bone ends. These joints are immobile. In other cartilaginous joints, such as the intervertebral discs, the hyaline cartilage fuses to an intervening plate of flexible fibrocartilage. This structural feature accounts for the flexibility of the vertebral column. Bones in synovial joints are enclosed by a cavity that is filled with synovial fluid, which is a filtrate of blood plasma. Synovial joints are freely moveable, and allow many kinds of movements. Synovial joints are found at all articulations of the limbs. They have several characteristics:
   - The articular surfaces are covered with articular cartilage.
   - The joint cavity is enclosed by a tough, fibrous, double-layered articular capsule; internally, the cavity is lined with a synovial membrane that covers all surfaces that are not covered by the articular cartilage.
   - Synovial fluid fills the free spaces of the joint capsule, which enhances the smooth movement of the articulating bones.

NCLEX Review Question Answers

1. Answer: 4
Rationale: The tissues and structures of the musculoskeletal system perform *many* functions, including support, protection, and movement. The musculoskeletal system is composed of bones of the skeletal system and ligaments, tendons, and

muscles of the muscular system, and joints. The bones serve as the framework for the body and for the attachment of muscles, tendons, and ligaments. The musculoskeletal system has two subsystems: the bones and joints of the skeleton, and the skeletal muscles.
Nursing Process: Assessment
Client Need: Physiologic Integrity

2. Answer: 2
   Rationale: The human skeleton is made up of 206 (not 226) bones. Bones store minerals. Bones of the skeletal system are divided into the axial and the appendicular skeleton. Bones protect vital organs from injury and serve to move body parts by providing points of attachment for muscles.
   Nursing Process: Assessment
   Client Need: Physiologic Integrity

3. Answer: 2
   Rationale: Long bones are longer than they are wide. Short bones, also called cuboid bones, are spongy bone that is covered by compact bone. Flat bones are thin and flat, and most are curved. Irregular bones are of various shapes and sizes and, like flat bones, are plates of compact bone with spongy bone between.
   Nursing Process: Assessment
   Client Need: Physiologic Integrity

4. Answer: 4
   Rationale: Short bones, also called cuboid bones, are spongy bone that is covered by compact bone. They include the bones of the wrist and ankle. Irregular bones are of various shapes and sizes and, like flat bones, are plates of compact bone with spongy bone between. Long bones are longer than they are wide. Flat bones are thin and flat, and most are curved.
   Nursing Process: Assessment
   Client Need: Physiologic Integrity

5. Answer: 1
   Rationale: Rough muscle is not a type of muscle tissue in the body. The three types of muscle tissue in the body are skeletal muscle, smooth muscle, and cardiac muscle.
   Nursing Process: Assessment
   Client Need: Physiologic Integrity

6. Answer: 3
   Rationale: The body has approximately 600 skeletal muscles.
   Nursing Process: Assessment
   Client Need: Physiologic Integrity

7. Answer: 4
   Rationale: Synovial joints are freely moveable, and allow many kinds of movements. Synovial joints are found at all articulations of the limbs. Fibrous joints permit little or no movement, because the articulating bones are joined either by short connective tissue fibers that bind the bones

together, as with the sutures of the skull, or by short cords of fibrous tissue called ligaments that permit slight give but no true movement. Some cartilaginous joints, such as the sternocostal joints of the rib cage, are composed of hyaline cartilage growths that fuse together the articulating bone ends. These joints are immobile. In other cartilaginous joints, such as the intervertebral discs, the hyaline cartilage fuses to an intervening plate of flexible fibrocartilage. This structural feature accounts for the flexibility of the vertebral column. Amphiarthroses is a slightly moveable joint. These joints are located in the vertebral joints and the joint of the pubic symphysis.
Nursing Process: Assessment
Client Need: Physiologic Integrity

8. Answer:3
   Rationale: The instruction to "spread your fingers" assess abduction. "Make a fist" assesses flexion. "Open your hand" assesses extension. "Close your fingers" assesses adduction.
   Nursing Process: Assessment
   Client Need: Physiologic Integrity

9. Answer: 2
   Rationale: A lateral, S-shaped curvature of the spine is called scoliosis. An increased lumbar curve is called lordosis. Kyphosis is an exaggerated thoracic curvature of the spine. Synovitis is inflammation of the synovial membrane lining the articular capsule of a joint.
   Nursing Process: Assessment
   Client Need: Physiologic Integrity

10. Answer: 3
    Rationale: Numbness and burning in the fingers during the Phalen's test may indicate carpal tunnel syndrome. The bulge test checks for small amounts of fluid on the knee. In the Thomas test, ask the client to lie down and extend one leg while bringing the knee of the opposite leg to the chest. In McMurray's test, the client reclines, then ask the client to turn the flexed knee toward the center of the body. Stabilize the knee with one hand, and apply pressure on the lower leg with the other hand.
    Nursing Process: Assessment
    Client Need: Physiologic Integrity

Chapter 41

Case Study Answers

1. *Define strain and sprain.* A strain is a stretching injury to a muscle or a muscle-tendon unit caused by mechanical overloading. A muscle that is forced to extend past its elasticity will become strained. A sprain is a stretch and/or tear of one or more ligaments that surround a joint. Forces going in opposite directions cause the ligament to overstretch and/or tear. The ligaments may be partially or completely torn.

2. *Give examples of how a strain or sprain could occur.* Lifting heavy objects without bending the knees, or a sudden acceleration-deceleration, as in a motor vehicle crash, can cause strains. The most common sites for a muscle strain are the lower back and cervical regions of the spine. Although any joint may be involved, sprains of the ankle and knee are most common; more than 25,000 people sprain an ankle each day in the United States.

3. *What are the manifestations of a strain and a sprain?* The manifestations of a strain include pain, limited motion, muscle spasms, swelling, and possible muscle weakness. Severe strains that partially or completely tear the muscle or tendon are very painful and disabling. Manifestations include loss of the ability to move or use the joint, a feeling of a "pop" or tear, discoloration, pain, and rapid swelling. Motion increases the joint pain. The intensity of the manifestations depends on the severity of the sprain.

4. *Explain RICE therapy.* The goal of the initial stage of treating soft-tissue trauma is to reduce swelling and pain. Clients should follow a regimen of rest, ice, compression, and elevation (RICE) for the first 24 to 48 hours.

NCLEX Review Question Answers

1. Answer: 2
   Rationale: A strain is a stretching injury to a muscle or a muscle-tendon unit caused by mechanical overloading. A sprain is a stretch and/or tear of one or more ligaments that surround a joint. The most common sites for a muscle strain are the lower back and cervical regions of the spine. The manifestations of a strain include pain, limited motion, muscle spasms, swelling, and possible muscle weakness. Severe strains that partially or completely tear the muscle or tendon are very painful and disabling.
   Nursing Process: Assessment
   Client Need: Physiologic Integrity

2. Answer: 1
   Rationale: RICE (rest, ice, compression, elevation) therapy for musculoskeletal injuries.
   Nursing Process: Evaluation
   Client Need: Physiologic Integrity

3. Answer: 1
   Rationale: A dislocation is an injury of a joint in which the ends of bones are forced from their normal position. A strain is a stretching injury to a muscle or a muscle-tendon unit caused by mechanical overloading. A sprain is a stretch and/or tear of one or more ligaments that surround a joint. Forces going in opposite directions cause the ligament to overstretch and/or tear. A fracture is any break in the continuity of a bone.
   Nursing Process: Assessment
   Client Need: Physiologic Integrity

4. Answer: 4
   Rationale: Any of the 206 bones in the body can be fractured. Fractures vary in severity according to the location and the type of fracture. A fracture occurs when the bone is subjected to more kinetic energy than it can absorb. Two basic mechanisms produce fractures: direct force and indirect force.
   Nursing Process: Assessment
   Client Need: Physiologic Integrity

5. Answer: 1
   Rationale: Compartment syndrome usually develops within the first 48 hours of injury, when edema is at its peak. Compartment syndrome occurs when excess pressure in a limited space constricts the structures within a compartment, which reduces circulation to muscles and nerves. Acute compartment syndrome may result from hemorrhage and edema within the compartment following a fracture or from a crush injury, or from external compression of the limb by a cast that is too tight. Increased pressure within the confined space of the compartment results in entrapment of nerves, blood vessels, and muscles.
   Nursing Process: Evaluation
   Client Need: Physiologic Integrity

6. Answer: 2
   Rationale: Skeletal traction is the application of a pulling force through placement of pins into the bone. Skin traction (also called straight traction) is used to control muscle spasms and to immobilize a part of the body before surgery, with traction exerting its grabbing and pulling force through the client's skin. Balanced suspension traction involves more than one force of pull. In manual traction, the hand directly applies the pulling force.
   Nursing Process: Assessment
   Client Need: Physiologic Integrity

7. Answer: 1
   Rationale: A plaster cast may require up to 48 (not 24) hours to dry; whereas a fiberglass cast dries in less than 1 hour (not 2 hours). The cast is applied to immobilize the joint above and the joint below the fractured bone so that the bone will not move during healing. Casts are applied on clients who have relatively stable fractures. The cast must be allowed to dry before any pressure is applied to it; simply palpating a wet cast with the fingertips will leave dents that may cause pressure sores.
   Nursing Process: Evaluation
   Client Need: Physiologic Integrity

8. Answer: 2
   Rationale: One should never break off any rough edges from the cast. Do not try to scratch under a cast with a sharp or dull object. Do not get a plaster cast wet. Elevate the injured extremity above the level of the heart.
   Nursing Process: Planning
   Client Need: Physiologic Integrity

9. Answer: 1

    Rationale: Put the amputated part in a plastic bag and put the bag on ice. Do not let the amputated part come into direct contact with the ice or water. Apply firm pressure to the bleeding area with a towel or article of clothing. Send the amputated part to the emergency department with the injured person, and be sure the emergency personnel know what it is. Wrap the amputated part in a clean cloth.

    Nursing Process: Implementation
    Client Need: Physiologic Integrity

10. Answer: 4

    Rationale: Healing of a fractured hip may take from 12 to 16 weeks (not 8 to 10 weeks). An uncomplicated fracture of the arm or foot can heal in 6 to 8 weeks. A fractured vertebra will take at least 12 weeks to heal. The age, physical condition of the client, and the type of fracture sustained influence the healing of fractures.

    Nursing Process: Assessment
    Client Need: Physiologic Integrity

Chapter 42

Case Study Answers

1. *What are the unmodifiable risk factors for osteoporosis?*
   - Both men and women are susceptible to osteoporosis
   - European Americans and Asians are at a higher risk for osteoporosis than African Americans
   - Premature osteoporosis is increasing in female athletes
   - Poor nutrition
   - Intense physical training
   - Decreased estrogen
   - Lack of calcium and vitamin D
   - Clients who have an endocrine disorder

2. *What are the modifiable risk factors for osteoporosis?* Modifiable risk factors include behaviors that place a person at risk for developing osteoporosis, as well as physical changes such as menopause whose contribution to osteoporosis can be modified by preventive strategies.
   - Calcium deficiency
   - A high intake of diet soda
   - With menopause and decreasing estrogen levels, bone loss accelerates in women.
   - Cigarette smoking
   - Excess alcohol
   - Sedentary lifestyle
   - Prolonged use of medications that increase calcium excretion

3. *What are the most common signs and symptoms of osteoporosis?* The most common manifestations of osteoporosis are loss of height, progressive curvature of the spine, low back pain, and fractures of the forearm, spine, or hip. Osteoporosis is often called the "silent disease," because bone loss occurs without symptoms. The loss of height occurs as vertebral bodies collapse. Acute episodes generally are painful, and pain radiates around the flank into the abdomen. Vertebral collapse can occur with little or no stress; minimal movements such as bending, lifting, or jumping may precipitate the pain. In some clients, vertebral collapse may occur slowly, accompanied by little discomfort. Along with loss of height, characteristic dorsal kyphosis and cervical lordosis develop, accounting for the "dowager's hump" often associated with aging. The abdomen tends to protrude and knees and hips flex as the body attempts to maintain its center of gravity.

4. *Are there complications of osteoporosis?* Fractures are the most common complication of osteoporosis; the disease is responsible for more than 1.5 million fractures each year. These include 700,000 vertebral compression fractures, 300,000 hip fractures, 250,000 wrist fractures, and 300,000 fractures at other sites (National Osteoporosis Foundation, 2004). There may be no obvious manifestations of osteoporosis until fractures occur. Some fractures are spontaneous; others may result from everyday activities. While wrist and vertebral fractures have not been shown to increase disability or mortality, persistent pain and associated posture changes may restrict the client's activities or interfere with ADLs.

NCLEX Review Question Answers

1. Answer: 2

    Rationale: Calcium, not vitamin D, deficiency is an important modifiable risk factor that contributes to osteoporosis. The most common manifestations of osteoporosis are loss of height, progressive curvature of the spine, low back pain, and fractures of the forearm, spine, or hip. Fractures are the most common complication of osteoporosis. Osteoporosis is both preventable and treatable

    Nursing Process: Assessment
    Client Need: Physiologic Integrity

2. Answer: 4

    Rationale: Carrots are not a food source of calcium. Milk and milk products are the best sources of calcium. Other food sources of calcium include sardines, clams, oysters, salmon, and dark green, leafy vegetables such as broccoli, collard greens, bok choy, and spinach.

    Nursing Process: Assessment
    Client Need: Physiologic Integrity

3. Answer: 2

    Rationale: In Paget's disease, also called osteitis deformans, the bones increase in size and thickness. The most common manifestation of Paget's disease is localized pain of the long bones, spine, pelvis, and cranium. Paget's disease is a progressive metabolic skeletal disorder of the

osteoclast that results from excessive metabolic activity in bone, with excessive bone resorption followed by excessive bone formation.
Nursing Process: Evaluation
Client Need: Physiologic Integrity

4. Answer: 2
Rationale: Gout has an acute onset, usually at night, and often involves the first metatarsophalangeal joint (great toe). Over time, urate deposits in subcutaneous tissues cause the formation of small white nodules called tophi. Kidney disease may occur in clients with untreated gout, particularly when hypertension is also present. Serum uric acid is nearly always elevated (usually above 7.5 mg/dL).
Nursing Process: Evaluation
Client Need: Physiologic Integrity

5. Answer: 3
Rationale: The primary causes of osteomalacia are vitamin D deficiency and hypophosphatemia. Osteomalacia may be difficult to differentiate from osteoporosis because the manifestations are very similar. The manifestations of osteomalacia include bone pain and tenderness Osteomalacia is a metabolic bone disorder characterized by inadequate or delayed mineralization of bone matrix in mature compact and spongy bone, which results in softening of bones.
Nursing Process: Planning
Client Need: Physiologic Integrity

6. Answer: 4
Rationale: Men (not women) are affected more than women at an earlier age, but the rate of osteoarthritis (OA) in women (not men) exceeds men by the middle adult years. The onset of OA is usually gradual and insidious, and the course slowly progressive. OA (also called degenerative joint disease) is the most common of all forms of arthritis, and is a leading cause of pain and disability in older adults. The onset of osteoarthritis is usually gradual and insidious.
Nursing Process: Evaluation
Client Need: Physiologic Integrity

7. Answer: 2
Rationale: A white skin discoloration, especially on the face, is not a manifestation of systemic lupus erythematosus (SLE). Manifestations of SLE include: painful or swollen joints and muscle pain; unexplained fever; red rash, especially on the face; unusual loss of hair; pale, cyanotic fingers or toes; sensitivity to the sun; edema in legs and around eyes; ulcers in the mouth; enlarged glands; and extreme fatigue.
Nursing Process: Assessment
Client Need: Physiologic Integrity

8. Answer: 1
Rationale: Hallux valgus, commonly called a bunion, is the enlargement and lateral

displacement of the first metatarsal (the great toe). Hammertoe (claw toe) is the dorsiflexion of the first phalanx with accompanying plantar flexion of the second and third phalanges. Morton's neuroma is a tumor-like mass formed within the neurovascular bundle of the intermetatarsal spaces
Nursing Process: Assessment
Client Need: Physiologic Integrity

9. Answer: 1
Rationale: Scoliosis is a lateral curvature of the spine. Kyphosis is excessive angulation of the normal posterior curve of the thoracic spine. The manifestations of kyphosis include moderate back pain and increased curvature of the thoracic spine as viewed from the side ("hunchback"). Along with loss of height, characteristic dorsal kyphosis and cervical lordosis develop, which accounts for the "dowager's hump" often associated with aging.
Nursing Process: Assessment
Client Need: Physiologic Integrity

10. Answer: 2
Rationale: Fibromyalgia is a common rheumatic syndrome characterized by musculoskeletal pain, stiffness, and tenderness. Osteomyelitis is an infection of the bone. Polymyositis is a systemic connective-tissue disorder characterized by inflammation of connective tissue and muscle fibers that leads to muscle weakness and atrophy. Sjögren's syndrome is an autoimmune disorder that causes inflammation and dysfunction of exocrine glands throughout the body.
Nursing Process: Assessment
Client Need: Physiologic Integrity

Chapter 43

Case Study Answers

1. *What are the four major regions of the brain?* The brain has four major regions: the cerebrum, the diencephalon, the brainstem, and the cerebellum.

2. *What does the brainstem consist of?* The brainstem consists of the midbrain, pons, and medulla oblongata.

3. *What protects and surrounds the spinal cord?* The spinal cord is protected by the vertebrae, the meninges, and cerebrospinal fluid (CSF). The spinal cord is surrounded and protected by 33 vertebrae, including 7 cervical, 12 thoracic, 5 lumbar, 5 sacral, and 4 fused vertebrae that form the coccyx.

4. *How many pairs of spinal nerves are there and where are they located?* There are 31 pairs of spinal nerves and they are named by their location:
- Cervical nerves: 8 pairs
- Thoracic nerves: 12 pairs
- Lumbar nerves: 5 pairs
- Sacral nerves: 5 pairs
- Coccygeal nerves: 1 pair

NCLEX-RN Review Question Answers

1. Answer: 4

    Rationale: A nucleus is not part of a neuron. A nucleus is part of a cell. Each neuron consists of a dendrite, a cell body, and an axon.
    Nursing Process: Assessment
    Client Need: Physiologic Integrity

2. Answer: 3

    Rationale: The dendrite is a short process (projection) from the cell body that conducts impulses toward (afferent) the cell body. Many axons are covered with a myelin sheath, which is a white lipid substance. Cell bodies, most of which are located within the CNS, are clustered in ganglia or nuclei. The myelin sheath serves to increase the speed of nerve impulse conduction in axons and is essential for the survival of larger nerve processes.
    Nursing Process: Assessment
    Client Need: Physiologic Integrity

3. Answer: 2

    Rationale: The excitatory (not inhibitory) neurotransmitter is almost always acetylcholine (ACh). The neurotransmitter may either be inhibitory or excitatory. Norepinephrine (NE), which may be either excitatory or inhibitory, is another major neurotransmitter. Neurotransmitters are the chemical messengers of the nervous system.
    Nursing Process: Assessment
    Client Need: Physiologic Integrity

4. Answer: 2

    Rationale: The brain weighs an average of 3 to 4 lbs (48 to 64 ounces). The brain is the control center of the nervous system and also generates thoughts, emotions, and speech. The brain has four major regions: the cerebrum, the diencephalon, the brainstem, and the cerebellum. The brain is surrounded by the skull.
    Nursing Process: Assessment
    Client Need: Physiologic Integrity

5. Answer: 4

    Rationale: The brainstem consists of the midbrain, pons, and medulla oblongata. The brain contains four ventricles, which are chambers filled with cerebrospinal fluid (CSF).
    Nursing Process: Assessment
    Client Need: Physiologic Integrity

6. Answer: 3

    Rationale: The brain contains four ventricles, which are chambers filled with cerebrospinal fluid (CSF).
    Nursing Process: Assessment
    Client Need: Physiologic Integrity

7. Answer: 3

    Rationale: The usual amount of cerebrospinal fluid (CSF) ranges from 80 to 200 mL, and averages about 150 mL. CCSF, a clear and colorless liquid, is formed by the choroid plexus, which are groups of specialized capillaries located in the brain ventricles. CSF is normally produced and absorbed in equal amounts.
    Nursing Process: Assessment
    Client Need: Physiologic Integrity

8. Answer: 4

    Rationale: Potassium does not affect cerebral blood flow. At least three metabolic factors affect cerebral blood flow: carbon dioxide, hydrogen ion, and oxygen concentrations.
    Nursing Process: Assessment
    Client Need: Physiologic Integrity

9. Answer: 3

    Rationale: The spinal cord is surrounded and protected by 33 vertebrae, including 7 cervical, 12 thoracic, 5 lumbar, 5 sacral, and 4 fused vertebrae that form the coccyx.
    Nursing Process: Assessment
    Client Need: Physiologic Integrity

10. Answer: 4

    Rationale: Cranial nerve VII allows the client to smile, frown, wrinkle forehead, show teeth, puff out cheek, purse lips, raise eyebrows, and close eyes against resistance. Additional cranial nerve testing results include: II corresponds to vision 40/20 in both eyes, and the client has full visual fields bilaterally; III, IV, VI corresponds to bilateral full extraocular movements, client's pupils are equally round and react to light and accommodation, and no ptosis is present in either eye; V corresponds to the client's ability to identify sharp, dull, and light touch to forehead, cheek, and chin, and the corneal reflex is present bilaterally, but decreased (the client wears contact lenses).
    Nursing Process: Assessment
    Client Need: Physiologic Integrity

Chapter 44

Case Study Answers

1. *Explain the stages of a classic migraine.* The classic migraine headache has several stages, which are as follows:
    *   The aura stage is characterized by sensory manifestations, usually visual disturbances such as bright spots or flashing lights zig-zagging across the visual fields. This stage lasts from 5 to 60 minutes. Less common sensory symptoms include numbness or tingling of the face or hand, paresis of an arm or leg, mild aphasia, confusion, drowsiness, and lack of coordination. Additionally, some clients experience a premonition the day prior to an attack. They may feel nervous or have other mood changes. The aura period corresponds with the initial physiologic change of vasoconstriction.

- The headache stage is characterized by vasodilation, a decline in serotonin levels, and the onset of throbbing headache. It appears that the pain is related to increased vessel permeability and polypeptide exudation by perivascular nerve endings rather than the vasodilation itself. Cerebral arteries are dilated and distended, with walls that are edematous and rigid. Beginning unilaterally, the headache eventually may involve both sides as it increases in intensity during the next several hours. Nausea and vomiting often occur. The client may be acutely ill and is often extremely irritable. The sensory organs often become hypersensitive, and the client withdraws from sound and light. The scalp is tender. The headache may last from several hours to a day or two.
- During the post-headache phase, the headache area is sensitive to touch, and a deep aching is present. The client is exhausted. Vessel size and serotonin levels return to normal.

2. *What factors are believed to trigger an onset of a migraine?* A variety of factors are believed to trigger the onset of a migraine headache. Rapid changes in blood glucose levels, stress, emotional excitement, fatigue, hormonal changes due to menstruation, stimuli such as bright lights, and foods high in tyramine or other vasoactive substances (e.g., aged cheese, nuts, chocolate, and alcoholic beverages) have been associated with migraine attacks. Hypertension and febrile states may make the disorder worse.

3. *Discuss the therapeutic management of migraines.* Therapeutic management for migraine headache includes a combination of client teaching, medications, and measures to control contributing factors. Dietary changes such as eliminating caffeine, cured meats, monosodium glutamate (MSG), and foods that contain tyramine (red wine, aged cheese, and others) may be necessary. Stress management or biofeedback are also part of the overall strategy. Treatment protocols for cluster headache include eliminating aggravating factors (e.g., consumption of alcohol) and using medications and oxygen inhalation. The management of tension headaches is directed toward reducing the client's level of stress and relieving pain with ice and aspirin or NSAIDs.

NCLEX Review Question Answers

1. Answer: 3
   Rationale: With compression of cranial nerve III at the midbrain, the pupils may become oval or eccentric (off center).
   Nursing Process: Assessment
   Client Need: Physiologic Integrity

2. Answer: 1
   Rationale: Doll's eye movements are reflexive movements of the eyes in the opposite direction of head rotation; they are an indicator of brainstem function. As a result of the oculocephalic reflex, the eyes move upward with passive flexion of the neck and downward with passive neck extension. As brainstem function deteriorates, this reflex is lost. The eyes fail to turn together and, eventually, remain fixed in the midposition as the head is turned.
   Nursing Process: Assessment
   Client Need: Physiologic Integrity

3. Answer: 1
   Rationale: The electroencephalogram (EEG)—not the electrocardiogram (EKG)—may be used to establish the absence of brain activity when brain death is suspected. Brain death is the cessation and irreversibility of all brain functions, including the brainstem. The exact criteria for establishing brain death may vary somewhat from state to state. It is generally agreed that brain death has occurred when there is no evidence of cerebral or brainstem function for an extended period (usually 6 to 24 hours) in a client who has a normal body temperature and is not affected by a depressant drug or alcohol poisoning.
   Nursing Process: Assessment
   Client Need: Physiologic Integrity

4. Answer: 1
   Rationale: Cerebral edema increases ICP, which in turn decreases cerebral blood flow.
   Nursing Process: Assessment
   Client Need: Physiologic Integrity

5. Answer: 2
   Rationale: There are two types of migraine headaches: common migraine (*without* an aura) and classic migraine (*with* an aura; most often experienced as a visual disturbance prior to the pain). Tension headache is characterized by bilateral pain, with a sensation of a band of tightness or pressure around the head. Migraine headache is a recurring vascular headache that lasts from 4 to 72 hours, often initiated by a triggering event and usually accompanied by a neurologic dysfunction. A cluster headache is an extremely severe, unilateral, burning pain located behind or around the eyes.
   Nursing Process: Planning
   Client Need: Physiologic Integrity

6. Answer: 3
   Rationale: It is inappropriate to place a tongue blade in the client's mouth because it can obstruct the airway. First aid for a seizure includes: cushion the head; loosen anything tight around the neck; turn on the side; nothing in the mouth; and do not hold down.
   Nursing Process: Implementation
   Client Need: Physiologic Integrity

7. Answer: 1
   Rationale: It is not necessary to call for medical assistance if the seizure lasts for less than

4 minutes. Teach family members when to call for medical assistance when a person is experiencing a seizure: if the seizure lasts for more than 5 minutes; if there is slow recovery, a second seizure, or difficulty breathing after the seizure; and if there are signs of injury (such as bleeding from the mouth).
Nursing Process: Assessment
Client Need: Health Promotion and Maintenance

8. Answer: 2
Rationale: *Chronic* subdural hematomas develop over weeks or months. An epidural hematoma (also called an extradural hematoma) develops in the potential space between the dura and the skull, which normally adhere to one another. Subdural hematoma is a localized mass of blood that collects between the dura mater and the arachnoid mater. Intracerebral hematomas may be single or multiple, and are associated with contusions.
Nursing Process: Assessment
Client Need: Physiologic Integrity

9. Answer: 1
Rationale: The dura mater is not involved in meningitis. Meningitis is an inflammation of the pia mater, the arachnoid, and the subarachnoid space.
Nursing Process: Assessment
Client Need: Physiologic Integrity

10. Answer: 4
Rationale: In order to decrease incidents of migraine headaches, the client should not consume caffeine. Appropriate teaching to decrease incidents of migraine headaches includes: wake up at the same time each morning; exercise at least three times a week; no smoking or caffeine after 3:00 p.m.; no artificial sweeteners; no MSG (monosodium glutamate); reduce or eliminate red wine, cheese, alcohol, chocolate, and caffeine; and try a gluten-free diet.
Nursing Process: Planning
Client Need: Health Promotion and Maintenance

Chapter 45

Case Study Answers

1. *What is a stroke?* A stroke (cerebral vascular accident, CVA, or brain attack), is a condition in which neurologic deficits result from a sudden decrease in blood flow to a localized area of the brain.

2. *What type of complications can occur from a stroke?* Typical complications include sensoriperceptual deficits, cognitive and behavioral changes, communication disorders, motor deficits, and elimination disorders. These may be transient or permanent, depending on the degree of ischemia and necrosis as well as time of treatment. As a result of the neurologic deficits, the client with a stroke has complications that involve many different body systems. The disabilities that result from a stroke often cause serious alterations in functional health status.

3. *What are the manifestations of a stroke?* Manifestations of a stroke vary according to the cerebral artery involved and the area of the brain affected. Manifestations are always sudden in onset, focal, and usually one-sided. The most common manifestation is weakness that involves the face and arm, and sometimes the leg. Other common manifestations are numbness on one side, loss of vision, speech difficulties, a sudden severe headache, and difficulties with balance. The various deficits associated with involvement of a specific cerebral artery are collectively referred to as stroke syndromes, although the deficits often overlap.

NCLEX Review Question Answers

1. Answer: 4
Rationale: The term *heart attack* is not used to mean stroke. A stroke is also referred to as cerebral vascular accident, CVA, or brain attack. It is a condition in which neurologic deficits result from a sudden decrease in blood flow to a localized area of the brain.
Nursing Process: Assessment
Client Need: Physiologic Integrity

2. Answer: 3
Rationale: Ischemic strokes result from blockage of a cerebral artery, which decreases or stops blood flow and ultimately causes a brain infarction. An embolic stroke occurs when a blood clot or clump of matter traveling through the cerebral blood vessels becomes lodged in a vessel that is too narrow to permit further movement. A thrombotic stroke is caused by occlusion of a large cerebral vessel by a thrombus (blood clot). A hemorrhagic stroke, or intracranial hemorrhage, occurs when a cerebral blood vessel ruptures.
Nursing Process: Assessment
Client Need: Physiologic Integrity

3. Answer: 1
Rationale: Receptive aphasia is a sensory speech problem in which one cannot understand the spoken (and often written) word. Speech may be fluent but with inappropriate content; it is also called Wernicke's aphasia. Dysarthria is any disturbance in muscular control of speech. Expressive aphasia is a motor speech problem in which one can understand what is being said but can respond verbally only in short phrases; it is also called Broca's aphasia.
Nursing Process: Assessment
Client Need: Physiologic Integrity

4. Answer: 2
Rationale: The Hunt-Hess classification of subarachnoid manifestations is frequently used to classify nontraumatic subarachnoid hemorrhages.

A grade 2 severity indicates moderate to severe headache, neck rigidity, and cranial nerve deficits. The other grades of severity include: grade 1 is asymptomatic, or minimal headache and slight neck rigidity; grade 3 is drowsy, lethargic, and mild neurologic deficits; grade 4 is stuporus, moderate to severe hemiparesis, and early decerebrate rigidity; and grade 5 is deep coma, decerebrate rigidity, and moribund appearance.
Nursing Process: Assessment
Client Need: Physiologic Integrity

5. Answer: 3
   Rationale: To prevent aneurysm rebleeding, elevate the head of the bed 30 to 45 degrees. Elevating the head of the bed promotes venous return from the brain and thus decreases intracranial pressure. Decreasing activity reduces the likelihood of increases in blood pressure. Other aneurysm precautions to prevent rebleeding include: keep the client in a private, quiet, darkened room; limit visitors to two family members at any one time, and limit the duration of visits; allow reading, watching television, or listening to the radio to promote relaxation; and prevent constipation and straining to have a bowel movement.
   Nursing Process: Implementation
   Client Need: Physiologic Integrity

6. Answer: 3
   Rationale: Although SCIs occur in people of all ages, they are most often seen in young adults age 16 to 30. The three major risk factors for SCIs are age, gender, and alcohol or drug abuse. The major causes of SCI are contusion, laceration, transection, hemorrhage, and damage to blood vessels that supply the spinal cord. The most common cause of abnormal spinal column movements are acceleration and deceleration (forces that are applied to the body, for example, in automobile crashes and falls).
   Nursing Process: Assessment
   Client Need: Physiologic Integrity

7. Answer: 2
   Rationale: Paraplegia is paralysis of the lower portion of the body, which sometimes involves the lower trunk. Quadriplegia, also called tetraplegia, occurs when cervical segments of the cord are injured, which impairs function of the arms, trunk, legs, and pelvic organs. Autonomic dysreflexia (also called autonomic hyperreflexia) is an exaggerated sympathetic response that occurs in clients with SCIs at or above the T6 level.
   Nursing Process: Assessment
   Client Need: Physiologic Integrity

8. Answer: 4
   Rationale: All people who have sustained trauma to the head or spine, or who are unconscious, should be treated as though they have a spinal cord injury. The client should not be maintained in the prone position, but in the supine position. Other guidelines for emergency care are as follows: avoid flexing, extending, or rotating the neck; immobilize the neck, using rolled towels or blankets, or apply a cervical collar before moving the client onto a backboard; secure the head by placing a belt or tape across the forehead and securing it to the stretcher; maintain the client in the supine position; and transfer the client directly from the stretcher with backboard still in place to the type of bed that will be used in the hospital.
   Nursing Process: Implementation
   Client Need: Physiologic Integrity

9. Answer: 1
   Rationale: A bowel retraining program should include a high-fluid, high-fiber diet (not a low-fluid, low-fiber diet). Other aspects of a bowel retraining program include: assess usual patterns of bowel elimination to establish best times for an individualized program; use stool softeners as prescribed; rectal suppositories and enemas may be used 30 minutes after meals to stimulate stronger peristalsis and facilitate evacuation; maintain an upright position if at all possible and ensure privacy; and if the client is unable to evacuate, digital stimulation or manual removal on a regular basis may be the most effective long-term management.
   Nursing Process: Implementation
   Client Need: Health Promotion and Maintenance

10. Answer: 1
    Rationale: The intervertebral disks, located between the vertebral bodies, are made of an *inner* nucleus pulposus and an *outer* collar. A herniated intervertebral disk is also called a ruptured disk, herniated nucleus pulposus, or a slipped disk. A herniated intervertebral disk may occur at any adult age. The herniation may be abrupt or gradual.
    Nursing Process: Assessment
    Client Need: Physiologic Integrity

Chapter 46

Case Study Answers

1. *What are the risk factors of Alzheimer's disease?*
   The risk factors for Alzheimer's disease (AD) are older age, family history, and female gender.

2. *What are the warning signs of Alzheimer's disease?*
   Warning signs of AD are:
   - Memory loss that affects job skills
   - Difficulty performing familiar tasks
   - Problems with language
   - Disorientation to time and place
   - Poor or decreased judgment
   - Problems with abstract thinking
   - Misplacing things
   - Changes in mood or behavior

- Changes in personality
- Loss of initiative

3. *What are the stages of Alzheimer's disease?* In stage 1, a client typically appears physically healthy and alert, and cognitive deficits can go undetected unless thorough and periodic evaluations are performed. Clients may seem restless, forgetful, or uncoordinated; lack spontaneity; and be disoriented as to time and date. Usually, family members are the first to notice lapses in memory, subtle changes in personality, or problems in doing simple calculations. AD clients and families may consciously or unconsciously compensate for cognitive deficits by adjusting schedules and routines.

In stage 2, memory deficits are more apparent, and the client is less able to behave spontaneously. Clients may wander and get lost, even in their own homes. Although progression of manifestations continues and orientation to place and time deteriorates, AD clients may still have periods of mental lucidity and engage in time-oriented conversations. Generally, however, clients become more confused and lose their sense of time, which leads to changes in sleeping patterns, agitation, and stress. They may demonstrate repetitive behavior and eat ravenously. AD clients are less able to make even simple decisions and to adapt to environmental changes, and are often unable to carry out activities of daily living. Sundowning is another behavioral change, and it is characterized by increased agitation, time disorientation, and wandering behaviors during afternoon and evening hours; it is accelerated on overcast days. Language deficits are common in stage II. They include *paraphasia* (using the wrong word), *echolalia* (repetition of words or phrases), and *scanning speech,* in which the client appears to search for words. Eventually, total *aphasia* (absence of speech) may occur. Frustration and depression are common among AD clients as the full extent and implications of the deficits become obvious. The AD client slowly loses the ability to perform simple tasks required for hygiene or eating because sequencing of tasks is lost. For example, the client may open a can of soup but not remember to pour it into a pan to heat it. Instead, the client might place the can directly on the burner and leave the heat on high even after a smoke alarm sounds. The AD client may falsely interpret the smoke alarm as a telephone ringing, a tornado warning siren, or an ambulance siren. Thus, safety is a high priority for the client in stage 2. Sensorimotor deficits in stage 2 include *apraxia,* the inability to perform purposeful movements and use objects correctly; *astereognosis,* the inability to identify objects by touch; and *agraphia,* the inability to write properly. Problems related to malnutrition and decreased fluid intake, such as anemia and constipation, may be evident. Sleep pattern disturbances are also common and are related to the loss of time orientation, sundowning phenomenon, and depression.

Stage 3 brings increasing dependence, with inability to communicate, loss of urinary and fecal continence, and progressive loss of cognitive abilities. Common complications include pneumonia, dehydration, malnutrition, falls, depression, delusions, seizures, and paranoid reactions. The person is indifferent to food and loses weight. They are unable to recognize family or friends, or even themselves. The average life expectancy is for 1 to 2 years from the onset of stage 3, although the individual may live as long as 10 years. Most people with AD are institutionalized during this final stage of the disease. Death frequently occurs from pneumonia secondary to aspiration.

NCLEX Review Question Answers

1. Answer: 3
   Rationale: Clients with Alzheimer's disease have difficulty performing familiar tasks. Additional warning signs of Alzheimer's disease include: memory loss that affects job skills; problems with language; disorientation to time and place; poor or decreased judgment; problems with abstract thinking; misplacing things; changes in mood or behavior; changes in personality; and loss of initiative.
   Nursing Process: Assessment
   Client Need: Physiologic Integrity

2. Answer: 1
   Rationale: The onset of multiple sclerosis (MS) is usually between 20 and 50 years of age, with a peak at age 30. It is a chronic demyelinating neurologic disease of the central nervous system (brain, optic nerves, and spinal cord) associated with an abnormal immune response to an environmental factor. The initial onset may be followed by a total remission, which makes diagnosis difficult. The manifestations of MS vary according to the area of the nervous system affected.
   Nursing Process: Evaluation
   Client Need: Physiologic Integrity

3. Answer: 4
   Rationale: Parkinson's disease is one of the *most* common neurologic disorders that affect older adults. The disorder usually develops after the age of 65 years, but 15% of those diagnosed are under 40 years of age. Men and women are affected equally. Parkinson's disease begins with subtle manifestations.
   Nursing Process: Planning
   Client Need: Physiologic Integrity

4. Answer: 2
   Rationale: Parkinson's disease has five stages. In Parkinson's disease, neurons in the cerebral cortex atrophy and are lost, the dopaminergic nigrostriatal (pigmented) pathway degenerates, and the number of specific dopamine receptors in

the basal ganglia decreases. Both depression and dementia are pathologies associated with Parkinson's disease. Clients with Parkinson's disease commonly have sleep disturbances, although they may experience decreased manifestations during sleep in the early stages.
Nursing Process: Assessment
Client Need: Physiologic Integrity

5. Answer: 4
   Rationale: Obesity related to dysphagia is not a complication associated with Parkinson's disease. Complications associated with Parkinson's disease include: oculogyric crisis, in which the eyes become fixed with a lateral and upward gaze; paranoia and hallucinations that may accompany dementia; impaired communication due to changes in speech, handwriting, and expressiveness; falls from balance, posture, and motor changes; infections, such as pneumonia, related to immobility; malnutrition related to dysphagia and inability to prepare meals; altered sleep patterns due to loss of dopamine, l-dopa side effects (nightmares, dreams), or side effects of anticholinergics (hyperreflexia, muscle twitching), and depression; skin breakdown and pressure ulcers associated with urinary incontinence, malnutrition, and sweat reflex changes; and depression and social isolation.
   Nursing Process: Assessment
   Client Need: Physiologic Integrity

6. Answer: 3
   Rationale: Huntington's disease (HD) is a familial disease; each child of an HD parent has a *50%* chance of inheriting the HD gene and, if inherited, will eventually develop the disease. HD is a progressive, degenerative, inherited neurologic disease characterized by increasing dementia and chorea (jerky, rapid, involuntary movements). HD is a single-gene autosomal-dominant inherited disease that causes localized death of neurons of the basal ganglia. HD causes destruction of cells in the caudate nucleus and putamen areas of the basal ganglia.
   Nursing Process: Evaluation
   Client Need: Physiologic Integrity

7. Answer: 4
   Rationale: Amyotrophic lateral sclerosis (ALS) is not known as Babe Ruth's disease. ALS, or Lou Gehrig's disease, is a rapidly progressive and fatal degenerative neurologic disease characterized by weakness and wasting of muscles that are under voluntary control, without any accompanying sensory or cognitive changes. ALS is the most common motor neuron disease in the United States. ALS results from the degeneration and demyelination of both upper and lower motor neurons in the anterior horn of the spinal cord, brainstem, and cerebral cortex.

Nursing Process: Planning
Client Need: Physiologic Integrity

8. Answer: 1
   Rationale: Myasthenia gravis is a chronic autoimmune neuromuscular disorder characterized by fatigue and severe weakness of skeletal muscles. Guillain-Barré syndrome (GBS), not myasthenia gravis, is an acute inflammatory demyelinating disorder of the peripheral nervous system characterized by an acute onset of motor paralysis that is usually ascending. The manifestations of myasthenia gravis correspond to the muscles involved. Initially, the eye muscles are affected and the client experiences either diplopia (unilateral or bilateral double vision) or ptosis (drooping of the eyelid). In myasthenia gravis, antibodies destroy or block neuromuscular junction receptor sites, which results in a decreased number of acetylcholine receptors. Myasthenia gravis is sometimes associated with a tumor of the thymus, thyrotoxicosis (hyperthyroidism), rheumatoid arthritis, and lupus erythematosus.
   Nursing Process: Evaluation
   Client Need: Health Promotion and Maintenance

9. Answer: 4
   Rationale: Trigeminal neuralgia, also called *tic douloureux*, is a chronic disease of the trigeminal cranial nerve (V) that causes severe facial pain. Bell's palsy is also called facial paralysis, and is a disorder of the seventh cranial (facial) nerve, characterized by unilateral paralysis of the facial muscles. Trigeminal neuralgia occurs more commonly in middle and older adults and affects women more often than men. There are no specific diagnostic tests for trigeminal neuralgia. Trigeminal neuralgia is characterized by brief (lasting a few seconds to a few minutes), repetitive episodes of sudden severe (usually unilateral) facial pain.
   Nursing Process: Evaluation
   Client Need: Physiologic Integrity

10. Answer: 4
    Rationale: SE is not an abbreviation used to describe a rapidly progressive, degenerative neurologic disease that causes brain degeneration without inflammation. Creutzfeldt-Jakob disease (CJD or spongiform encephalopathy) is a rapidly progressive, neurologic disease that causes brain degeneration without inflammation.
    Nursing Process: Assessment
    Client Need: Physiologic Integrity

Chapter 47

Case Study Answers

1. *What is the colored part of the eye? What is its function?* The colored part of the eye is the iris. The iris is a disc of muscle tissue that surrounds the pupil

and lies between the cornea and the lens. The iris gives the eye its color and regulates light entry by controlling the size of the pupil. The pupil is the dark center of the eye through which light enters. The pupil constricts when bright light enters the eye and when it is used for near vision; it dilates when light conditions are dim and when the eye is used for far vision. In response to intense light, the pupil constricts rapidly in the pupillary light reflex.

2. *What does the external ear consist of?* The external ear consists of the auricle (or pinna), the external auditory canal, and the tympanic membrane.

3. *Explain equilibrium.* The inner ear provides information about the position of the head. This information is used to coordinate body movements so that equilibrium and balance are maintained. The types of equilibrium are static balance (affected by changes in the position of the head) and dynamic balance (affected by the movement of the head). Receptors called maculae in the utricle and the saccule of the vestibule detect changes in the position of the head. Maculae are groups of hair cells; these cells have protrusions that are covered with a gelatinous substance. Embedded in this gelatinous substance are tiny particles of calcium carbonate called otoliths (ear stones), which make the gelatin heavier than the endolymph that fills the membranous labyrinth. As a result, when the head is in the upright position, gravity causes the gelatinous substance to bear down on the hair cells. When the position of the head changes, the force on the hair cells also changes, bending them and altering the pattern of stimulation of the neurons. Thus, a different pattern of nerve impulses is transmitted to the brain, where stimulation of the motor centers initiates actions that coordinate various body movements according to the position of the head. The receptor for dynamic equilibrium is in the crista, a crest in the membrane that lines the ampulla of each semicircular canal. The cristae are stimulated by rotatory head movement (acceleration and deceleration) as a result of changes in the flow of endolymph and of movement of hair cells in the maculae. The direction of endolymph and hair cell movement is always opposite to the motion of the body.

NCLEX Review Question Answers

1. Answer: 3
   Rationale: The iris gives the eye its color and regulates light entry by controlling the size of the pupil. The pupil is the dark center of the eye through which light enters. The pupil constricts when bright light enters the eye and when it is used for near vision; it dilates when light conditions are dim and when the eye is used for far vision. In response to intense light, the pupil constricts rapidly in the pupillary light reflex. The

white sclera lines the outside of the eyeball, and protects and gives shape to the eyeball. The sclera gives way to the cornea over the iris and pupil. The cornea is transparent, avascular, and sensitive to touch. The cornea forms a window that allows light to enter the eye and is a part of its light-bending apparatus.
Nursing Process: Assessment
Client Need: Physiologic Integrity

2. Answer: 4
   Rationale: Aqueous humor, a *clear* fluid, is constantly formed and drained to maintain a relatively constant pressure of 15 to 20 mmHg in the eye. Aqueous humor provides nutrients and oxygen to the cornea and the lens. The anterior cavity is filled with aqueous humor.
   Nursing Process: Assessment
   Client Need: Physiologic Integrity

3. Answer: 1
   Rationale: When the eye focuses on an image, it is called accommodation. Refraction is the bending of light rays as they pass from one medium to another medium of different optical density. Convergence (which is the medial rotation of the eyeballs so that each is directed toward the viewed object) allows the eye to focus on the image in the retinal fovea of each eye. In the pupillary light reflex, the pupil constricts rapidly in response to intense light.
   Nursing Process: Assessment
   Client Need: Physiologic Integrity

4. Answer:1
   Rationale: To measure visual fields, sit directly opposite the client at a distance of 18 to 24 inches. Ask the client to cover one eye with the opaque cover while you cover your own eye opposite to the client (for example, if the client covers the right eye, you cover your left eye). Ask the client to look directly at you. Move the penlight from the periphery toward the center from right to left, above and below, and from the middle of each of these directions. Both you and the client should see the penlight enter the field of vision at the same time, if the examiner has normal peripheral vision.
   Nursing Process: Implementation
   Client Need: Physiologic Integrity

5. Answer: 4
   Rationale: The *bottom* number is the distance (in feet) at which a person with normal vision can read the line. The Snellen chart contains rows of letters in various sizes, with standardized numbers at the end of each row. The number at the end of the row indicates the visual acuity of a client who can read the row at a distance of 20 feet. A person with normal vision can read the row marked 20/20.
   Nursing Process: Assessment
   Client Need: Physiologic Integrity

6. Answer: 4

Rationale: The tympanic membrane is a part of the external ear, not the middle ear. The middle ear contains three auditory ossicles: the malleus, the incus, and the stapes. The external ear consists of the auricle (or pinna), the external auditory canal, and the tympanic membrane.
Nursing Process: Assessment
Client Need: Physiologic Integrity

7. Answer: 2

Rationale: The malleus attaches to the tympanic membrane and articulates with the incus, which in turn articulates with the stapes. The inner ear, also called the labyrinth, is a maze of bony chambers located deep within the temporal bone, just behind the eye socket. Within the chambers of the membranous labyrinth is a fluid called endolymph. The bony labyrinth has three regions: the vestibule, the semicircular canals, and the cochlea.
Nursing Process: Assessment
Client Need: Physiologic Integrity

8. Answer: 4

Rationale: The human ear is most sensitive to sound waves with frequencies between 1000 and 4000 cycles per second, but can detect sound waves with frequencies between 20 and 20,000 cycles per second. Hearing is the perception and interpretation of sound. Sound is produced when the molecules of a medium are compressed, which results in a pressure disturbance evidenced as a sound wave. Sound waves enter the external auditory canal and cause the tympanic membrane to vibrate at the same frequency.
Nursing Process: Assessment
Client Need: Physiologic Integrity

9. Answer: 4

Rationale: The tympanic membrane should be pearly gray, shiny, and translucent without bulging or retraction.
Nursing Process: Assessment
Client Need: Physiologic Integrity

10. Answer: 1

Rationale: To conduct the Weber test, place the base of a vibrating tuning fork on the midline vertex of the client's head. For the Rinne test, place the base of a vibrating tuning fork on the client's mastoid bone. To perform the whisper test, ask the client to occlude one ear with a finger. Stand 1 to 2 feet away from the client, on the side of the unoccluded ear. Softly whisper numbers and ask the client to repeat them. The caloric test is used to assess vestibular system function. Cold or warm water is used to irrigate the ear canals one at a time and the client is observed for nystagmus (repeated abnormal movements of the eyes). Normally, the nystagmus occurs opposite to the ear being irrigated. If no nystagmus occurs, the client has further testing for brain lesions.
Nursing Process: Assessment
Client Need: Physiologic Integrity

Chapter 48

Case Study Answers

1. *Is conjunctivitis the same thing as 'pink eye'?* Yes, bacterial conjunctivitis is also known as "pink eye."

2. *Is pink eye contagious?* Bacterial conjunctivitis, also known as "pink eye," is highly contagious, and often is caused by *Staphylococcus* and *Haemophilus*.

3. *What are the signs and symptoms of conjunctivitis?* Redness and itching of the affected eye are common manifestations of acute conjunctivitis. The client may also complain of a scratchy, burning, or gritty sensation. Pain is not common; however, photophobia may occur. Tearing and discharge accompany the inflammatory process. The discharge may be watery, purulent, or mucoid, depending on the cause of conjunctivitis. The client may have associated manifestations such as pharyngitis, fever, malaise, and swollen preauricular lymph nodes.

NCLEX Review Question Answers

1. Answer: 3

Rationale: In myopia (nearsightedness) the objects in close range are seen clearly and those at a distance are blurred. The eyeball is too short in hyperopia (farsightedness), which causes the image to focus behind the retina. People with this condition see objects clearer at a distance than objects close to them. Nystagmus is rapid involuntary eye movements. A cataract is an opacification (clouding) of the lens of the eye.
Nursing Process: Assessment
Client Need: Physiologic Integrity

2. Answer: 4

Rationale: Infectious conjunctivitis may be bacterial, viral, or fungal in origin. Bacterial conjunctivitis, also known as "pink eye" (not "red eye") is highly contagious, and often is caused by *Staphylococcus* and *Haemophilus*.
Nursing Process: Assessment
Client Need: Physiologic Integrity

3. Answer: 4

Rationale: LKT is not a type of laser eye surgery. Laser eye surgery is commonly performed to correct refractive errors such as myopia, hyperopia, and astigmatism. Several surgical procedures are available: laser in-situ keratomileusis (LASIK); photorefractive keratectomy (PRK); laser epithelial keratomileusis (LASEK); and laser thermokeratoplasty (LTK).
Nursing Process: Assessment
Client Need: Physiologic Integrity

4. Answer: 4

Rationale: Education is a vital strategy for preventing many corneal disorders. Teach all clients about proper eye care, including the importance of not sharing towels and makeup, avoiding rubbing or scratching the eyes, and preventing trauma and infection. Teach contact lens users appropriate care and cleaning techniques. Stress the importance of periodic removal of lenses, even extended-wear lenses.
Nursing Process: Evaluation
Client Need: Health Promotion and Maintenance

5. Answer: 2

Rationale: A chalazion is a granulomatous cyst or nodule of the lid. Infection of one or more of the sebaceous glands of the eyelid may cause a hordeolum (sty). Hyphema, which is bleeding into the anterior chamber of the eye, is a potential result of blunt eye trauma. A cataract is an opacification (clouding) of the eye lens.
Nursing Process: Assessment
Client Need: Physiologic Integrity

6. Answer: 4

Rationale: Critical proliferative retinopathy is not a stage of diabetic retinopathy. Diabetic retinopathy progresses through four stages: (1) mild nonproliferative or background retinopathy; (2) moderate nonproliferative retinopathy; (3) severe nonproliferative retinopathy; and (4) proliferative retinopathy.
Nursing Process: Assessment
Client Need: Physiologic Integrity

7. Answer: 2

Rationale: Otitis externa is inflammation of the ear canal. Commonly known as swimmer's ear (not diver's ear), it is most prevalent in people who spend significant time in the water. Competitive athletes, including swimmers, divers, and surfers, are particularly prone to otitis externa. Wearing a hearing aid or ear plugs, which hold moisture in the ear canal, is an additional risk factor.
Nursing Process: Evaluation
Client Need: Physiologic Integrity

8. Answer: 3

Rationale: Otosclerosis occurs most commonly in Caucasians and in females, not males. Otosclerosis is a common cause of conductive hearing loss. Otosclerosis is a hereditary disorder with an autosomal dominant pattern of inheritance. The progressive hearing loss typically begins in adolescence or early adulthood and seems to be accelerated by pregnancy.
Nursing Process: Assessment
Client Need: Physiologic Integrity

9. Answer: 3

Rationale: Ménière's disease, also known as endolymphatic hydrops, is a chronic disorder characterized by recurrent attacks of vertigo with tinnitus and a progressive unilateral hearing loss. Labyrinthitis, also called otitis interna, is inflammation of the inner ear. An acoustic neuroma or schwannoma is a benign tumor of cranial nerve VIII. Otitis externa is inflammation of the ear canal.
Nursing Process: Assessment
Client Need: Physiologic Integrity

10. Answer: 2

Rationale: In presbycusis, which is gradual hearing loss associated with aging, hearing acuity begins to decrease in early adulthood and progresses as long as the individual lives. Higher-pitched (not lower-pitched) tones and conversational speech are lost initially. Hearing aids and other amplification devices are useful for most clients with presbycusis. Because the hearing loss of presbycusis is gradual, the client and family may not realize the extent of the deficit.
Nursing Process: Planning
Client Need: Physiologic Integrity

Chapter 49

Case Study Answers

1. *What is the ovarian cycle?* The ovarian cycle has three consecutive phases that occur cyclically each 28 days (although the cycle normally may be longer or shorter), as follows:

- The follicular phase lasts from the 1st to the 10th day of the cycle.
- The ovulatory phase lasts from the 11th to the 14th day of the cycle and ends with ovulation.
- The luteal phase lasts from the 14th to the 28th days.

2. *Why do I need estrogen?* Estrogens are essential for the development and maintenance of secondary sex characteristics; and in conjunction with other hormones, they stimulate the female reproductive organs to prepare for growth of a fetus. Estrogens are responsible for the normal structure of skin and blood vessels. They also decrease the rate of bone resorption, promote increased high-density lipoproteins, reduce cholesterol levels, and enhance the clotting of blood. Estrogens also promote the retention of sodium and water.

3. *What is the difference between the vagina and cervix?* The vagina is a fibromuscular tube about 3 to 4 inches (8 to 10 cm) in length that is located posterior to the bladder and urethra and anterior to the rectum. The upper end contains the uterine cervix in an area called the fornix. The walls of the vagina are membranes that form folds, called rugae. These membranes are composed of mucus-secreting stratified squamous epithelial cells. The vagina serves as a route for the excretion of secretions, including menstrual fluid, and also is an organ of sexual response. The walls of the vagina are usually moist and maintain a pH that ranges from 3.8 to 4.2. This pH is bacteriostatic and is maintained by the action of estrogen and normal vaginal flora. Estrogen stimulates the growth of vaginal mucosal cells so that they thicken and have increased glycogen content. The glycogen is fermented to lactic acid by Döderlein's bacilli (lactobacilli that normally inhabit the vagina), which slightly acidifies the vaginal fluid. The cervix projects into the vagina and forms a pathway between the uterus and the vagina. The uterine opening of the cervix is called the internal os; the vaginal opening is called the external os. The space between these openings, which is the endocervical canal, serves as a route for the discharge of menstrual fluid and the entrance for sperm. The cervix is a firm structure, protected by mucus that changes consistency and quantity during the menstrual cycle and during pregnancy.

NCLEX Review Question Answers

1. Answer: 1

   Rationale: The testes develop in the abdominal cavity of the fetus and then descend through the inguinal canal into the scrotum. They are homologous to the female's ovaries. These paired organs are each about 1.5 inches (4 cm) long and 1 inch (2.5 cm) in diameter. They are suspended in the scrotum by the spermatic cord. Each is surrounded by two coverings: an outer tunica vaginalis and an inner tunica albuginea. Each testis is divided into 250 to 300 lobules, and each lobule contains one to four seminiferous tubules. The testes produce sperm and testosterone.
   Nursing Process: Assessment
   Client Need: Physiologic Integrity

2. Answer: 4

   Rationale: The prostate gland is about the size of a walnut (not a pea). It encircles the urethra just below the urinary bladder (see Figure 49–1). It is made of 20 to 30 tubuloalveolar glands surrounded by smooth muscle. Secretions of the prostate gland make up about one-third of the volume of semen. These secretions enter the urethra through several ducts during ejaculation.
   Nursing Process: Assessment
   Client Need: Physiologic Integrity

3. Answer: 3

   Rationale: The optimum temperature for sperm production is about 2 to 3 degrees below body temperature. The scrotum is a sac or pouch made of two layers. The scrotum hangs at the base of the penis, anterior to the anus, and regulates the temperature of the testes. When the testicular temperature is too low, the scrotum contracts to bring the testes up against the body.
   Nursing Process: Assessment
   Client Need: Physiologic Integrity

4. Answer: 2

   Rationale: Seminal fluid does not decrease alkalinity; it increases alkalinity. Seminal fluid also nourishes the sperm and provides bulk.
   Nursing Process: Assessment
   Client Need: Physiologic Integrity

5. Answer: 2

   Rationale: The labia majora, which are folds of skin and adipose tissue covered with hair, are outermost; they begin at the base of the mons pubis and end at the anus. The labia minora, which are located between the clitoris and the base of the vagina, are enclosed by the labia majora. The external genitalia collectively are called the vulva. It includes the mons pubis, the labia, the clitoris, the vaginal and urethral openings, and glands. The clitoris is an erectile organ that is analogous to the penis in the male. After puberty, the mons is covered with hair with a diamond-shaped distribution.
   Nursing Process: Assessment
   Client Need: Physiologic Integrity

6. Answer: 4

   Rationale: The walls of the vagina are usually moist and maintain a pH ranging from 3.8 to 4.2. The vagina is a fibromuscular tube about 3 to 4 inches (8 to 10 cm) in length that is located posterior to the bladder and urethra and anterior to the rectum. The walls of the vagina are membranes that form folds, called rugae. The vagina serves as a route for the excretion of secretions, including menstrual fluid, and also is an organ of sexual response.
   Nursing Process: Assessment
   Client Need: Physiologic Integrity

7. Answer: 3

   Rationale: The luteal phase does not last from the 5th to the 10th day of the cycle. The ovarian cycle has three consecutive phases that occur cyclically each 28 days (although the cycle normally may be longer or shorter), as follows: the follicular phase lasts from the 1st to the 10th day of the cycle; the ovulatory phase lasts from the 11th to the 14th day of the cycle and ends with ovulation; and the luteal phase lasts from the 14th to the 28th days.
   Nursing Process: Assessment
   Client Need: Physiologic Integrity

8. Answer: 1

   Rationale: Prostate specific antigen (PSA) is a blood test used to diagnose prostate cancer and to monitor treatment of prostate cancer. Venereal disease research laboratory (VDRL), rapid plasma reagin (RPR), and fluorescent treponemal antibody absorption (FTA-ABS) are blood tests conducted to screen for syphilis.
   Nursing Process: Assessment
   Client Need: Physiologic Integrity

9. Answer: 2

    Rationale: The ovaries in the adult woman are flat, almond-shaped structures located on either side of the uterus below the ends of the fallopian tubes. They are homologous to the male's testes. The other answer selections are not found in males and are not homologous to the male's testes.
    Nursing Process: Assessment
    Client Need: Physiologic Integrity

10. Answer: 3

    Rationale: The ovaries in the adult woman are flat, almond-shaped structures located on either side of the uterus below the ends of the fallopian tubes. A woman's total number of ova is present at birth. Each ovary contains many small structures called ovarian follicles. The ovaries store the female germ cells and produce the female hormones estrogen and progesterone.
    Nursing Process: Assessment
    Client Need: Physiologic Integrity

Chapter 50

Case Study Answers

1. *What is the cause of testicular cancer?* The cause of testicular cancer is unknown, but both congenital and acquired factors have been associated with tumor development. About 5% of testicular cancers develop in a man with a history of undescended testicle (*cryptorchidism*). Testicular cancer is more common on the right side, which parallels the incidence of cryptorchidism (Tierney et al, 2004).

2. *What are the risk factors for testicular cancer?* Risk factors for testicular cancer are listed below:
   - Age
   - Cryptorchidism
   - Genetic predisposition, especially in identical twins and brothers
   - Cancer of the other testicle
        Other risk factors under investigation include occupational risks, presence of multiple atypical nevi, HIV infection, cancer in situ, body size, and maternal hormone use (ACS, 2004).

3. *What are the manifestations of testicular cancer?* The first sign of testicular cancer may be a slight enlargement of one testicle with some discomfort. The man may also have an abdominal ache and a feeling of heaviness in the scrotum. Local spread of the cancer to the epididymis or spermatic cord is inhibited by the outer covering of the testicles, the tunica albuginea. Therefore, spread by lymphatic and vascular channels to other organs often causes distant disease before large masses develop in the scrotum. Lymphatic dissemination usually leads to disease in retroperitoneal lymph nodes, whereas vascular dissemination can lead to metastasis in the lungs, bone, or liver. Bilateral presentation of testicular cancer is unusual. Manifestations of metastasis include lower extremity edema, back pain, cough, hemoptysis, or dizziness. Tumors that produce HCG may cause breast enlargement (*gynecomastia*).

NCLEX Review Question Answers

1. Answer: 4

    Rationale: Erectile dysfunction (ED) is the inability of the male to attain and maintain an erection sufficient to permit satisfactory sexual intercourse. It has many possible causes. Impotence, a term often used synonymously with erectile dysfunction, may involve a total inability to achieve erection, an inconsistent ability to achieve erection, or the ability to sustain only brief erections. ED can be treated with oral medications, or medications injected directly into the penis or inserted into the urethra at the tip of the penis.
    Nursing Process: Assessment
    Client Need: Physiologic Integrity

2. Answer: 3

    Rationale: Minoxidil (Rogaine) is used to treat hair loss in men and women. The oral medications used to treat erectile dysfunction (ED) include sildenafil citrate (Viagra), vardenafil hydrochloride (Levitra), or tadalafil (Cialis).
    Nursing Process: Assessment
    Client Need: Physiologic Integrity

3. Answer: 2

    Rationale: Phimosis is constriction of the foreskin that it cannot be retracted over the glans penis. In paraphimosis, the foreskin is tight and constricted and is not able to cover the glans penis. Priapism is an involuntary, sustained, painful erection that is not associated with sexual arousal. A hydrocele, which is the most common cause of scrotal swelling, is a collection of fluid within the tunica vaginalis.
    Nursing Process: Assessment
    Client Need: Physiologic Integrity

4. Answer: 3

    Rationale: A hydrocele, which is the most common cause of scrotal swelling, is a collection of fluid within the tunica vaginalis. A spermatocele is a mobile, usually painless, mass that forms when efferent ducts in the epididymis dilate and form a cyst. Testicular torsion, which is twisting of the spermatic cord with scrotal swelling and pain, is a potential medical emergency. A varicocele is an abnormal dilation of a vein within the spermatic cord.
    Nursing Process: Assessment
    Client Need: Physiologic Integrity

5. Answer: 2

    Rationale: The most common infectious cause of orchitis in postpubertal men is mumps (not the measles). Orchitis is an acute inflammation or

infection of the testes. It most commonly occurs as a complication of a systemic illness or as an extension of epididymitis. The manifestations have a sudden onset, usually within 3 to 4 days after the swelling of the parotid glands.
Nursing Process: Assessment
Client Need: Physiologic Integrity

6. Answer: 1
   Rationale: Testicular cancer is more common on the right side, which parallels the incidence of cryptorchidism. Testicular cancer accounts for only 1% of all cancers in men; however, it is the most common cancer in men between the ages of 15 and 40. The first sign of testicular cancer may be a slight enlargement of one testicle with some discomfort.
   Nursing Process: Assessment
   Client Need: Physiologic Integrity

7. Answer: 2
   Rationale: Benign prostatic hyperplasia (BPH), an age-related, nonmalignant enlargement of the prostate gland, is a common disorder of the aging male. Testicular torsion, which is the twisting of the spermatic cord with scrotal swelling and pain, is a potential medical emergency. The two necessary preconditions for BPH are age of 50 or greater and the presence of testes. The exact cause of BPH is unknown. Risk factors of BPH include age, family history, race (highest in African Americans and lowest in native Japanese), and a diet high in meat and fats.
   Nursing Process: Assessment
   Client Need: Physiologic Integrity

8. Answer: 3
   Rationale: Gynecomastia is usually bilateral. If it is unilateral, biopsy may be necessary to rule out breast cancer. Gynecomastia, the abnormal enlargement of the male breast, is thought to result from a high ratio of estradiol to testosterone. Drugs such as digitalis, opiates, and chemotherapeutic agents are also associated with gynecomastia. No treatment is necessary for the transient gynecomastia of puberty.
   Nursing Process: Assessment
   Client Need: Physiologic Integrity

9. Answer: 1
   Rationale: A spermatocele is a mobile, usually painless, mass that forms when efferent ducts in the epididymis dilate and form a cyst. A hydrocele, which is the most common cause of scrotal swelling, is a collection of fluid within the tunica vaginalis. Testicular torsion, which is the twisting of the spermatic cord with scrotal swelling and pain, is a potential medical emergency. A varicocele is an abnormal dilation of a vein within the spermatic cord.
   Nursing Process: Assessment
   Client Need: Physiologic Integrity

10. Answer: 3
    Rationale: Testicular torsion may occur spontaneously, or it may follow trauma or physical exertion. Testicular torsion, which is the twisting of the spermatic cord with scrotal swelling and pain, is a potential medical emergency. Orchitis is an acute inflammation or infection of the testes. Epididymitis is an infection or inflammation of the epididymis, which is the structure that lies along the posterior border of the testis.
    Nursing Process: Assessment
    Client Need: Physiologic Integrity

Chapter 51

Case Study Answers

1. *How often does the American Cancer Society recommend Pap tests?* The American Cancer Society (2005) recommends that women should begin annual screening for cervical cancer with the Pap test about 3 years after a woman begins having vaginal intercourse, but no later than 21 years of age. Screening should be done every year with regular Pap tests or every 2 years using liquid-based tests. At or after the age of 30, after three consecutive normal Pap tests, screening can be performed every 2 to 3 years, at the discretion of the healthcare provider. Alternately, cervical cancer screening with HPV DNA tests and Pap tests may be performed every 3 years. Women 70 years of age and older who have had 3 or more normal Pap smears in the last 10 years may choose to stop cervical cancer screening. Screening for women who have had a total hysterectomy (including the cervix) is not recommended unless the surgery was done as a treatment for cancer. Women who have had a hysterectomy without removal of the cervix should continue to follow ACS guidelines (ACS, 2006a).

2. *What are risk factors for cervical cancer?* It is vital that nurses educate women of all ages about controlling risk factors for cervical cancer and about the importance of screening for this cancer throughout the life span. Teach young women about the relationship between early sexual activity, multiple partners, and risk for sexually transmitted diseases and cervical cancer. Discuss safer sex alternatives and using condoms for protection. Emphasize the importance of continued screening exams for the older woman who may not see a gynecologic specialist on a regular basis.

3. *What are the instructions for how to perform a breast self-examination?* Provide the following instructions to the client for performing a breast self-examination (BSE):
   - Lie down on your back and place your right arm behind your head. (BSE should be done while lying down because this position spreads breast

tissue evenly over the chest wall, which makes it easier to feel all the breast tissue.)

- Use the finger pads of the middle fingers on your left hand to feel for lumps in the right breast. Use overlapping dime-sized circular motions of the finger pads to feel the breast tissue.
- Use three different levels of pressure to feel all the breast tissue. Light pressure is needed to feel the tissue closest to the skin; medium pressure to feel a little deeper; and firm pressure to feel the tissue closest to the chest and ribs. A firm ridge in the lower curve of each breast is normal. Use each pressure level to feel the breast tissue before moving on to the next spot.
- Move around the breast in an up–and-down pattern starting at an imaginary line drawn straight down your side from the underarm and moving across the breast to the middle of the chest bone (sternum, breastbone). Be sure to check the entire breast area before going down until you feel only ribs and up to the neck or collar bone.
- Repeat the exam on your left breast, using the finger pads of your right hand.
- Stand in front of the mirror with your hands pressing firmly down on your hips. Look at your breasts for any changes in size, shape, contour, or dimpling.
- Examine your underarm while sitting or standing and with your arm only slightly raised.
- If you find any changes, see your healthcare provider as soon as possible.

NCLEX Review Question Answers

1. Answer: 4

   Rationale: The sexual response cycle has four phases: excitement, plateau, orgasm, and resolution. These phases always occur in the same sequence; however, the duration of each phase may vary. Multiple orgasms are physically possible in all women. Sexual stimulation results in vasocongestion of the blood vessels that surround the vagina, which causes engorgement, increased lubrication, and genital swelling and enlargement.
   Nursing Process: Assessment
   Client Need: Physiologic Integrity

2. Answer: 2

   Rationale: Menopause is neither a disease nor a disorder, but a normal physiologic process. Menopause is the permanent cessation of menses. Earlier menopause is associated with genetics, smoking, higher altitude, and obesity. The average woman will live one-third of her life after menopause.
   Nursing Process: Planning
   Client Need: Health Promotion and Maintenance

3. Answer: 2

   Rationale: Metrorrhagia is bleeding between menstrual periods. Menorrhagia is excessive or prolonged menstruation. Oligomenorrhea is scant menses. Amenorrhea is the absence of menstruation.
   Nursing Process: Assessment
   Client Need: Physiologic Integrity

4. Answer: 3

   Rationale: Anteversion is an exaggerated forward tilting of the uterus. Retroversion of the uterus is a backward tilting of the uterus toward the rectum. Retroflexion involves a flexing or bending of the uterine corpus in a backward manner toward the rectum. Anteflexion is a flexing or folding of the uterine corpus upon itself.
   Nursing Process: Assessment
   Client Need: Physiologic Integrity

5. Answer: 3

   Rationale: Use overlapping dime-sized (not quarter-sized) circular motions of the finger pads to feel the breast tissue. Lie down on your back and place your right arm behind your head. Use three different levels of pressure to feel all the breast tissue. Look at your breasts for any changes in size, shape, contour, or dimpling.
   Nursing Process: Evaluation
   Client Need: Health Promotion and Maintenance

6. Answer: 3

   Rationale: An enlarged abdomen with ascites signals *later*-stage disease. Ovarian cancer is the fourth most common gynecologic cancer in women in the United States. There are several types of ovarian cancers: epithelial tumors, germ cell tumors, and gonadal stromal tumors. In early stages, ovarian cancer generally causes no warning signs or manifestations.
   Nursing Process: Planning
   Client Need: Physiologic Integrity

7. Answer: 2

   Rationale: FCC is most common in women 30 to 50 years of age, and is rare in postmenopausal women who are not taking hormone replacement. Fibrocystic changes (FCC), or fibrocystic breast disease, is the physiologic nodularity and breast tenderness that increases and decreases with the menstrual cycle. FCC includes many different lesions and breast changes. Women with fibrocystic changes experience bilateral or unilateral pain or tenderness in the upper, outer quadrants of their breasts, and report that their breasts feel particularly thick and lumpy the week prior to menses.
   Nursing Process: Assessment
   Client Need: Physiologic Integrity

8. Answer: 4

   Rationale: Premenstrual syndrome (PMS) can be a factor in absenteeism at school or work, decreased productivity, interpersonal relationship difficulties, and lifestyle disruption. Manifestations of PMS occur during the *luteal*

phase of the menstrual cycle (7 to 10 days prior to the onset of the menstrual flow), and abate when the menstrual flow begins. The treatment of PMS integrates a self-monitored record of manifestations, regular exercise, avoiding caffeine, and a diet low in simple sugars and high in lean proteins. Alternative and complementary therapies that the woman with PMS may find helpful focus on diet, exercise, relaxation, and stress management.
Nursing Process: Assessment
Client Need: Physiologic Integrity

9. Answer: 4
Rationale: A third-degree prolapse, or procidentia, is complete prolapse of the uterus outside the body, with inversion of the vaginal canal. First-degree, or mild, prolapse involves a descent of less than half the uterine corpus into the vagina. Second-degree, or marked, prolapse involves the descent of the entire uterus into the vaginal canal, so that the cervix is at the introitus to the vagina.
Nursing Process: Assessment
Client Need: Physiologic Integrity

10. Answer: 1
Rationale: A polyp is a highly vascular, solid tumor attached by a pedicle or stem. A cyst is a fluid-filled sac. A fistula is an abnormal opening or passage between two organs or spaces that are normally separated or an abnormal passage to the outside of the body. Displacement or prolapse of the uterus, bladder, or rectum can be a congenital or an acquired condition.
Nursing Process: Assessment
Client Need: Physiologic Integrity

Chapter 52

Case Study Answers

1. *What cause genital herpes?* Genital herpes is caused by the herpes simplex viruses HSV-1 and HSV-2.

2. *What are the three clinical stages of syphilis?* Syphilis is generally characterized by three clinical stages: primary, secondary, and tertiary.

3. *Which STIs are reportable?* Gonorrhea, syphilis, and AIDS are reportable diseases in every state, and chlamydial infections are reportable in most states.

NCLEX Review Question Answers

1. Answer: 1
Rationale: Many STIs are more easily transmitted from a man to a woman than from a woman to a man. Sexually transmitted infections (STIs) have reached epidemic proportions in the United States and continue to increase worldwide. The incidence of STIs is highest in young adults ages 15 to 24. Sexually transmitted infections

include those caused by bacteria, chlamydiae, viruses, fungi, protozoa, and parasites. Infections that are transmitted by vaginal, oral, and anal intimate contact and intercourse are referred to as sexually transmitted infections (STIs).
Nursing Process: Assessment
Client Need: Physiologic Integrity

2. Answer: 3
Rationale: HSV-1 is associated with cold sores, but may be transmitted to the genital area by oral intercourse or by self-inoculation through poor hand-washing practices. HSV-2 is transmitted by sexual activity or during childbirth to an infected woman, and is the virus that causes genital herpes. Genital warts are caused by human papillomavirus (HPV), and are transmitted by vaginal, anal, or oral-genital contact. Gonorrhea, also known as "GC" or "the clap," is caused by *Neisseria gonorrhoeae,* a gram-negative diplococcus.
Nursing Process: Assessment
Client Need: Physiologic Integrity

3. Answer: 1
Rationale: Genital warts are not a reportable disease. Gonorrhea, syphilis, and AIDS are reportable diseases in every state, and chlamydial infections are reportable in most states.
Nursing Process: Assessment
Client Need: Physiologic Integrity

4. Answer: 2
Rationale: Chlamydia may be present for months or years without producing noticeable symptoms in women. Because chlamydia is asymptomatic in most women until the uterus and fallopian tubes have been invaded, treatment may be delayed, which results in devastating long-term complications. The infections caused by chlamydia include acute urethral syndrome, nongonococcal urethritis, mucopurulent cervicitis, and pelvic inflammatory disease (PID). Complications of chlamydial infections in men include epididymitis, prostatitis, sterility, and Reiter's syndrome.
Nursing Process: Assessment
Client Need: Physiologic Integrity

5. Answer: 3
Rationale: Humans are the only host for the organism that causes gonorrhea. Gonorrhea, also known as "GC" or "the clap," is caused by *Neisseria gonorrhoeae,* a gram-negative diplococcus. Gonorrhea is the most common reportable communicable disease in the United States.
Nursing Process: Evaluation
Client Need: Physiologic Integrity

6. Answer: 3
Rationale: The primary stage of syphilis is characterized by the appearance of a chancre and

by regional enlargement of lymph nodes; little or no pain accompanies these warning signs. Manifestations of secondary syphilis may appear any time from 2 weeks to 6 months after the initial chancre disappears. These symptoms can include a skin rash, especially on the palms of the hands or soles of the feet, mucous patches in the oral cavity; sore throat; generalized lymphadenopathy; condyloma lata (flat, broad-based papules, unlike the pedunculated structure of genital warts) on the labia, anus, or corner of the mouth; flu-like symptoms; and alopecia. The latent stage of syphilis begins 2 or more years after the initial infection and can last up to 50 years. During this stage, no symptoms of syphilis are apparent, and the disease is not transmissible by sexual contact. It can be transmitted by infected blood, however; thus, all prospective blood donors must be screened for syphilis.
Nursing Process: Assessment
Client Need: Physiologic Integrity

7. Answer: 1
   Rationale: Pelvic inflammatory disease (PID) is not a reportable disease in the United States. PID is usually polymicrobial (caused by more than one microbe) in origin; gonorrhea and chlamydia are common causative organisms. Manifestations of PID include fever, purulent vaginal discharge, severe lower abdominal pain, and a painful cervical movement. Complications include pelvic abscess, infertility, ectopic pregnancy, chronic pelvic pain, pelvic adhesions, dyspareunia, and chronic pelvic pain. Abscess formation is common.
   Nursing Process: Assessment
   Client Need: Physiologic Integrity

8. Answer: 3
   Rationale: Flat warts are slightly raised lesions that are often invisible to the naked eye, and also develop on keratinized skin. Condyloma acuminata are cauliflower-shaped lesions that appear on moist skin surfaces such as the vagina or anus. Keratotic warts are thick, hard lesions that develop on keratinized skin such as the labia

major, penis, or scrotum. Papular warts are smooth lesions that also develop on keratinized skin.
Nursing Process: Assessment
Client Need: Physiologic Integrity

9. Answer: 1
   Rationale: Trichomoniasis is caused by *Trichomonas vaginalis,* a protozoan parasite. It is the most common curable STI in young, sexually active women. Symptoms usually appear within 5 to 28 days of exposure. Women have a frothy, green-yellow vaginal discharge with a strong fishy odor that is often accompanied by itching and irritation of the genitalia.
   Nursing Process: Assessment
   Client Need: Physiologic Integrity

10. Answer: 4
    Rationale: The venereal disease research laboratory (VDRL) and rapid plasma reagin (RPR) blood tests measure antibody production. People with syphilis become positive about 4 to 6 weeks after infection. However, these tests are not specific for syphilis, and other diseases may also cause positive results. Additional tests are required for definitive diagnosis. The fluorescent treponemal antibody absorption (FTA-ABS) test is specific for *T. pallidum* and can be used to confirm VDRL and RPR findings. It may be used for clients whose clinical picture indicates syphilis but who have negative VDRL results. In immunofluorescent staining, a specimen obtained from early lesions or aspiration of lymph nodes is specially treated and examined microscopically for the presence of *T. pallidum.* Darkfield microscopy involves examining a specimen from the chancre for the presence of *T. pallidum* using a darkfield microscope. Diagnosis of gonorrhea is based on cultures from the infected mucous membranes (cervix, urethra, rectum, or throat), examination of urine from an infected person, and a Gram stain to visualize the bacteria under the microscope.
    Nursing Process: Assessment
    Client Need: Physiologic Integrity